Frontiers in Drug Design & Discovery

(Volume 8)

Edited by:

Atta-ur-Rahman, *FRS*
Kings College, University of Cambridge, Cambridge, UK

&

M. Iqbal Choudhary
H.E.J. Research Institute of Chemistry, International Center for Chemical and Biological Sciences, University of Karachi, Karachi, Pakistan

Bentham Science Publishers Ltd.
Executive Suite Y - 2
PO Box 7917, Saif Zone
Sharjah, U.A.E.
Email: subscriptions@benthamscience.org

BENTHAM
SCIENCE

CONTENTS

PREFACE i

LIST OF CONTRIBUTORS iv

CHAPTER 1 CANCER CHEMOTHERAPY: RECENT DEVELOPMENTS IN HEMATOLOGY ONCOLOGY 1

Sapna Parmar, Rebecca Nelson and *Erica Hochard*

INTRODUCTION 1

CHRONIC LEUKEMIAS 2

Background 2

BOSUTINIB 4

PONATINIB 5

OMACETAXINE MEPESUCCINATE 6

OFATUMUMAB 7

OBINUTUZUMAB 9

IBRUTINIB 11

IDELALISIB 13

FUTURE DIRECTIONS 15

Chronic Myeloid Leukemia 15

Chronic Lymphocytic Leukemia 15

KEY CONCEPTS 16

HODGKIN LYMPHOMA AND ANAPLASTIC LARGE CELL LYMPHOMA 16

Background 16

BRENTUXIMAB VEDOTIN 18

FUTURE DIRECTIONS 19

KEY CONCEPTS 20

MANTLE CELL LYMPHOMA 20

Background 20

LENALIDOMIDE 22

IBRUTINIB 23

FUTURE DIRECTIONS 23

KEY CONCEPTS 23

ACUTE LYMPHOBLASTIC LEUKEMIA 24

Background 24

BLINATUMOMAB 26

ASPARAGINASE ERWINIA CHRYSANTHEMI 27

VINCRISTINE SULFATE LIPOSOME 28

FUTURE DIRECTIONS 29

KEY CONCEPTS 31

T-CELL LYMPHOMAS, MULTIPLE MYELOMA, MYELOFIBROSIS 31

Background 31

Therapies Used in T-cell Lymphomas 33

PRALATREXATE 33

ROMIDEPSIN 33

BELINOSTAT 35

Therapies Used in Multiple Myeloma 36

CARFILZOMIB 36

POMALIDOMIDE 38

Latest Therapies in Multiple Myeloma 39

Therapies Used in Myelofibrosis 39

RUXOLITINIB 39
FUTURE DIRECTIONS 42
Multiple Myeloma 42
Myelofibrosis 42
KEY CONCEPTS 43
CONCLUDING REMARKS 44
CONFLICT OF INTEREST 44
ACKNOWLEDGEMENTS 44
REFERENCES 44

CHAPTER 2 CURRENT INNOVATIONS IN MANAGEMENT OF ESOPHAGEAL CARCINOMA 52
Julie H. Rowe, Fathima Kamil, Melissa Yan, Curtis J. Wray and *Atilla Ertan*
EPIDEMIOLOGY 53
Age, Gender, and Race 53
Risk Factors 54
HEREDITARY CANCER SYNDROME 55
Genetic Mutations 56
Bloom Syndrome 56
Familial Barrett's Esophagus 57
Fanconi Anemia 57
Tylosis Esophageal Cancer 58
PATHOLOGY 59
Anatomy 59
Siewert Classification and EGJ 60
Precursor Lesions 61
Barrett's Esophagus 62
Screening and Surveillance of Barrett's Esophagus 66
Treatment of GERD and Barrett's Esophagus 67
Other Rare Histologies 67
SIGNALING PATHWAYS IN ESOPHAGEAL CANCER 68
SCREENING 71
PREVENTION 72
STAGING AND WORKUP OF ESOPHAGEAL CANCER 72
Clinical Presentation 72
Diagnostic Evaluation 72
PATHOLOGY EVALUATION 77
HER-2-Neu Evaluation 77
ASSESSMENT OF TREATMENT RESPONSE 78
Role of PET Scans in Treatment Response 79
Role of Micro-RNAs in Treatment Response 80
MANAGEMENT OF EARLY STAGE ESOPHAGEAL CANCER 81
Endoscopic Procedures 81
MANAGEMENT OF SURGICALLY RESECTABLE ESOPHAGEAL CANCER 84
Criteria for Surgery 84
Surgical Techniques 85
Comparison Between TTE and THE 85
Minimally Invasive Esophagectomy 86
Lymph Node Dissection 86
Timing of Surgery 87

Postoperative Complications ... 87
THE DEVELOPMENT OF CHEMORADIOTHERAPY ... 88
Definitive Chemoradiation ... 88
Current and Novel Radiotherapy Techniques ... 89
Choice of Chemotherapeutic Agent ... 89
COMBINED TRIMODALITY TREATMENTS ... 91
Preoperative Chemoradiotherapy ... 91
Postoperative Treatment ... 93
PERIOPERATIVE CHEMOTHERAPY ... 95
HOW TO APPROACH A NON-RESECTABLE ESOPHAGEAL CANCER PATIENT ... 96
Definitive Treatment ... 97
Radiation ... 97
Chemoradiation ... 97
SURVEILLANCE AND FOLLOW UP ... 99
Role of Surveillance ... 99
Surveillance Strategy ... 102
MANAGEMENT OF METASTATIC DISEASE: ... 103
Current Strategies with First-Line Chemotherapy ... 103
Monotherapy ... 105
Second Line Therapy ... 105
Radiation ... 106
TARGETED THERAPIES IN ESOPHAGEAL CANCER ... 106
Trastuzumab ... 107
Ramucirumab ... 108
FUTURE AND NOVEL THERAPEUTIC AGENTS ... 110
THE PALLIATIVE APPROACH TO PATIENT ... 111
Supportive Care ... 111
Dysphagia ... 111
Nausea and Vomiting ... 113
Bleeding ... 113
Mucositis ... 113
Radiation Esophagitis ... 114
Pain ... 114
Cachexia ... 114
CONCLUSION ... 115
ABBREVIATIONS ... 115
CONFLICT OF INTEREST ... 117
ACKNOWLEDGEMENTS ... 117
REFERENCES ... 117

CHAPTER 3 ANDROGEN DEPRIVATION THERAPY FOR PROSTATE CANCER ... 134
Patricia Tai, Evgeny Sadikov, Asim Amjad, Nelson Leong, Arbind Dubey, Wojciech Dolata, Miroslav Jancewicz and *Rashmi Koul*
INTRODUCTION ... 134
WHAT ARE THE INDICATIONS OF ADT? ... 135
Chemoprevention ... 135
Treatment of Prostate Cancer (Fig. 1) ... 136
ADT as Primary Treatment ... 137
ADT Combined with Surgery ... 137
ADT Combined with Radiotherapy ... 138
Hormonal Therapy Combined with Chemotherapy ... 139

Other Adjunctive Treatments 139
WHICH ADT TO USE? 140
Bilateral Orchiectomy 140
Estrogen and Progesterone 140
Steroidal Anti-androgen: Cyproterone Acetate (Androcur) 141
Non-steroidal Anti-androgens 141
LHRH Agonist 143
GnRH Antagonist 144
WHAT ARE THE SECOND LINE ADT? 146
Castrate-Resistant Prostate Cancer (CRPC) 147
Ketoconazole (Nizoral) Plus Steroid 148
Enzalutamide (Xtandi) 148
Abiraterone (Zytiga, Abiratas, Abretone, Abirapro) 149
TAK-700 (Orteronel) 149
WHAT ARE THE CONTROVERSIES OF ADT? 149
Maximum Androgen Blockade (MAB) 150
Timing of ADT 152
Neoadjuvant ADT and Radiotherapy 152
Total Duration of ADT with Radiotherapy 152
Early Versus Late ADT for Metastatic Prostate Cancer 153
Intermittent ADT (IHT) 154
Recovery of Testosterone in Intermittent ADT 155
More Cardiovascular Complications with IHT- A Surprise 156
SIDE EFFECTS OF ADT 156
Cardiovascular Toxicity 156
Gynecomastia 157
Osteoporosis and Fractures 157
WHAT WOULD PATIENTS ASK THEIR DOCTOR? 157
FUTURE RESEARCH 158
Androgen Receptor Signaling Pathway 158
Genetic Mutation 159
CONCLUSIONS 159
CONFLICT OF INTEREST 160
ACKNOWLEDGEMENTS 160
REFERENCES 160

CHAPTER 4 CANCER AND ITS TREATMENT: DEVELOPMENT OF ANTICANCER CHEMOTHERAPEUTIC AGENTS FROM NATURAL PRODUCTS 172
S.K. Mishra, S. Tiwari, A.A. Mahdi, S.K. Agarwal and *V. Lakshmi*
INTRODUCTION 173
CANCER 174
TYPES OF CANCER 175
1. Carcinomas 175
2. Sarcomas 175
3. Myelomas 175
4. Lymphomas 175
5. Leukemias 176
6. Mixed Types 176
CLINICAL FEATURES/SYMPTOMS 176
TUMOR CELL MARKERS 177
PATHOPHYSIOLOGY 177

CHARACTERISTIC FEATURES OF CANCER CELLS 178
Morphological Changes 178
Biochemical Changes 179
Genetics of Cancer 180
ETIOLOGY OF CANCER 183
1. Predisposing Factors 183
Life Style 183
Dietary 184
Occupational 184
Iatrogenic 184
2. Carcinogenic Agents 185
a. Physical Agents 185
b. Chemical Agents 186
c. Biological Factors 186
3. Major Classes of Virus Causing Cancer Involve 187
A. DNA Viruses 187
B. RNA Viruses 188
Incidence of a Second Cancer in Survivors 188
ROLE OF APOPTOSIS IN CANCER 188
OXIDATIVE STRESS AND CANCER 189
Primary Defense Against ROS: Catalytic Removal of ROS 190
Superoxide Dismutases (SOD) 190
Catalase (CAT) 191
Glutathione Peroxidases (GPx) 191
Peroxiredoxins (Prdx) 191
Secondary Defense Against ROS: Free Radical Scavengers 192
Genetic Landmarks in Cancer Research 192
DIAGNOSIS OF CANCER 192
CANCER THERAPY 193
Surgery 193
Radiation Therapy 194
Chemotherapy 194
DRUGS DAMAGING THE NUCLEAR DNA 196
DRUGS INHIBITING THE REPLICATION OF DNA 196
DRUGS AFFECTING THE SYNTHESIS AND BREAKDOWN OF THE MITOTIC SPINDLES (ANTIMITOTIC AGENTS) 196
1. Taxanes 196
2. Vinca Alkaloids 197
..... 198
3. Colchicine 198
ALKYLATING AGENTS (NITROGEN MUSTARDS) 198
ANTIMETABOLITES 199
PLANT ALKALOIDS 199
Vinca Alkaloids 199
Taxanes 199
Podophyllotoxin 199
Camptothecin Analogues 200
DRUGS INHIBITING ANGIOGENESIS 201
HORMONAL AGENTS 201
MISCELLANEOUS AGENTS 202
DEVELOPMENT OF ANTICANCER DRUGS 202

Historical Background ... 202
ANTICANCER DRUGS ACTING THROUGH FACILITATING THE APOPTOSIS ... 205
ANTICANCER DRUG DEVELOPMENT BASED ON MOLECULAR TARGETS ... 205
ANTICANCER DRUGS ACTING THROUGH INHIBITION OF METASTASIS ... 206
ANTICANCER DRUGS ACTING THROUGH INHIBITION OF ANGIOGENESIS ... 207
DEVELOPMENT OF ANTIBODIES AGAINST TUMOR-SPECIFIC ANTIGENS ... 208
ROLE OF METABOLOMICS AND PHARMACOGENETICS IN TREATMENT OF CANCER ... 208
OTHER ANTICANCER AGENTS ACTING THROUGH INDIRECT MECHANISMS ... 209
Drugs Reversing the Multidrug Resistance ... 209
Vaccines or Immunomodulators ... 209
Chemoprotective Agents ... 209
Drugs Restoring Hormonal Balance ... 209
Photosensitizers ... 210
Supportive Cancer-Care Agents ... 210
PROCESS OF ANTICANCER DRUG DEVELOPMENT ... 210
1. Identification of Biologically Active Compounds ... 210
2. Screening of Biological Activity and Preclinical Pharmacology ... 211
3. Clinical Development ... 211
NATURAL PRODUCTS AS SOURCE OF THERAPEUTIC AGENTS ... 211
Azadirachta Indica Juss (Neem) ... 214
Thymus Vulgaris (Ajowan) ... 214
Ocimum Sanctum Linn (Tulsi) ... 214
Garlic ... 215
BIOASSAY GUIDED DRUG DISCOVERY ... 217
MECHANISM-BASED ASSAYS ... 218
CELL-BASED ASSAYS ... 219
POTENTIAL ANTICANCER AGENTS OBTAINED FROM NATURAL PRODUCTS ... 220
Alvaradoin E ... 225
Psammaplin A ... 225
Pancratistatin ... 225
Didemnin B ... 226
Neopeltolide ... 226
Bryostatin 1 ... 226
Palmerolide A ... 226
Dolastatin 10 ... 227
Pericosine A ... 228
Dolastatin 15 ... 228
Silvestrol ... 228
Ecteinascidin-743 ... 229
Symplocamide A ... 229
Spiruchostatin A ... 229
Halichondrin B ... 229
Flavopiridol ... 230
CONCLUSION ... 231
CONFLICT OF INTEREST ... 231
ACKNOWLEDGEMENTS ... 231
REFERENCES ... 231

CHAPTER 5 POLYHYDROXYALKANOATES AS PROMISING MATERIALS IN BIOMEDICAL SYSTEMS ... 242

Michał Michalak, Sebastian Jurczyk, Katarzyna Jelonek, Minna Hakkarainen and *Piotr Kurcok*
INTRODUCTION 243
BIODEGRADABILITY AND BIOCOMPATIBILITY OF PHAs 246
BIOMEDICAL DEVICES 252
Cartilage Tissue Regeneration 252
Bone Tissue Engineering 253
Surgical Applications 254
Nerve Tissue Engineering 255
Heart Valve Engineering 256
Dermal Tissue Regeneration 257
Miscellaneous Medical Applications 258
DRUG RELEASING MEDICAL DEVICES 259
POLYMER–DRUG CONJUGATES 262
MICRO- AND NANOPARTICLES FOR DRUG DELIVERY 265
Polyhydroxyalkanoate Particles – Model Study 265
Evaluation of PHA Particles in Drug Delivery 266
Targeted Therapy Based on PHA Particles 269
CONCLUSIONS AND OUTLOOK 271
CONFLICT OF INTEREST 272
ACKNOWLEDGEMENTS 272
REFERENCES 272

SUBJECT INDEX 289

PREFACE

Drug discovery and development against prevailing and emerging diseases is one of the most important areas of modern health care research. This interdisciplinary area requires consistent well coordinated efforts of scientists with diverse expertise. It starts from target identification that underlies a particular disease process. It often takes years of study in order to characterize the targets for a potential drug. Once a receptor target has been characterized and validated, the most challenging task of identifying appropriate ligands from natural or synthetic sources begins. The study of the biochemical mechanism of the receptor-ligand interaction is the next step in this process. Often the ligands need to be modified to achieve greater specificity and affinity, requiring skills of medicinal chemists. This is followed by pre-clinical and clinical studies for safety, efficacy and specificity, often leading to frustrating failures, and re-initiation of the whole process. Finally, there are other considerations in the development of new drugs, termed ADMET (absorption, desorption, metabolism, excretion, and toxicity). Despite the challenges associated with the drug discovery and development, it is a fascinating and much needed scientific research which continues unabated.

The 8th volume of the ebook series entitled, "*Frontiers in Drug Design and Discovery*", is a compilation of five exhaustively written reviews focussing on various aspects of drug discovery and development in key therapeutic areas. These reviews provide a wealth of information about topics of great interest in this field.

Parmer *et al.*, have contributed a comprehensive review on the development of new chemotherapautic agents against haematological cancers. Hematological malignancies are among the most common cancer types. They affect the blood and lymph systems and include chronic and acute leukaemia, non-Hodgkin lymphoma, Hodgkin lymphoma, and multiple myeloma. There has been a major gap between the needs of treatment for haematological cancers and the current pace of drug development in this field. The authors have skilfully dealt with the subject by highlighting major developments in this important area along with pharmacology, pharmacokinetics, and clinical studies on various classes of drugs, including targeted therapies.

In chapter 2, Rowe *et al.* review the recent literature on the current developments in the management of esophageal carcinoma. The review begins with the description of two major types of esophageal carcinoma i.e. squamous cell carcinoma and adenocarcinoma. Different therapeutic interventions at various stages of esophageal carcinoma, as well as the health status and age of patients are described. This review presents treatment options for squamous cell cancer such as chemotherapy and radiation therapy as the first lines of treatment followed by surgery. Studies showing that chemoradiotherapy before surgery is better than surgery alone are presented. For adenocarcinoma, the most common treatment is chemotherapy and radiation therapy, followed by surgery. For advanced stage esophageal cancer, chemotherapy and radiation therapy remain the only options. Most importantly, the review describes advances in endoscopic treatments of early stage esophageal cancers such as endoscopic mucosal resection (EMR), endoscopic submucosal dissection (ESD) as well as endoscopic ablation procedures, including photodynamic therapy (PDT) and radio frequency ablation (RFA). These advances have proven to be safe and effective for the treatment of esophageal dysplasia and early stage neoplasia.

Androgen hormones stimulate prostate cancer cells to grow faster. The most important among them are testosterone and dihydrotestosterone (DHT). Lowering androgen levels or stopping them from getting into prostate cancer cells have been used to slow down the growth of prostate cancers. This is called androgen deprivation therapy (ADT). However, there are a lot of controversies associated with ADT. Tai *et al* in chapter 3 have reviewed past uses, and recent scientific evidences concerning the ADT in the treatment of prostate cancer. Current trends of the use of ADT in combination with radiotherapy to avoid recurrence of cancer are discussed.

Secondary metabolites from natural sources such as plants, microorganisms, and marine organisms have played an important role in world's healthcare systems from ancient times till to date. Many cancer chemotherapeutic drugs have been obtained from nature and modified for optimal activity and safety. As cancers continue to take heavy toll of human life, the search for natural products with anti-neoplastic activities has continued in recent years with large scale screenings of marine fauna and flora, terrestrial microorganisms and plants in many laboratories of the world. Several new classes of natural products and their derivatives have been developed with the potential to be used as cancer chemotherapeutic agents. Lakshmi *et al.* comprehensively review the most notable discoveries of anti-cancer natural products in the last 5 decades in chapter 4. Most importantly, they describe the mechanism of action of key classes of natural anti-cancer agents at molecular levels, such as inhibition of enzymes and signalling pathways. The structure-activity relationships and results of pre-clinical studies add further value to this chapter.

Finally, chapter 5 by Kurcok *et al* is focussed on the tremendous new and well known biomedical and pharmaceutical applications of natural biopolymers, polyhydroxyalkanoates (PHAs). These natural linear polyesters are produced intercellularly by various species of bacteria through the fermentation of sugars or lipids. Many PHAs have also been prepared by chemical synthesis. PHAs are generally biocompatible and biodegradable in nature, and are used in the production of bioplastics. PHAs and their copolymers have found extensive applications in biomedical systems, including tissue engineering, orthopaedic materials, drug-loaded implants, drug careers, transdermal administration drugs and cosmetics, *etc*. Recent research studies on the conjugation of drugs with low molecular weight PHAs have shown to improve the bioavailability and safety profiles of drugs.

The above chapters are contributed by leading researchers and experts in the fields making volume 8 of the *Frontiers in Drug Design and Discovery* an interesting and useful reading for both young and established scientists, as well as students of biomedical and health sciences, and medicinal and pharmaceutical chemistry. We wish to express our gratitude to them for their excellent scholarly contributions for this reputed ebook series. We also greatly appreciate the efforts of the entire team of Bentham Science Publishers for efficient and timely processing of the publication. The skills, efforts and commitment of Mr. Omer Shafi (Assistant Manager Publications), Mr. Shehzad Naqvi (Manager Publications) and leadership of Mr. Mahmood Alam (Director Publications) are especially praiseworthy. We also hope that like the previous volumes of this internationally recognized book series, volume 8 will also receive wide readership, and appreciation.

Atta-ur-Rahman, *FRS*
Kings College,
University of Cambridge,
Cambridge,
UK

M. Iqbal Choudhary
H.E.J. Research Institute of Chemistry,
International Center for Chemical and
Biological Sciences,
University of Karachi,
Karachi,
Pakistan

List of Contributors

A.A. Mahdi	Department of Biochemistry, King George's Medical University, Lucknow 226001, India
Arbind Dubey	Departments of Radiation Oncology (PT, ES, AA, NL), and Medical Oncology (WD, MJ), Allan Blair Cancer Centre, Regina, Canada Department of Radiation Oncology (AD, RK), CancerCare Manitoba, Winnipeg, Canada
Asim Amjad	Departments of Radiation Oncology (PT, ES, AA, NL), and Medical Oncology (WD, MJ), Allan Blair Cancer Centre, Regina, Canada Department of Radiation Oncology (AD, RK), CancerCare Manitoba, Winnipeg, Canada
Atilla Ertan	University of Texas Health Science Center-McGovern Medical School, Houston, USA Department of Internal Medicine, Division of Gastroenterology, Hepatology, and Nutrition, University of Texas Health Science Center, Houston, USA
Curtis J. Wray	University of Texas Health Science Center-McGovern Medical School, Houston, USA Department of Surgery, Division of Minimally Invasive and Elective General Surgery, University of Texas Health Science Center, Street no., Houston, USA
Erica Hochard	NewYork-Presbyterian Hospital/Weill Cornell Medical Center, New York, USA
Evgeny Sadikov	Departments of Radiation Oncology (PT, ES, AA, NL), and Medical Oncology (WD, MJ), Allan Blair Cancer Centre, Regina, Canada Department of Radiation Oncology (AD, RK), CancerCare Manitoba, Winnipeg, Canada
Fathima Kamil	University of Texas Health Science Center-McGovern Medical School, Houston, USA Department of Internal Medicine, University of Texas Health Science Center, Houston, USA
Julie H. Rowe	University of Texas Health Science Center-McGovern Medical School, Houston, USA Department of Internal Medicine, Division of Oncology, University of Texas Health Science Center, Houston, USA
Katarzyna Jelonek	Centre of Polymer and Carbon Materials, Polish Academy of Sciences, 34, M. Curie-Skłodowskiej St., 41-819 Zabrze, Poland
Melissa Yan	University of Texas Health Science Center-McGovern Medical School, Houston, USA Department of Internal Medicine, University of Texas Health Science Center, Houston, USA
Michał Michalak	Centre of Polymer and Carbon Materials, Polish Academy of Sciences, 34, M. Curie-Skłodowskiej St., 41-819 Zabrze, Poland
Minna Hakkarainen	Department of Fibre and Polymer Technology, KTH Royal Institute of Technology, Stockholm, Sweden

Miroslav Jancewicz	Departments of Radiation Oncology (PT, ES, AA, NL), and Medical Oncology (WD, MJ), Allan Blair Cancer Centre, Regina, Canada Department of Radiation Oncology (AD, RK), CancerCare Manitoba, Winnipeg, Canada
Nelson Leong	Departments of Radiation Oncology (PT, ES, AA, NL), and Medical Oncology (WD, MJ), Allan Blair Cancer Centre, Regina, Canada Department of Radiation Oncology (AD, RK), CancerCare Manitoba, Winnipeg, Canada
Patricia Tai	Departments of Radiation Oncology (PT, ES, AA, NL), and Medical Oncology (WD, MJ), Allan Blair Cancer Centre, Regina, Canada Department of Radiation Oncology (AD, RK), CancerCare Manitoba, Winnipeg, Canada
Piotr Kurcok	Centre of Polymer and Carbon Materials, Polish Academy of Sciences, 34, M. Curie-Skłodowskiej St., 41-819 Zabrze, Poland Institute of Chemistry, Environment Protection and Biotechnology, Jan Długosz Academy, 13/15 Armii Krajowej Ave., 42-200 Czestochowa, Poland
Rashmi Koul	Departments of Radiation Oncology (PT, ES, AA, NL), and Medical Oncology (WD, MJ), Allan Blair Cancer Centre, Regina, Canada Department of Radiation Oncology (AD, RK), CancerCare Manitoba, Winnipeg, Canada
Rebecca Nelson	NewYork-Presbyterian Hospital/Weill Cornell Medical Center, New York, USA
S. Tiwari	Pesticide Toxicology Division, Indian Institute of Toxicology Research, Lucknow 226001, India
S.K. Agarwal	Department of Biochemistry, King George's Medical University, Lucknow 226001, India
S.K. Mishra	Medicinal and Process Chemistry Division, Central Drug Research Institute, Lucknow 226001, India
Sapna Parmar	NewYork-Presbyterian Hospital/Weill Cornell Medical Center, New York, USA
Sebastian Jurczyk	Paint and Plastics Department in Gliwice, Institute for Engineering of Polymer Materials and Dyes, 50A, Chorzowska St., 44-100 Gliwice, Poland
V. Lakshmi	Medicinal and Process Chemistry Division, Central Drug Research Institute, Lucknow 226001, India Department of Biochemistry, King George's Medical University, Lucknow 226001, India
Wojciech Dolata	Departments of Radiation Oncology (PT, ES, AA, NL), and Medical Oncology (WD, MJ), Allan Blair Cancer Centre, Regina, Canada Department of Radiation Oncology (AD, RK), CancerCare Manitoba, Winnipeg, Canada

CHAPTER 1

Cancer Chemotherapy: Recent Developments in Hematology Oncology

Sapna Parmar*, **Rebecca Nelson** and **Erica Hochard**

NewYork-Presbyterian Hospital/Weill Cornell Medical Center, New York, USA

Abstract: Research specialized in the field of hematology oncology over relatively recent years has revolutionized patient care and led to an array of chemotherapeutic agents approved by the Food and Drug Administration. Both oral and intravenous drug formulations have been marketed, including targeted therapies, for several hematologic disorders including acute and chronic leukemias, Hodgkin and non-Hodgkin's lymphomas, multiple myeloma, and myelofibrosis. The primary focus of this chapter will include latest chemotherapy developments in hematology covering critical topics of pharmacology, pharmacokinetics/pharmacodynamics, and pivotal clinical studies addressing both labeled and off-labeled indications. Lastly, future directions will be addressed, where applicable, in this continuously evolving clinical field.

Keywords: Acute lymphoblastic leukemia, Anaplastic large cell lymphoma, Bone marrow transplant, Cancer, Chemotherapy, Chronic lymphocytic leukemia, Chronic myeloid leukemia, Hematology, Hodgkin lymphoma, Mantle cell lymphoma, Multiple myeloma, Myelofibrosis, Non-Hodgkin's lymphoma, Oncology, T-cell lymphoma.

INTRODUCTION

Substantial strides have been made in recent years in the diagnosis, prevention, and treatment of hematological malignancies due to ongoing specialized research. A multitude of chemotherapeutic agents have been made available in the United States, revolutionizing patient care and resulting in improved response rates and median survival. Both oral and intravenous drug formulations have been marketed, including targeted therapies, for several hematologic disorders including acute and chronic leukemias, Hodgkin and non-Hodgkin's lymphomas, multiple myeloma, and . The chapter will focus on state-of-the-art drug developments in malignant hematology, covering crucial topics of pharmacology,

* **Corresponding author Sapna Parmar**: NewYork-Presbyterian Hospital/Weill Cornell Medical Center, New York, NY, USA; Tel: 212-746-0723; Fax: 212-746-8506; E-mail: sap9074@nyp.org

Atta-ur-Rahman and M. Iqbal Choudhary (Eds.)

pharmacokinetics/pharmacodynamics, and pivotal clinical trials addressing both labeled and off-labeled purposes. Finally, advances and possible future directions in the treatment of chosen hematological malignancies will be presented.

CHRONIC LEUKEMIAS

Background

The chronic leukemias are a group of malignancies involving the hematopoietic system. They can be broadly classified into two types: chronic myelogenous leukemia (CML) and chronic lymphocytic leukemia (CLL). CML is a myeloproliferative disorder characterized by increased proliferation of the granulocytic cell line without the loss of their capacity to differentiate [1]. The median age at diagnosis is 67 years and it accounts for approximately 15% of all leukemias in adults. CML is rarely seen in the pediatric population. The estimated number of new cases in both males and females for the year 2015 is projected to be 6,660, with 1,140 predicted deaths [2]. CML was the first neoplastic process where a single chromosomal abnormality, the Philadelphia chromosome, was demonstrated as fundamental to the etiology of the disease. The Philadelphia chromosome results from a reciprocal chromosomal translocation consisting of juxtaposition of the ABL (Abelson Murine Leukemia) gene from chromosome 9 and the BCR (Breakpoint Cluster Region) gene from chromosome 22, consequently leading to unusual tyrosine kinase activity (see Fig. **1**). CML occurs in three distinct phases (chronic, accelerated, and blast phase); nearly 90% of patients are diagnosed in the chronic phase. Patients in the chronic phase of disease often have splenomegaly and thrombocytosis with elevated white cell counts and circulating immature precursors. Typical symptoms at presentation include fatigue, night sweats, abdominal fullness, anorexia, and weight loss; however, up to 50% of patients are asymptomatic due to the initial indolent phase of the disease. Untreated CML inescapably progresses to the more aggressive accelerated and blast phases. The median survival of patients in blast phase is less than 6 months, with the most common causes of death being infection and hemorrhage [3]. Until the 1980s, CML was regarded as incurable and inevitably fatal [4]. Management of this disease has undergone a radical change in a very short period of time. The introduction of the tyrosine kinase inhibitors revolutionized the treatment of CML subsequently improving the ten year overall survival (OS) from 20% up to 90% [5]. Imatinib (Gleevec®) was the first tyrosine kinase inhibitor introduced for patients with CML, initially marketed in the United States in 2001. Since then, multiple options have emerged for this patient population. This review will focus on the latest therapies approved for the management of this disease [4].

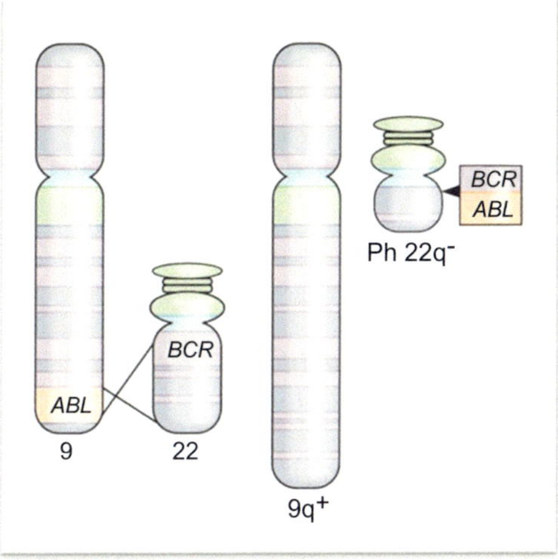

Fig. (1). Philadelphia chromosome shown.

Unlike the rarity of CML, chronic lymphocytic leukemia remains the most prevalent adult leukemia in Western countries [6]. In the United States alone, an estimated 14,620 new cases of CLL and 4,650 deaths will occur in 2015 [2]. CLL is a neoplasm characterized by proliferation and accumulation of small lymphocytes in the peripheral blood, lymph nodes, spleen, and bone marrow [7]. It is important to note that both CLL and small lymphocytic lymphoma (SLL) are essentially the same disease of B-cell lymphomas, with the only difference being where the malignancy predominantly occurs. In the simplest sense, in patients with CLL, majority of the malignant cells are located in the bloodstream and bone marrow; however, lymph nodes and spleen are also frequently involved. In SLL, malignant cells are merely isolated to the lymph nodes [8]. CLL is most common in the elderly, with a median age at diagnosis of 72 years. The disease is twice as common in males as females and occurs more frequently in Caucasians compared with African-Americans. CLL is considered an indolent disease however, it can be extremely heterogeneous in its clinical course. Some patients survive for decades without treatment, whereas others may suffer a rapidly progressive course despite aggressive therapy, eventually leading to fatality. In such cases, patient experience deteriorating blood counts (*e.g.,* anemia and thrombocytopenia) and organomegaly. Typical "B" symptoms of lymphoma may be present (*e.g.,* unintentional weight loss, fever, drenching night sweats, and significant fatigue). Recurrent infections and hypogammaglobulinemia are typical due to inherent impairment in cellular and humoral immunity [6]. Outside of the context of a clinical trial, in general practice, newly diagnosed patients with asymptomatic, low risk, early stage disease should be monitored without therapy unless they have evidence of disease progression. Those with advanced stage or high risk

CLL commonly present with symptomatic disease and require immediate treatment. The current standard of care has evolved from single agent alkylating agents, through the introduction of purine analogs, to chemoimmunotherapy combinations. Choice of therapy is stratified based on patient age and genetic mutations present [9]. Several novel therapeutic options have developed in recent years for the management of this disease state and will be reviewed here.

BOSUTINIB

Pharmacology/Pharmacokinetics/Pharmacodynamics

Noted previously, the treatment landscape for CML dramatically changed after the advent of the tyrosine kinase inhibitors. Although clinical outcomes are favorable in patients who receive first-line tyrosine kinase inhibitor therapy with imatinib, dasatinib (Sprycel®), and nilotinib (Tasigna®), relapse or disease progression may occur generating the need for second-line therapy [10]. Bosutinib (Bosulif®) is an orally available, once-daily dual Src and Abl kinase inhibitor, approved by the United States Food and Drug Administration (FDA) in September 2012. It is indicated for the treatment of chronic, accelerated, or blast phase Philadelphia chromosome-positive CML in patients resistant or intolerant to previous therapies. Bosutinib shows potent inhibitory activity against Bcr-abl and Src family of kinases and has minimal activity against c-KIT and platelet-derived growth factor receptor; both which are non-specific targets associated with toxicity in other agents in its class. It is mainly metabolized by cytochrome P450 (CYP) 3A4 in the liver, primarily to inactive metabolites and excreted in the feces (>90%). In healthy adult patients, median time to peak plasma concentration is generally 4-6 hours and half-life elimination is 22-27 hours [11, 12].

Pivotal Clinical Studies

Bosutinib was evaluated as frontline therapy in the phase III Bosutinib Efficacy and Safety in Newly Diagnosed Chronic Myeloid Leukemia ("BELA") trial [13]. A total of 502 patients with chronic phase CML were randomly assigned 1:1 to bosutinib or imatinib. At 12 months, bosutinib treated patients had a statistically significant higher major molecular response (MMR) rate (41% vs. 27%, respectively; $P < 0.001$) and faster time to both MMR and complete cytogenetic response (CCyR). However, the study did not meet its primary endpoint of improved CCyR at 12 months (70% for bosutinib vs. 68% for imatinib, $P= 0.601$). On-treatment transformation to accelerated phase or blast phase occurred in only four patients (2%) treated with bosutinib vs. 4% of patients in the imatinib treated arm (N=10). The safety profiles of both agents were relatively dissimilar with gastrointestinal and liver-related events being more common with bosutinib; and neutropenia, musculoskeletal disorders, and edema seen more frequently with imatinib treated patients. Three CML-related fatalities ensued on the bosutinib arm *vs.* eight on the imatinib arm. With the present data, bosutinib is currently not recommended in the first-line setting. Bosutinib has been studied in the second-line and beyond settings with promising results. It is a safe and effective treatment option for select patients who are intolerant or resistant to prior tyrosine kinase inhibitor therapy [14, 15].

PONATINIB

Pharmacology/Pharmacokinetics/Pharmacodynamics

Although bosutinib has demonstrated activity against many Bcr-abl kinase domain mutations that are resistant to first and second-generation tyrosine kinase inhibitors (*e.g.,* imatinib, dasatinib, and nilotinib), it cannot overcome T315I and V299 mutants. T315I currently remains the most troublesome mutation and is associated with a highly aggressive disease phenotype and poor outcome. Ponatinib (Iclusig®) received accelerated approval by the FDA in December 2012 based on disease response. It is an orally available, pan-Bcr-abl tyrosine kinase inhibitor and due to its unique structure, it is the only inhibitor with the capability to counter the T315I mutation. The FDA issued a Drug Safety Communication in October 2013 reporting increased frequency of life-threatening blood clots and narrowing of blood vessels in the extremities. These safety concerns likely emerged from ponatinib's ability to cause pan-vascular endothelial growth factor (VEGF) inhibition. As a result, labeled indications include treatment of CML in chronic, accelerated, or blast phase for whom no other tyrosine kinase inhibitor therapy is indicated or for those who are T315I positive. Ponatinib is also FDA approved for patients with Philadelphia chromosome-positive acute lymphoblastic leukemia (ALL). It undergoes both phase I and II hepatic metabolism primarily through CYP3A4 and its half-life elimination is approximately 24 hours (range 12-66 hours). Ponatinib is largely excreted in the feces (~90%) [16, 17].

Pivotal Clinical Studies

The PACE ("The Ponatinib Ph+ ALL and CML Evaluation") trial was a pivotal phase 2 study evaluating the efficacy of ponatinib in patients who are resistant or intolerant to dasatinib or nilotinib or had the T315I mutation [18]. Investigators enrolled 449 heavily pretreated patients with CML (any phase) or Philadelphia chromosome-positive ALL. Among the 267 patients with chronic phase CML, 56% had a major cytogenetic response (MCyR), 46% had a CCyR, and 34% had a MMR. No single Bcr-abl mutation conferring resistance to ponatinib was detected. Among 83 patients with accelerated phase CML and 62 patients with blast phase CML, 55% and 31% had a major hematologic response, respectively;

and 39% and 23% had a MCyR, respectively. Commonly seen adverse events were thrombocytopenia, rash, dry skin, and abdominal pain. Serious arterial thrombotic events were observed in 9% of patients, one-third of these events were considered to be related to ponatinib. The PACE trial demonstrated response rates to ponatinib regardless of mutation. Patients previously treated with fewer tyrosine kinase inhibitors established higher response rates to ponatinib.

Activity and safety of ponatinib as first-line treatment for patients with chronic phase CML was recently published by Jain P and colleagues [19]. Of the 46 evaluable patients, 94% (N=43) achieved a CCyR at 6 months. The most common toxicities included dermatological and elevated lipase. Hypertension occurred in approximately half of the patient population and grade ¾ myelosuppression occurred in 29% (N=15). Five patients developed cerebrovascular or vaso-occlusive disease. Due to concerns from the FDA regarding risk of thromboembolism, the study was terminated in June 2014. Authors concluded other therapies should be considered initially in the frontline setting due to thrombotic toxicities associated with ponatinib.

Existing data demonstrates that ponatinib has substantial activity in patients with advanced disease. It stands as an important therapeutic option for patients resistant or intolerant to prior therapies. Current clinical practice supports consideration of ponatinib only for patients with a T315I mutation and for those who have failed 2 or more prior tyrosine kinase inhibitors. General use in the community along with ongoing clinical studies will further define the role of ponatinib in the management of patients with CML as well as incidence and management of its severe side effects [17].

OMACETAXINE MEPESUCCINATE

Pharmacology/Pharmacokinetics/Pharmacodynamics

Omacetaxine mepesuccinate (omacetaxine hereafter; brand name Synribo®) was granted accelerated approval by the FDA in October 2012 for the treatment of chronic or accelerated phase CML with resistance and/or intolerance to $\geq$ 2 tyrosine kinase inhibitors [20]. Omacetaxine, also known as homoharringtonine, is a natural cephalotaxine alkaloid and is the only effective natural therapeutic agent used in patients with CML. Interestingly, it has been studied for more than 30 years and was initially used in the early 1980s to treat CML patients in China. It functions as a reversible inhibitor of protein synthesis by binding to the A-site cleft of the ribosomal subunit to interfere with chain elongation and inhibit protein synthesis. Unique to this agent, omacetaxine acts independently of Bcr-abl kinase-binding activity and has demonstrated activity against tyrosine kinase inhibitor-resistant Bcr-abl mutations. Omacetaxine is administered subcutaneously (different from the tyrosine kinase inhibitors which are all taken orally by mouth) and maximum blood concentration is achieved within one hour of injection. It is rapidly absorbed and widely distributed and subsequently, primarily hydrolyzed to 4'-DMHHT through plasma esterases with hepatic microsomal oxidative and/or esterase-mediated metabolism. Mean half-life following administration is approximately six hours and less than 15% is excreted unchanged in the urine [21].

Pivotal Clinical Studies

Cortes J and colleagues published a multicenter, single-arm, phase 2 study of omacetaxine after tyrosine kinase inhibitor failure in patients with chronic phase CML harboring the T315I mutation [22]. A total of 62 patients were enrolled in the study; all were heavily pretreated with conventional therapies for CML. All patients had failed therapy with imatinib and 74% (N=46) had failed treatment with at least two tyrosine kinase inhibitors. Patients received a median of 7 cycles of omacetaxine (range 1-41). Complete hematologic response was achieved in 77% (N=48) and median response duration was 9.1 months. With respect to cytogenetic response, 23% (N=14) achieved a major cytogenetic response, including a complete response in 16% (N=10). Therapy with omacetaxine was generally well tolerated in this study however; hematologic events were common in the initial cycles of treatment. Grade 3/4 hematologic toxicity comprised of thrombocytopenia (76%), neutropenia (44%), and anemia (39%); all of which were managed by dose reduction. Non-hematologic adverse events included infection (42%), diarrhea (40%), and nausea (34%). Injection site reactions were common, with erythema reported in 21% (N=13). Progression-free survival was noted to be 7.7 months.

Omacetaxine provides a unique mechanism of action in our fight against cancers. It offers an innovative treatment alternative for those patients with CML with the T315I mutation who have failed prior tyrosine kinase inhibitor therapy. Literature suggests that there is a favorable benefit/risk profile in this subset of patients who otherwise have a poor prognosis and no proven treatment options.

OFATUMUMAB

Pharmacology/Pharmacokinetics/Pharmacodynamics

As alluded to earlier, CLL is a neoplasm of lymphoid origin; more specifically, it is a malignancy of mature B-lymphocytes. CD20 is expressed on normal and malignant B cells, but not on hematopoietic stem cells, and therefore considered to be a favorable target in the development of monoclonal antibodies used to treat B cell malignancies [6]. Ofatumumab (Arzerra®) is a second generation, fully human, cytolytic monoclonal antibody that is specific for CD20. It binds specifically the extracellular, large and small, loops of the CD20 molecule which results in potent complement-dependent cell lysis and antibody-dependent cell-mediated toxicity in cells that overexpress CD20. In October 2009, the FDA announced the approval of ofatumumab for its use in patients with refractory or relapsed CLL who have failed fludarabine and alemtuzumab-based regimens [23]. In April 2014, labeled indications were further expanded to include previously untreated CLL, in combination with chlorambucil, when fludarabine-based therapy was not feasible due to advanced age and/or co-morbidities [24]. The specifics of the clinical trial (COMPLEMENT 1 study) leading to this approval will be discussed below.

Ofatumumab is administered intravenously; pre-medications (*e.g.*, aceta-mino--phen, anti-histamine, corticosteroid) are recommended prior to doses due to its potential to cause serious, including fatal, infusion reactions. Ofatumumab is eliminated through both a target-independent route and a B cell-mediated route. Due to the depletion of B cells, the clearance of ofatumumab decreases substantially after second and greater infusions compared with the first infusion. Following repeated doses, the half-life of ofatumumab is approximately 15.6 days [25].

Pivotal Clinical Studies

Use of Ofatumumab as Front-line Therapy in CLL

Hillmen P and colleagues [26] carried out the COMPLEMENT 1 study which investigated the efficacy and safety of ofatumumab added to chlorambucil compared with chlorambucil monotherapy in patients with previously untreated CLL for whom fludarabine-based regimens were considered unsuitable due to presence of comorbidities and/or advanced age. This prospective, randomized, phase 3 study consisted of 447 patients; median age was 69 years and majority (N=391 or 87%) of patients reported at least one comorbidity. Median progression-free survival was 22.4 months for the combination treatment arm compared to 13.1 months for patients receiving single-agent chlorambucil ($P< 0.001$). Ofatumumab plus chlorambucil also resulted in higher overall response rate (82% *versus* 69%, $P= 0.001$) and superior complete response rate (12% *versus* 1%) compared to chlorambucil alone. The most common adverse reactions in the combination group were infusion reactions, neutropenia, asthenia, headache, leukopenia, herpes simplex, lower respiratory tract infection, arthralgia, and upper abdominal pain. Authors concluded that chlorambucil plus ofatumumab is an important treatment option for those patients who cannot tolerate more intensive therapy.

Novel Uses of Ofatumumab

Due to the unique mechanism of action of ofatumumab and its ability to exert potent complement-dependent cell lysis, its use is being explored for disorders other than CLL. Pidala J and colleagues [27] investigated its potential in management of chronic graft-*versus*-host disease (cGVHD) since multiple observations implicate B-lymphocytes in the pathogenesis of this disease. This major late complication of allogeneic hematopoietic cell transplantation (HCT) is primarily treated with ≥ 1 mg/kg/day of prednisone with or without a calcineurin inhibitor and results in complete resolution of cGVHD by 6-9 months in only 30% of patients.

Patients aged ≥ 18 years with moderate-to-severe cGVHD affecting various organs and requiring ≥ 1 mg/kg/day prednisone were treated at three escalating dose levels of intravenous ofatumumab (300mg, 700mg, and 1000mg) on days 1 and 14 of initial glucocorticoid therapy in this phase 1 trial. A total of 12 patients were treated; four possibly related adverse events were observed and included: grade 1 fatigue, grade 1 transaminitis, and 2 infusion reactions (grades 2 and 3). There were no cases of hepatitis B reactivation or progressive multifocal leukoencephalopathy. A phase 2 examination of efficacy is ongoing.

A case series of the use of ofatumumab for rituximab-resistant nephrotic syndrome in children was published in 2014 [28]. Rituximab was found to be a promising agent during the past decade in management of steroid-resistant nephrotic syndrome that was resilient to alkylating agents and calcineurin inhibitors. Due to now increasing rituximab resistance, innovative strategies are being tested such as the role of ofatumumab in this disorder. Five children were treated with a total of six doses of ofatumumab; all patients had been treated with ≥ 3 previous therapies. Remission was achieved after the fourth dose in three patients and after the sixth dose in two patients. No serious adverse events were observed during the study period; one transient infusion reaction was reported. Further studies are necessary to define the role of ofatumumab in managing rituximab-resistant nephrotic syndrome.

OBINUTUZUMAB

Pharmacology/Pharmacokinetics/Pharmacodynamics

Obinutuzumab (Gazyva®) is a glycoengineered, humanized, type II antibody targeted against CD20 that is administered intravenously. Type II antibodies, as obinutuzumab, bind in a different orientation than type I antibodies (*e.g.*, ofatumumab) and are more potent in generating direct cell death. Upon binding to CD20, obinutuzumab activates complement-dependent cytotoxicity, antibody-dependent cellular cytotoxicity, and antibody-dependent cellular phagocytosis. Obinutuzumab was approved by the FDA in November 2013 for the treatment of patients with previously untreated CLL in combination with chlorambucil.

Similar to ofatumumab, pre-medication is recommended prior obinutuzumab to reduce the risk of infusion reactions. From a pharmacokinetic perspective, obinutuzumab is largely restricted to the plasma and interstitial fluid. Its metabolism has not been studied directly; however, it is known that antibodies are predominantly cleared *via* catabolism. Age and creatinine clearance do not affect the pharmacokinetics of obinutuzumab, however data are limited in patients with severe renal impairment (creatinine clearance < 30 ml/min). The half-life of obinutuzumab is approximately 30 days [29, 30].

Pivotal Clinical Studies

Goede V and colleagues [31] investigated obinutuzumab *versus* rituximab, each combined with chlorambucil, in patients with previously untreated CLL and concomitant medical conditions in the CLL 11 trial. A total of 781 patients, median age 73 years, were randomized to receive chlorambucil, obinutuzumab plus chlorambucil, or rituximab plus chlorambucil. The combination of obinutuzumab plus chlorambucil resulted in a higher overall response rate (78.4% *versus* 65.1%), complete response (20.7% *versus* 7%), and significantly improved progression-free survival (26.7 months *versus* 15.2 months; P< 0.001) when compared to rituximab-chlorambucil. Neutropenia (35%), infusion related reactions (21%), thrombocytopenia (11%), and infections (11%) comprised the most frequent grade 3 or higher toxicities with the obinutuzumab-chlorambucil treatment arm. Results of the CLL 11 study established obinutuzumab plus chlorambucil as the new standard of care for both elderly patients and for patients with coexisting conditions, lacking del(17p). Based on the results of this trial, obinutuzumab in combination with chlorambucil was approved by the FDA for frontline therapy in CLL patients.

Cartron G and colleagues [32] conducted the phase 1/2 GAUGUIN study to evaluate the safety and efficacy of obinutuzumab monotherapy in patients with relapsed/refractory CLL. Infusion related reactions occurred in nearly all patients; however only a few were grade 3 or higher reactions. Grade 3/4 neutropenia occurred in seven patients in phase 1 and in four patients in phase 2. Best overall response was 62% and 30% in phase 1 *versus* phase 2, respectively. Median progression-free survival in phase 2 was 10.7 months and median duration of response was 8.9 months.

In conclusion, GAUGUIN demonstrated that obinutuzumab is active as monotherapy in patients with heavily pretreated relapsed/refractory CLL. Clinical application of obinutuzumab monotherapy would be useful in scenarios where rituximab or ofatumumab monotherapy are currently used, due to its higher propensity for B cell depletion, and in patients not suitable for cytotoxic, aggressive chemotherapy.

IBRUTINIB

Pharmacology/Pharmacokinetics/Pharmacodynamics

A number of critical signaling pathways including the B cell receptor (BCR), CXCR4/5, CD40, integrin, and interleukin-6 that signal *via* phosphatidylinositol 3-kinase (PI3K), Bruton's tyrosine kinase (BTK), and/or spleen tyrosine kinase are implicated in the pathogenesis of CLL. In an effort to optimize treatment outcomes, novel molecularly targeted therapies are being evaluated in this patient population. In February 2014, the FDA granted accelerated approval to ibrutinib (Imbruvica®) for patients with CLL who have received at least one prior therapy and expanded its use in July 2014 for treatment of CLL patients with 17p deletion (as first-line therapy). Ibrutinib is also FDA approved for patients with relapsed/refractory mantle cell lymphoma and Waldenström macroglobulinemia.

As alluded to earlier, the BCR pathway regulates multiple cellular processes that are essential for the functioning and survival of both normal and malignant B cells. Aberrant BCR signaling plays a critical role in the evolution of CLL. The BCR pathway is responsible for the phosphorylation of numerous protein tyrosine kinases, including BTK. Ibrutinib is an orally administered, highly potent, selective, and irreversible small molecular inhibitor of BTK. This inhibition subsequently prevents downstream activation of the BCR pathway and blocks cell growth, proliferation, and survival of malignant B cells (see Fig. **2**).

After oral administration, ibrutinib is rapidly absorbed with peak plasma concentrations observed one to two hours after dosing. It is converted in the liver to several metabolites, primarily by CYP3A4 and to a minor extent by CYP2D6. The active metabolite, the dihydrodiol PCI-45227, has inhibitory activity towards BTK approximately 15 times lower than that of ibrutinib. Plasma concentrations follow a biphasic elimination pattern, resulting in an apparent terminal half-life of four to six hours. Ibrutinib is eliminated primarily *via* the feces (~80%), mainly in the form of metabolites [6].

Pivotal Clinical Studies

Approval of ibrutinib was confirmed by the open label, randomized, phase 3 RESONATE trial [33]. Investigators randomized 391 patients with relapsed or refractory CLL or SLL to receive oral ibrutinib, until disease progression or unacceptable toxicity, or intravenous ofatumumab (latter for up to 24 weeks). Median age in both groups was 67 years. At a median follow-up of 9.4 months, ibrutinib significantly improved progression-free survival; median duration was not reached in the ibrutinib arm (88% noted at 6 months), as compared with a median of 8.1 months in the ofatumumab arm. Overall survival was also markedly improved in the ibrutinib treatment arm (hazard ratio for death, 0.43; P= 0.005). The overall response rate was 42.6% *versus* 4.1% in the ibrutinib and ofatumumab groups, respectively (P< 0.001). It is important to point out that similar effects were seen regardless of whether patients had high-risk disease (*e.g.,* 17p deletion) or history of resistance to purine analogues. The most frequent non-hematologic adverse events that occurred in at least 20% of patients were diarrhea, fatigue, pyrexia, and nausea in the ibrutinib group. Phase 3 studies examining the benefit of ibrutinib in previously untreated CLL or SLL patients are ongoing.

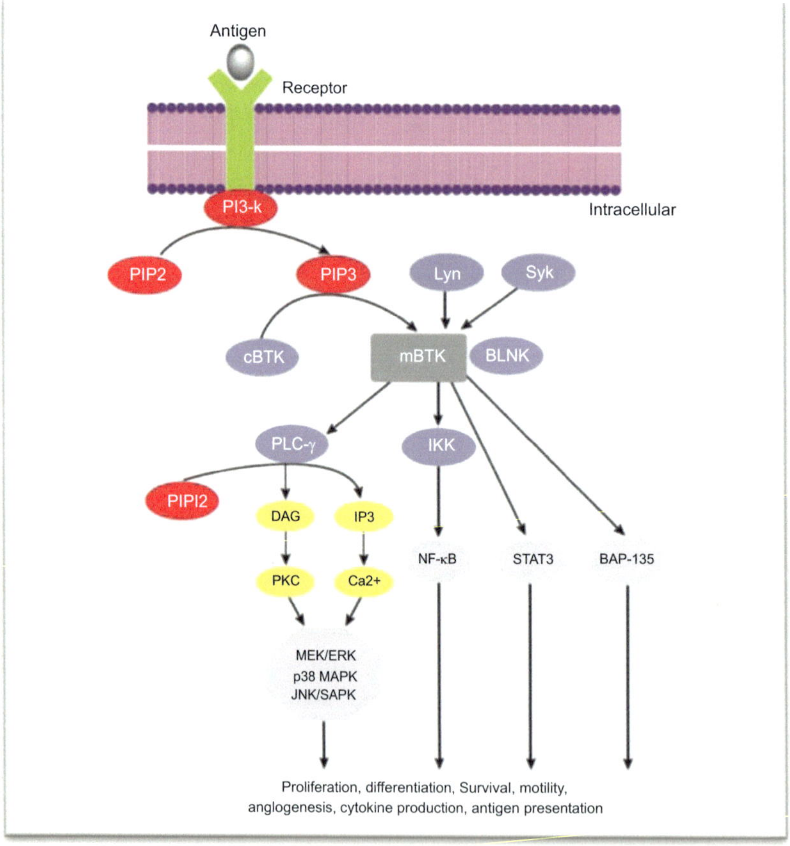

Fig. (2). BTK signaling pathway shown.

The results of the phase 2 study (RESONATE-17) further confirmed the efficacy of ibrutinib in 144 patients with relapsed or refractory CLL/SLL with 17p deletion [34]. At a median follow-up of 13 months, the overall response rate and progression-free survival were 82.6% and 79.3%, respectively.

Novel Uses of Ibrutinib

Dubovsky J and colleagues [35] hypothesized that ibrutinib may be ideally suited in the treatment of cGVHD due to its ability to block activation of B cells *via* BTK inhibition as well as specific T helper subsets that drive the development of this disease *via* interleukin-2 inducible T cell kinase (ITK) inhibition. Two different murine models (one imitating a T cell-driven sclerodermatous process and the other simulating an alloantibody-driven bronchiolar obliterans process) demonstrated that ibrutinib treatment delayed progression, improved survival, and ameliorated clinical and pathological manifestations of cGVHD and restored pulmonary function in the T and B cell-driven processes, respectively. Interestingly, animals lacking BTK and ITK did not develop cGVHD, signifying that these kinases are crucial in the pathogenesis of cGVHD.

Subsequently, Miklos DB and colleagues [36] described an ongoing phase 1b/2 study designed to evaluate the safety and efficacy of ibrutinib in patients with steroid-dependent/refractory cGVHD. Patients should have received no more than three prior regimens for their cGVHD to be eligible for the study. To date, six patients are evaluable for phase 1b. Median age is 56 years and median time from HCT was 23 months. Initial dose being evaluated is 420mg and median time on ibrutinib was 19.3 weeks. With respect to safety profile, most frequent mild adverse events included fatigue (N=5), diarrhea (N=4), bruising (N=3), and stomatitis (N=2); all reported to be grade 1 or 2. Serious adverse events, all grade 3, occurred in two patients (one with pneumonia and another with pyrexia and fungal brain abscess; the latter event leading to discontinuation of ibrutinib). A preliminary analysis of efficacy revealed that the remaining 5 patients achieved a partial response after at least 3 months of treatment. Phase 2 enrollment is ongoing to confirm these results in a greater number of patients.

IDELALISIB

Pharmacology/Pharmacokinetics/Pharmacodynamics

Idelalisib (Zydelig®) is an oral, first-in-class, potent small molecule inhibitor of the delta isoform of PI3K. It has been established that the PI3K protein plays a key role in the activation, proliferation, and viability of B cells. It is the most critical isoform involved in the malignant phenotype in CLL and is highly expressed in lymphoid cells. Additionally, idelalisib inhibits several signaling pathways, including BCR and CXCR4/5; all which may play key roles in pathophysiology of CLL. It was approved by the FDA in July 2014 for treatment of relapsed CLL (in combination with rituximab) when rituximab alone is appropriate therapy due to other comorbidities (*e.g.*, reduced renal function defined by creatinine clearance <60 ml/min or grade 3 or higher neutropenia/ thrombocytopenia from previous cytotoxic chemotherapy). Idelalisib also carries indications for follicular B-cell non-Hodgkin lymphoma (NHL) and SLL.

Following administration, maximum idelalisib plasma concentrations are reached at a median of 1.5 hours. Idelalisib is hepatically metabolized to its major inactive metabolite GS-563117 primarily *via* aldehyde oxidase and CYP3A4. It incurs minor metabolism through UDP-glucuronosyltransferase (UGT) 1A4. At steady state, idelalisib has a terminal elimination half-life of 8.2 hours. It is largely excreted in the feces (78%) [37].

Pivotal Clinical Studies

The FDA approval was based on a phase 3, placebo-controlled, randomized trial of rituximab monotherapy plus placebo (N=110) or idelalisib in combination with rituximab (N=110) in heavily, pre-treated relapsed CLL patients [38]. The majority of patients (78%) were 65 years or older; 40% had moderate renal dysfunction (defined as creatinine clearance <60 ml/min); 35% had grade 3 or higher cytopenias. At the first planned interim analysis, the trial was stopped early due to the tremendous efficacy of idelalisib plus rituximab. The median progression-free survival was 5.5 months in the placebo group and was not reached in the idelalisib group. Improved rates of overall response (81% *versus* 13%; P< 0.001) were seen in the idelalisib/rituximab group. Overall survival at 12 months was also greater in this arm (92% *versus* 80%; P= 0.02). In the idelalisib group, the most common adverse events were pyrexia, fatigue, nausea, chills, and diarrhea. Grade 3 or 4 adverse events (*e.g.*, pneumonia, pyrexia, and febrile neutropenia) were reported in 40% of patients in the idelalisib group and 35% in the placebo group.

In conclusion, idelalisib is an important addition to the armamentarium of CLL management. The combination of idelalisib to rituximab in a population of fragile and difficult-to-treat patients, including those with adverse prognostic features, was superior to rituximab monotherapy (a commonly used treatment in such patients). As the results from various ongoing studies become available (*e.g.*, idelalisib monotherapy and in combination with other agents in previously untreated and relapsed/refractory CLL patients), the role of idelalisib will likely continue to expand.

FUTURE DIRECTIONS

Chronic Myeloid Leukemia

Future directions in the management of patients with CML will focus on the possibility of discontinuation of tyrosine kinase inhibitor therapy and potential cure of this disease.

Tyrosine kinase inhibitors are unquestionably the standard frontline therapy for patients with newly diagnosed CML. However, allogeneic HCT remains a potentially curative treatment in CML and is recommended for patients who are intolerant to all oral therapies (albeit unusual); those with the T315I mutation; as well as for the rare patients who present with or progress to accelerated or blast phase. Of concern, relapse after HCT is still a problem for patients who undergo transplant in advanced phase disease and those undergoing a T-cell depleted transplant. Therefore, post-transplant tyrosine kinase inhibitor therapy should be considered following HCT.

Most of the existing data consists of experience with imatinib or dasatinib as either prophylaxis (*e.g.,* maintenance therapy) or treatment of relapse post-HCT. There are still many questions that remain ambiguous such as "trigger" point of time and disease burden for starting tyrosine kinase inhibitors post-HCT. It is unknown if all patients should be treated prophylactically or only started when a molecular relapse is detected. Which therapies should be used and for what duration post-HCT? Clinical research should continue to evaluate these therapeutic concerns in order to maximize treatment outcomes for patients with CML [39, 40].

Chronic Lymphocytic Leukemia

Management of patients with CLL has changed significantly over the recent years. A plethora of novel therapeutic agents have been developed and approved for clinical use, resulting in improved response rates and increased progression-free/OS for this patient population. Both intravenous (*e.g.,* CD20 targeted antibodies such ofatumumab and obinutuzumab) and oral directed therapies (*e.g.,* ibrutinib and idelalisib) are available currently.

Although obinutuzumab has produced impressive results (either in combination with chlorambucil or as monotherapy), the most exciting development will lie in its potential for combination with new kinase inhibitors such as ibrutinib or idelalisib. Unlike cytotoxic chemotherapy, both ibrutinib and idelalisib have the strong ability to induce the migration of clonal cells from lymph node and bone marrow to the blood. Thus, combination with such abilities may allow agents such as obinutuzumab to act synergistically in eliminating circulating B cells [32].

KEY CONCEPTS

Key Concepts in Chronic Myelogenous Leukemia
• CML is a myeloproliferative disorder which results from a single chromosomal abnormality, the Philadelphia chromosome.
• The introduction of the tyrosine kinase inhibitors revolutionized the treatment of CML, improving the ten year overall survival from 20% up to 90%.
• Notable recent therapies approved for CML include the Bcr-abl kinase inhibitors, bosutinib and ponatinib; and omacetaxine, a reversible inhibitor of protein synthesis.
• Future directions in the management of patients with CML will focus on the possibility of discontinuation of tyrosine kinase inhibitor therapy and potential cure of this disease.
Key Concepts in Chronic Lymphocytic Leukemia
• CLL is a neoplasm characterized by proliferation and accumulation of small lymphocytes and it remains the most prevalent adult leukemia in Western countries.
• The current standard of care has evolved from single agent alkylating agents, through the introduction of purine analogs, to chemoimmunotherapy combinations.
• Several novel therapeutic options have been developed in recent years, including monoclonal antibodies directed against CD20, ofatumumab and obinutuzumab; ibrutinib, BTK inhibitor; and idelalisib, inhibitor of PI3K.
• Management of patients with CLL has changed significantly over the recent years, with the plethora of new agents resulting in improved response rates and increased progression-free and overall survival for this patient population.

In addition to ibrutinib and idelalisib, several other BTK and PI3K inhibitors are in development along with spleen tyrosine kinase inhibitors. Another class of promising agents is the BCL-2 inhibitors. Venetoclax, the first in this class, is in registration phase 3 trials. It has demonstrated complete responses in patients with relapsed/refractory CLL. It also has activity in patients with very high risk CLL (*e.g.*, 17p deletion) [41].

HODGKIN LYMPHOMA AND ANAPLASTIC LARGE CELL LYMPHOMA

Background

Hodgkin lymphoma (HL), also known as Hodgkin disease, is a lymphoma of the white blood cells, specifically the lymphocytes which play a major role in the immune system. Lymphoid tissue can be found in many parts of the body but major sites are the lymph nodes, bone marrow, and spleen. The most common sites of lymph node involvement are the chest, neck, or under the arms. It occurs in both children and adults and is most common during the ages of 15 to 40 years and after the age of 55 years. There are two main types of HL: classic (nodular sclerosing, mixed cellularity, lymphocyte-rich, lymphocyte-depleted) accounting for 95% of cases; and nodular lymphocyte-predominant, accounting for 5% of cases. An abnormal B lymphocyte called Reed-Sternberg cells are found in classic HL and express CD30.

The American Cancer Society estimates that there will be 9,050 new cases in 2015 with an estimated 1,150 deaths [42]. Risk factors include Epstein-Barr viral infection, also known as mononucleosis, ages 15-40 years and ≥ 55 years of age, male gender, living in a developed country (United States, Canada, and northern Europe), brother or sister with HL (especially an identical twin), HIV infection, and higher socioeconomic status [42]. The disease is staged I-IV, bulky *versus* non-bulky, and as A (no B symptoms present) or B (B symptoms present, *e.g.*, ≥ 10% weight loss over the last six months, unexplained fever, drenching night sweats). Later stage disease, as well as bulky stage disease may require more intensive treatment. Resistant or recurrent HL is especially difficult to treat and presents many challenges to the healthcare team.

Over the past several decades, survival rates have continued to improve. The 1-year survival rate is now an estimated 92% and 5-year survival is approximately 85%. Based on stage, the 5-year survival rates are stage I 90%, stage II 90%, stage III 80%, and stage IV 65% [42]. There are four main modalities for treatment which include radiation, chemotherapy, monoclonal antibodies, and high dose chemotherapy followed by stem cell transplant. Radiation therapy is employed usually in early, localized disease and also may follow chemotherapy in some cases. Chemotherapy regimens are commonly multidrug regimens that exploit each drug's mechanism of action to increase synergy.

The most common regimen used in the United States is ABVD (doxorubicin, bleomycin, vinblastine, dacarbazine). Other regimens that can be utilized include BEACOPP (bleomycin, etoposide, doxorubicin, cyclophosphamide, vincristine, procarbazine, and prednisone) and the Stanford V regimen (doxorubicin, mechlorethamine, vincristine, vinblastine, bleomycin, etoposide, and prednisone). Stage I and IIA with favorable risk factors are treated with ABVD for 2 to 4 cycles followed by radiation or ABVD alone for 4 to 6 cycles. For stages I and II with unfavorable risk factors, the treatment usually consists of ABVD for 4 to 6 cycles. Patients with stage III and IV disease are often treated with ABVD for 6 cycles but BEACOPP and Stanford V may also be considered. If patients do not respond to chemotherapy or relapse, then salvage chemotherapy followed by a stem cell transplant is considered. An autologous stem cell transplant is the most utilized type of transplant but for those who still progress after an autologous transplant, an allogeneic transplant may be considered. Treatment options for patients who are relapsed or refractory are limited especially following transplant and outcomes are grim. Targeted therapy and immunotherapy are areas of interest for future treatment options for this patient population.

Anaplastic large cell lymphoma (ALCL) accounts for 12.1% of T-cell lymphomas and less than 5% of all NHL [43]. There are two distinct subtypes of ALCL which are systemic (ALK-negative or ALK-positive) and primary cutaneous. ALK-positive ALCL is most common in children and young adults and carries a better prognosis, whereas ALK-negative ALCL occurs in older patients and is associated with a worse prognosis. ALCL is an aggressive lymphoma but may be curable with chemotherapy alone. The most commonly used regimen is CHOP (cyclophosphamide, doxorubicin, vincristine, and prednisone). Following this anthracycline-based regimen, ALK-positive disease had superior results when compared to ALK-negative disease. Five-year failure-free survival (FFS) was 60% *versus* 36% and 5-year OS was 70% compared to 49% [43]. Unfortunately, about half of patients still develop recurrent disease. ALCL does strongly express CD30, which makes it a target for brentuximab which will be further discussed. Autologous stem cell transplant is an option but is often reserved for relapsed or refractory patients with chemotherapy-sensitive disease.

BRENTUXIMAB VEDOTIN

Pharmacology/Pharmacokinetics/Pharmacodynamics

Brentuximab vedotin (Adcetris®) was granted accelerated approval by the FDA in 2012. It is a CD30-directed antibody drug conjugate (ADC). The drug consists of 3 main parts: the chimeric antibody IgG1 cAC10 which is specific for CD30, the microtubule disrupting agent monomethyl auristatin E (MMAE), and a protease cleavable linker [44]. The antibody is produced from Chinese hamster ovaries while the small molecular components are produced *via* chemical synthesis. Brentuximab exerts its effects resulting in apoptosis of cancer cells. Apoptosis occurs when the ADC binds to CD30 positive cells and the entire complex is internalized. Upon internalization, the complex is cleaved resulting in release of MMAE. As a microtubule disrupting agent, MMAE functions by binding to tubulin and causing cell cycle arrest. Currently brentuximab is approved for HL after failure of autologous stem cell transplant or after two or more multidrug chemotherapy regimens in patients who are not transplant candidates [44]. An additional indication is for systemic ALCL following failure of a multidrug chemotherapy regimen.

The pharmacokinetics of brentuximab have been studied in phase 1 trials that included a total of 314 patients. When discussing the pharmacokinetics it is important to evaluate each of the drug's components including the ADC and

MMAE. The maximum concentration was observed towards the end of the infusion for ADC and for MMAE which ranged from 1 to 3 days. Steady-state was achieved for ADC within 21 days and the terminal half-life was about 4 to 6 days. MMAE steady-state was also achieved in 21 days but exposures decreased by 20-50% after the first dose. ADC revealed a high volume of distribution of approximately 6-10L. As expected, MMAE was highly protein bound with estimates ranging from 68-82% and it is a substrate for p-glycoprotein. Interestingly, only a small fraction of MMAE released from the drug complex is actually metabolized *via* CYP3A4/5. MMAE has been proven to be an inhibitor of CYP3A4/5 but does not affect other CYP enzymes. Only 24% of MMAE was recovered in the urine and approximately 72% eliminated in the feces.

Pivotal Clinical Studies

Accelerated approval of brentuximab was granted for both HL and systemic ALCL based on the overall response rate (ORR). A phase II, open-label, multicenter trial of 102 patients with HL treated with brentuximab 1.8mg/kg intravenously every 21 days was conducted [45]. Efficacy was evaluated based on ORR and duration of response. Patients in this study were heavily pretreated with a median of 3.5 prior therapies and all patients had previously undergone autologous stem cell transplant. The ORR was 75%, with 34% achieving a complete remission (CR) and the median duration of response for patients in CR was 20.5 months. Based on this study, brentuximab had manageable toxicities and an ORR of 75% in patients with relapsed or refractory HL.

A phase II, open-label, multicenter trial of 58 patients with relapsed ALCL were treated with brentuximab 1.8mg/kg intravenously every 21 days [46]. Efficacy was evaluated based on ORR and duration of response. On average, patients had received 2 prior therapies with 50% being relapsed and 50% refractory to their most recent therapy. The ORR was 86%, with 57% achieving a CR. Median duration of ORR was 12.6 months. Forty-two patients had ALK-negative ALCL and their results were similar to ALK-positive patients, ORR 88% *versus* 81% and CR 52% *versus* 69%, respectively. Progression-free survival (PFS) and median duration of response was also not different between ALK-negative and ALK-positive patients. Based on this study, over half of patients with relapsed or refractory ALCL achieved a CR making it a valuable treatment option.

FUTURE DIRECTIONS

Brentuximab is also being studied as maintenance post-transplant and as part of upfront regimens. A phase III randomized, placebo-controlled, multicenter trial evaluated the use brentuximab as a maintenance strategy post-autologous transplant to prevent disease progression in high risk HL patients [47]. There were a total of 327 patients enrolled and patients were to receive therapy for 1 year or approximately 16 cycles. The estimated 2-year PFS was 54% and 2-year OS was 88%. For upfront therapy, brentuximab is being evaluated in place of bleomycin.

Treatment strategies for relapse after autologous stem-cell transplant are limited for HL. Brentuximab is an option for those who have not received it but if a response is achieved the duration of that response is often short. In 2015, a small study was published evaluating the effects of PD-1 on relapsed or refractory HL [48]. Reed-Sternberg cells escape detection by the immune system by taking advantage of the PD-1 pathway resulting in overexpression of the associated ligands. It was hypothesized that nivolumab, a PD-1 inhibitor approved for the treatment of melanoma, may have activity in relapsed or refractory HL. Twenty-three heavily pretreated patients were enrolled with 78% having received prior autologous stem cell transplant as well as 78% having received prior brentuximab. Twenty patients (87%) achieved an objective response with 17% being a CR and 70% achieving a partial response (PR). The other 3 patients had stable disease (SD). Progression-free survival at 24 weeks was 86% and 6 patients were able to proceed with a stem cell transplant. Overall, nivolumab had therapeutic activity with an acceptable safety profile in relapsed or refractory HL. This drug is currently being used off-label for patients similar to those in the trial.

KEY CONCEPTS

Key Concepts in Hodgkin Lymphoma and Anaplastic Large Cell Lymphoma
• HL has an estimated 85% 5-year survival rate and is treated with four main modalities including radiation, chemotherapy, monoclonal antibodies, and high dose chemotherapy followed by stem cell transplant.
• Relapsed HL remains difficult to treat but the targeted agent, brentuximab has shown an ORR of 75% and immunotherapy continues to be an area of promising research.
• ALCL is a rare NHL and is difficult to treat especially in the relapsed setting. Brentuximab is a newly approved option for ALCL with an ORR of 86%.

MANTLE CELL LYMPHOMA

Background

Mantle cell lymphoma (MCL) is a subtype of NHL. The American Cancer Society estimates that there will be 71,850 new cases of NHL in 2015 and 19,790 deaths due to NHL [43]. It is a cancer of the lymphocytes which are part of the immune system. Most lymphocytes are found in lymph nodes but other lymphoid-containing tissues include the spleen and bone marrow. Lymphocytes are further divided into B and T lymphocytes. MCL is a B cell lymphoma and accounts for about 5% of all lymphomas. It occurs more frequently in men and the average age of onset is the early 60s. Risk factors for NHL in general include older age, male gender, Caucasian ethnicity, living in a developed country, chemical exposure (*e.g.*, benzene, certain herbicides or pesticides), radiation exposure, immune suppression or deficiency (prior organ transplant, human immunodeficiency virus (HIV), rheumatoid arthritis, lupus, Sjogren disease, celiac sprue), human T-cell lymphotropic virus (HTLV-1) infection, Epstein-Barr virus (EBV) infection, human herpes virus-8 (HHV8) infection, Heliobacter pylori infection, and hepatitis C infection [43].

Prognosis depends on several factors including the type and stage of NHL. The 5-year OS for all NHL is 69% and the 10-year rate is 59% [43]. To predict survival the revised international prognostic index is often used which differentiates patients into very good, good, and poor risk. Factors taken into consideration for scoring are age, stage, performance status, serum lactate dehydrogenase (LDH), and extent of lymphoma involvement.

MCL is an aggressive lymphoma that can be difficult to treat and cure. Although, patients may respond to frontline treatment, many patients relapse and die from their disease. Treatment of NHL, MCL included, may include chemotherapy, radiation, surgery, targeted therapy, immunotherapy, or stem cell transplant. Chemotherapy may be utilized alone or with radiation and regimens often consist of multiple chemotherapy agents. Early stage disease is often treatable with radiation with or without rituximab. For later stage disease, performance status heavily influences which regimens may be used. For patients with a poorer performance status, regimens that may be considered include bendamustine and rituximab, cladribine and rituximab, RCHOP (rituximab, cyclophosphamide, doxorubicin, vincristine, and prednisone), and modified HyperCVAD (cyclosphosphamide, vincristine, doxorubicin, and steroids alternating with methotrexate and cytarabine). When patients have a better performance status more intensive regimens may be used such as HyperCVAD, CALGB protocols, NORDIC regimen, RCHOP alternating with RDHAP (dexamethasone, cytarabine, cisplatin), or sequential RCHOP with RICE (rituximab, ifosfamide, carboplatin, etoposide). Targeted therapy options in MCL include bortezomib and ibrutinib. Immunotherapy options include rituximab and lenalidomide. Prior to the approval of lenalidomide and ibrutinib, bortezomib was the only FDA approved therapy for relapsed disease. An autologous stem cell transplant may be considered as consolidation strategy or for patients with relapsed disease. Allogeneic transplant may be considered for a second consolidation or for those patients who relapse particularly after an autologous transplant. Newer treatments recently approved are providing better chances of long-term survival.

LENALIDOMIDE

Pharmacology/Pharmacokinetics/Pharmacodynamics

Lenalidomide (Revlimid®) is an immunomodulating agent and is a direct derivative of thalidomide with both antineoplastic and antiangiogenesis properties. It acts by inhibiting proliferation thus resulting in apoptosis of the hematologic cancer cell. It affects the immune system inhibiting inflammatory cytokines, specifically IL-6 and TNF-alpha through activation of natural killer and T cells. Lenalidomide has several indications but most recently it was approved in 2013 for MCL in patients whose disease had relapsed or progressed after 2 prior therapies, including bortezomib.

Lenalidomide is taken orally without regard to food. Pharmacodynamic studies have shown that lenalidomide is rapidly absorbed *via* the oral route and AUC peaks within 0.5-6 hours [49]. The half-life varies from 3 to 5 hours. This drug is excreted largely unchanged in the urine so requires dose adjustments for moderate to severe renal dysfunction. Pharmacokinetic studies have shown that half-life increases and clearance decreases linearly with renal dysfunction. Lenalidomide is present in semen and is embryo-fetal toxic and thus contraindicated in pregnancy. Females should avoid pregnancy while taking lenalidomide and for 4 weeks after the last dose. Males should use protection during sex and for 4 weeks after the last dose. This drug has a risk evaluation and mitigation strategy (REMS) program requirement which requires patient-physician agreement forms as well as monthly pregnancy tests for females. Lenalidomide is only available through pharmacies that are certified in REVLIMID REMS™.

Pivotal Clinical Studies

The safety and efficacy of lenalidomide in the treatment of MCL was studied in a multicenter, single-arm, phase II trial [50]. All 134 patients had advanced disease with 53% of patients previously treated with 4 or more regimens and were relapsed after or were refractory to a bortezomib-containing regimen. These patients were treated with lenalidomide 25mg or 10mg, respectively depending on renal function, by mouth daily for days 1-21 of 28 day cycle until progression, toxicity, or withdrawal. The ORR was 28% consisting of CR and CRu (complete response unconfirmed) 7%, and PR 19%. Median time to response was 2.2 months with a median duration of response of 16.6 months. Median PFS was 4 months and median OS was 19 months. Overall, lenalidomide demonstrated a durable response in heavily pretreated MCL patients.

IBRUTINIB

<u>*Pivotal Clinical Studies*</u>

Ibrutinib, a Bruton's tyrosine kinase inhibitor, has been previously discussed in the CLL section but it was also approved in 2013 for MCL. The drug was an accelerated approval based on ORR. It is indicated in MCL patients who have received at least one prior therapy [51]. Accelerated approval was based on an open-label, multicenter, single-arm phase II trial consisting of 111 patients who had received at least one prior therapy for MCL. [52]. Patients were divided into 2 groups, those who had been treated with at least 2 cycles of bortezomib or patients treated with no or less than 2 cycles of bortezomib. Median number of prior treatments was 3 and 11% of patients had previously underwent a stem cell transplant. Dosing differed than in CLL, 560mg by mouth was administered once daily. The primary endpoint was ORR which was 68%. Of those that responded, 21% obtained a CR and 47% obtained a PR. Median duration of response was concluded to be 17.5 months. Prior treatment with bortezomib had no effect on response rate. At a follow-up of 15.3 months, median PFS was 13.9 months and OS was not reached. The estimated OS at 18 months was 58%. Overall, ibrutinib produced high, durable response rates in patients with relapsed or refractory MCL that had previously only been observed with multidrug, intensive regimens.

FUTURE DIRECTIONS

Future directions for the treatment of MCL are centered on combining chemotherapy with immunotherapy or targeted therapy. Some examples include ibrutinib with bendamustine and rituximab, lenalidomide with rituximab, rituximab with lenalidomide and bortezomib, rituximab and bortezomib with HyperCVAD, ibrutinib and bortezomib. ACP-196 is also another Bruton's tyrosine kinase inhibitor that is being investigated.

KEY CONCEPTS

Key Concepts in Mantle Cell Lymphoma
• MCL accounts for 5% of all NHL and often responds to frontline chemotherapy but relapse is common.
• Targeted therapy options in MCL include bortezomib and ibrutinib. Immunotherapy options include rituximab and lenalidomide.
• Future directions for the treatment of MCL consist of combining chemotherapy with immunotherapy or targeted therapy.

ACUTE LYMPHOBLASTIC LEUKEMIA

Background

Acute lymphocytic or lymphoblastic leukemia is an aggressive cancer of the bone marrow, specifically affecting the immature lymphocytes that is fatal within weeks if left untreated. Leukemia cells are aggressive, rapidly reproducing, and do not mature appropriately. There are two types of ALL based on the affected lymphocytes, B lymphocytes or T lymphocytes. B lymphocytes are important to the immune system as they protect the body from invaders (*e.g.*, viruses, bacteria, fungi) and make antibodies that tag these intruders and trigger the immune system to destroy them. T lymphocytes can directly destroy invaders but some types also boost or slow the immune system depending on their specific subtype [53]. ALL mainly affects the bone marrow but can also spread quickly to other sites such as the lymph nodes, spleen, testicles, and central nervous system (CNS).

The American Cancer Society estimates that there will be 6250 new cases of ALL in 2015 and 1450 deaths from ALL [53]. The highest incidence of ALL occurs in children less than 5 years of age. This risk then decreases until the mid-20s and begins to increase again after the age of 50. About 40% of cases are in adults, males are at a slightly higher risk than females, and it is more common in whites than African Americans. Even though only 40% of cases are in adults, about 80% of deaths due to ALL occurs in adults [53]. There are risk factors for ALL but the majority of patients diagnosed with ALL have no risk factors at all. Risk factors include high levels of radiation exposure, chemical exposure (*e.g.*, chemotherapy, benzene), inherited syndromes (Down syndrome, Klinefelter syndrome, Fanconi anemia, Bloom syndrome, ataxia-telangiectasia, and neurofibromatosis), white ethnicity, male gender, and an identical twin with ALL [53]. What causes ALL is still unknown but scientists do know that translocations are the most common form of mutation in ALL although deletions and inversions can also occur. The Philadelphia chromosome (Ph+), t(9;22), is an exchange of DNA between chromosomes 9 and 22 and is the most common translocation in ALL occurring in about 25% of adult ALL cases. Other translocations that occur in ALL but are less common are t(4;11) and t(8;14).

ALL is not staged like most other cancers, rather it is classified by the type of lymphocyte, cell maturity, and cytogenetics. B-cell ALL is divided into common ALL (50%), early pre-B ALL (10%), pre-B ALL (10%) and mature B-cell or Burkitt's leukemia (4%) [53]. T-cell ALL consists of mature T-cell ALL (15-20%) and pre-T cell ALL (5-10%). There are several prognostic factors that can affect outcomes. Patients diagnosed with ALL under the age of 50 tend to have better outcomes than those over the age of 60. Initial white blood cell count

(WBC) is also critical to prognosis. For B-cell ALL, a WBC less than 30,000 is a better prognosis and for those with T-cell ALL a WBC less than100,000 at diagnosis is a better prognostic indicator. The subtype also plays an important role in prognosis. Generally, mature B-cell ALL is the poorest prognosis while T-cell ALL has a better prognosis and all the other types are somewhere in the middle. Chromosome abnormalities are also important as t(4;11), trisomy 8, or deletion 7 are poor prognostic indicators. The Philadelphia chromosome used to be thought of as a poor prognostic indicator but now there are targeted drugs (*e.g.*, tyrosine kinase inhibitors) that can improve the overall prognosis. The response to initial chemotherapy also impacts prognosis as those who go into CR (>*e.g.*, less than 5% blasts in the marrow and normal blood counts) within 4-5 weeks have better a prognosis while those that do not go into CR have a poorer prognosis.

Treatment of ALL can consist of chemotherapy, targeted therapy, and stem cell transplant. The initial induction treatment is usually started urgently and is aggressive. Generally, 80-90% of patients will attain CR but roughly 50% relapse contributing to an overall cure rate of about 40%. Treatment usually consists of 3 phases: induction, consolidation, and maintenance with treatment lasting 2 to 3 years. ALL is treated with a combination of chemotherapy agents. Regimens consist of a combination of some of the following agents vincristine, anthracyclines, cytarabine, L-asparaginase, topoisomerase II inhibitors, 6-mercaptopurine, methotrexate, cyclophosphamide, steroids, and intrathecal chemotherapy as ALL is prone to relapse in the CNS.

Targeted therapy has evolved in the last several years especially in regards to treatment of Ph+ ALL. Several tyrosine kinase inhibitors have been approved for Ph+ ALL including imatinib, dasatinib, nilotinib, and ponatinib. These agents have been shown to increase remission rates and are important strategies for maintenance therapy. Asparaginase has also played a valuable role in the treatment of ALL in children and young adults. Monoclonal antibodies can also play an important role in treatment, especially in relapsed or refractory patients. Blinatumomab is one of those monoclonal antibodies that will be discussed in further details in the next section. Radiation therapy is generally not used but can be used in certain situations such as CNS disease, testicular involvement, part of the preparative regimen for transplant, and as palliation for pain [53]. When standard chemotherapy fails to cure patients or patients have high risk features, an allogeneic stem cell transplant may considered. Patients who relapse following an allogeneic transplant have limited treatment options.

BLINATUMOMAB

Pharmacology/Pharmacokinetics/Pharmacodynamics

Blinatumomab (Blincyta®) was approved *via* accelerated approval in 2014 for Ph-negative relapsed or refractory B-cell ALL. The drug is manufactured *via* Chinese hamster ovary cells. It is a CD19-directed CD3-targeted monoclonal antibody that binds to CD19 on B cells and CD3 on T cells. It causes lysis of CD19+ cells *via* a connection of CD3 with CD19 on benign and cancerous B cells (see Fig. **3**). This results in the upregulation of adhesion molecules, release of cytokines, and proliferation of T cells [54]. Cytokine elevation is the highest during the first 48 hours of the first cycle of blinatumomab.

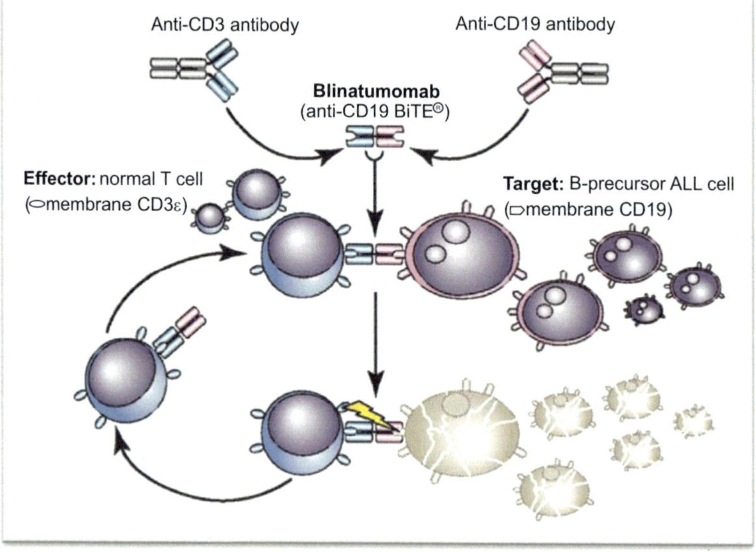

Fig. (3). Pharmacology of blinatumomab shown.

Blinatumomab is administered as a continuous infusion over 28 days. It is given as a 9 mcg/day infusion on days 1-7, increased to 28 mcg/day for days 8-28, and then a 2 week rest period. For the remaining cycles, blinatumomab is given as a 28 mcg/day continuous infusions on days 1-28. Initially there is a redistribution of T cells and a decrease in B cells, as well as the previously discussed cytokine release. T cell counts decrease within 1-2 days and return to baseline levels usually with 7 to 14 days. Drug interactions have not been formally evaluated but blinatumomab causes cytokine release which can suppress CYP450 enzymes. This theoretical interaction could affect CYP450 substrates especially during the first 9 days of the first cycle and the first 2 days of the second cycle. The metabolism of blinatumomab has not been well characterized as of yet but is likely degraded into small peptides and basic amino acids.

Pivotal Clinical Studies

The landmark study for blinatumomab was a phase II open-label, multicenter, single-arm study of 189 patients with relapsed or refractory B-cell ALL who were Ph-negative [55]. Sixty-three (34.1%) of patients had a previous HSCT and 17.3% had at least 2 prior salvage regimens. Blinatumomab was administered as a continuous infusion over 28 days. The beginning dose was 9mcg/day for 1 week then 28mcg/day for 3 weeks. For subsequent cycles, blinatumomab 28mcg/day was administered. At the end of 2 cycles, 43% of patients had achieved CR or CRh (CR with incomplete blood cell count recovery) and 40% of those patients went on to transplant. Most patients, 81%, achieved CR after the first cycle. The median duration of response was 5.9 months for patients in CR or CRh. In conclusion, this was one of the largest trials in patients with relapsed or refractory ALL and blinatumomab proved to be a viable option for this patient population.

In addition, there is a randomized, open-label phase III study of blinatumomab *versus* standard of care (one of four protocol defined regimens) for Philadelphia chromosome-negative relapsed or refractory B-cell ALL, also known as the TOWER study. The prespecified interim analysis showed that the primary endpoint of OS was met. This is the first immunotherapy study to show an OS benefit in this patient population. Final results are expected in August of 2016.

ASPARAGINASE ERWINIA CHRYSANTHEMI

Pharmacology/Pharmacokinetics/Pharmacodynamics

Pegaspargase (Oncaspar®) has been incorporated into many pediatric and young adult ALL treatment protocols but patients may experience hypersensitivity reactions. As an alternative to pegaspargase, E.coli asparaginase (Elspar®) was developed but hypersensitivity continued to be a hurdle to therapy. Asparaginase Erwinia chrysanthemi (Erwinaze®) was approved in 2011 as yet another alternative. The specific indication for asparaginase Erwinia is for patients with ALL who have developed a hypersensitivity reaction to E.coli asparaginase. It is an enzyme that is specific for the amino acid, asparagine. This enzyme causes the breakdown of asparagine *via* deamination to aspartic acid and ammonia. This results in a decrease of asparagine due to lack of asparagine synthetase which is essential to leukemia cells. Leukemia cells cannot synthesize asparagine, which is essential to survival specifically due to its involvement in protein metabolism.

There are specific dosage recommendations when substituting asparaginase Erwinia for pegaspargase or E.coli asparaginase. For each pegaspargase dose,

25,000 International Units (IU)/m2 of asparaginase Erwinia should be given intramuscularly or intravenously three times a week for 6 doses. To substitute for E.coli asparaginase, 25,000 IU/m2 of asparaginase Erwinia should be administered either intramuscularly or subcutaneously.

There are differences noted in pharmacokinetics when comparing intramuscular *versus* intravenous administration. The mean half-life of intravenous asparaginase was determined to be 7.51 hours *versus* 15.6 hours for intramuscular administration. This shorter half-life was documented when comparing 48 and 72 hour nadir serum asparaginase activity (NSAA). After intramuscular administration, a 48 hour NSAA greater than 0.4 IU/mL was achieved in 80% of patients and 38% at 72 hours. Whereas, following intravenous administration these numbers decreased dramatically to 29% and 0%, respectively [56].

Pivotal Clinical Studies

Two pertinent evaluations have been conducted to determine the safety of asparaginase Erwinia. The first study was a single-arm, multicenter, open-label trial to determine safety and the clinical efficacy. The main objective was to determine the amount of patients who obtained a trough asparaginase level greater than or equal to 0.1 IU/mL. Activity greater than or equal to 0.1 IU/mL has shown effective in depleting asparagine and predicts clinical efficacy. There were 48 evaluable patients treated on various cooperative ALL protocols that reacted to pegaspargase. Forty-four (76%) of patients were able to complete all therapy. Fourteen (24%) patients stopped therapy with 7 of those being due to allergic reactions. All of the patients were able to obtain the desired trough asparaginase activity.

The second evaluation was from the Erwinaze Master Treatment Protocol (EMTP) which is an expanded access program. This evaluation consisted of 940 patients with ALL or lymphoblastic lymphoma who received asparaginase after hypersensitivity to the native form. Of note, the doses ranged from 20,000 to 25,000 units/m2 and was given either intramuscularly or intravenously. 693 (78%) of patients were to receive all scheduled doses for their treatment regimen and there was a 14% incidence of systemic hypersensitivity which is comparable to what was elucidated in first study.

VINCRISTINE SULFATE LIPOSOME

Pharmacology/Pharmacokinetics/Pharmacodynamics

Vincristine sulfate has been previously approved for several types of cancer. It is a sulfate salt isolated from the periwinkle plant. The newly approved liposomal formulation is more than 95% encapsulated in sphingomyelin and cholesterol liposomes. Non-liposomal vincristine sulfate binds to tubulin, altering the tubulin polymerization equilibrium, resulting in altered microtubule structure and function. Non-liposomal vincristine sulfate stabilizes the spindle apparatus, preventing chromosome segregation, triggering metaphase arrest and inhibition of mitosis. Liposomal vincristine (Marqibo®) is indicated for patients with Ph-negative ALL in second or greater relapse whose disease has progressed following two or more other therapies. Approval was granted in 2012 based on ORR.

Liposomal vincristine is not immediately bioavailable after intravenous administration unlike non-liposomal vincristine. The plasma clearance of liposomal vincristine is much slower than non-liposomal vincristine, 345 mL/h *versus* 11,340 mL/h [57]. This results in a much higher AUC for liposomal vincristine. The main route of excretion is *via* the fecal route. Vincristine is a substrate for CYP3A so strong CYP3A inducers and inhibitors should be avoided. It is also a substrate for p-glycoprotein and therefore potent inhibitors and inducers should be avoided, although this interaction has not been thoroughly studied.

Pivotal Clinical Studies

The landmark trial for liposomal vincristine was a phase II open-label, multicenter, single-arm study in adult patients with Ph-negative ALL in second or greater relapsed or whose disease had progressed following at least two other therapies [58]. All patients must have achieved CR with at least one prior therapy for equal to or greater than 90 days. The treatment consisted of liposomal vincristine monotherapy dosed at 2.25 mg/m2 intravenously every 7 days. A total of 65 patients were enrolled and all had previously received non-liposomal vincristine, 48% had undergone prior stem cell transplant, 51% had received 3 or more prior therapies, 45% were refractory to their most recent treatment, and 80% had pre-existing neuropathy. CR or CRi (CR with incomplete hematologic recovery) was 20% and ORR was 35% with a median duration of response of 23 weeks. In conclusion, liposomal vincristine provided meaningful clinical outcomes in relapsed or refractory ALL patients and may serve as a bridge to transplant for some patients.

FUTURE DIRECTIONS

Patients with ALL who are chemo-refractory or who relapse after allogeneic stem cell transplant have a high mortality rate with limited treatment options. Over the past two decades, we have learned a great deal about the heterogeneity of ALL and its potential molecular weaknesses. These molecular targets have become a primary area of research. Several agents are under study but some of the most promising examples include inotuzumab ozogamicin and chimeric antigen receptor (CAR) T cells.

Inotuzumab ozogamicin, a humanized anti-CD22 antibody-drug conjugate, was recently granted breakthrough status by the FDA. Mature B cells and the majority of immature B cells express CD22. Mechanistically, inotuzumab binds to the CD22 target and is then internalized resulting in DNA strand breaks and apoptosis caused by the conjugated chemotherapy agent. The INO-VATE ALL trial was a phase III study for relapsed or refractory ALL patients in which patients received inotuzumab or chemotherapy [59]. One hundred and nine patients received inotuzumab at a dose of 0.8 mg/m2 on day 1 and then 0.5 mg/m2 on days 8 and 15. In the chemotherapy arm, there were 109 patients who received physicians' choice of fludarabine plus cytarabine, high dose cytarabine, or cytarabine with mitoxantrone.

The response rate for inotuzumab was 80.7% *versus* 33.3% for the chemotherapy arm, respectively ($P< 0.0001$). Results were also significantly different in favor of inotuzumab for responses in patients receiving inotuzumab as first or second line salvage therapy. The duration of first CR was durable with responses lasting 12 or more months in 43% of patients on the inotuzumab arm. At the time of the approval, data for OS was not yet available but the duration of response was significantly longer for inotuzumab, 4.6 months compared to 3.1 months ($P= 0.0169$). Forty percent of patients in the chemotherapy arm discontinued treatment due to resistant disease, while the most frequent reason for inotuzumab discontinuation was CR at 35%. Inotuzumab was utilized in 48 patients as a bridge to transplant, which is twice as many patients that received transplant in the chemotherapy arm. Veno-occlusive disease occurred more frequently in the inotuzumab arm, 15 *versus* 1, respectively but 10 of the cases were post-transplant. Further research is ongoing for inotuzumab in elderly ALL patients and also in other disease states.

CAR T cell therapy is an adoptive immunotherapy strategy currently being investigated in phase II studies for ALL and lymphomas. T cells are collected from the patient and genetically modified with synthetic chimeric antigen receptors. When the product is infused, these T cells are capable of selective binding to CD19 which is expressed on leukemia cells and limited nonmalignant cells. Binding results in stimulation of T cells and eventually exponential CAR T cell expansion and killing of the cancer cells. Preliminary results have been promising, demonstrating that this therapy can induce remissions in even those patients multiply relapsed. In phase I trials in both adults and children with relapsed ALL, 67-90% of patients have achieved morphologic remission [60].

Researchers are also conducting studies utilizing CAR T cells to target the CD22 antigen. CD22 is present on most B cells but in smaller quantities than CD19. Together, CD19 and CD22 could be used in conjunction to target both antigens. In some patients, CD19 expression can be lost but CD22 expression is maintained which could also prove to be another role for CD22 targeted therapy. Adverse effects of CAR T cell therapy include neurologic toxicity and cytokine release syndrome. These adverse effects thus far seem to be transient but can be life-threatening.

KEY CONCEPTS

Key Concepts in Acute Lymphoblastic Lymphoma
• ALL is an aggressive cancer of the bone marrow initially treated with intense chemotherapy.
• For Ph+ ALL, targeted therapy with tyrosine kinase inhibitors remains vital to treatment due to their ability to increase remission rates and serve as a maintenance therapy.
• Other agents approved in the last 5 years include blinatumomab, asparaginase Erwinia chrysanthemi, vincristine sulfate liposome, and inotuzumab ozogamicin.
• CAR T cell therapy is an adoptive immunotherapy strategy currently under investigation.

T-CELL LYMPHOMAS, MULTIPLE MYELOMA, MYELOFIBROSIS

Background

T-cell Lymphoma, a less frequent form of NHL, is often split into Cutaneous T-Cell Lymphoma (CTCL) and Peripheral T-cell Lymphoma (PTCL) subtypes. Cytogenetic abnormalities frequently involve translocations of antigens in T-cell receptor genes. HTLV-1 has also been associated with adult T-cell lymphoma [70]. CTCL consists of mycosis fungoides (MF) and Sezary syndrome (SS). CTCLs primarily develop in the skin, and at times progress to involve the lymph nodes, blood, and visceral organs. MF accounts for 50-70% of CTCL cases while SS accounts for only 1-3%. CD30 expression of tumor cells is associated with large cell transformation in 30-50% of cases of both MF and SS. Initial treatment in patients with patch or plaque disease consists of skin-directed therapies with milder systemic therapy for refractory, persistent, or progressive disease. PTCL can be further divided into Anaplastic Large Cell Lymphoma (ALK+, ALK negative), Angioimmunoblastic (AITL), Extranodal NK, and Peripheral T-cell Leukemia. PTCL has traditionally had a very poor prognosis, and often treated with B-cell Lymphoma type regimens, such as CHOP and ABVD. Other modalities imploded in the treatment of PTCL are antifolates, histone deacetylase inhibitors, monoclonal antibodies, nucleoside analogs, proteasome inhibitors, and signaling inhibitors [71].

Multiple myeloma (MM), a plasma cell disorder, is one of the most common hematological malignancies. MM is seen in the 7th decade of life, and often characterized by the progression of normal plasma cells to monoclonal gammopathy of undetermined significance (MGUS) [61]. There are several mutations associated with MM, these include t(14:16), t(11:14), and the poorest prognostic factors, deletion 13 and t(4:14) [62 - 64]. The cumulative probability of progression from MGUS to full blown MM after 25 years is approximately 30%. MM cells secrete IL-6 and IL-1 cytokines [65]. These cytokines contribute to many of the major symptoms often remembered by the acronym CRAB: elevated calcium, renal dysfunction, anemia, and bone disease. Plasma cell proliferation reduces normal hematopoiesis and enhances hyperviscosity often leading to bleeding, blurred vision, and confusion [66 - 68]. Lytic bone lesions are present in nearly 80% of cases and is thought to be caused by the activation of osteoclasts *via* soluble IL-6 receptors [69]. Unfortunately MM still remains incurable. The goal of therapy is to prolong and improve quality of life. Treatment therapies are largely determined by whether patients are transplant candidates. If a patient is transplant eligible, autologous HCT remains the treatment of choice.

Classified as a myeloproliferative neoplasm, myelofibrosis can arise on its own (primary myelofibrosis) or as a progression of polycythemia vera or essential thrombocythemia. Myelofibrosis is a chronic blood cancer with acquired mutations that target the hematopoietic stem cell and induce dysregulation of kinase signaling, clonal myeloproliferation, and abnormal cytokine expression. The pathogenetic processes create bone marrow stromal changes, extramedullary hematopoiesis, and ineffective erythropoiesis [72]. The abnormal stem cells produce more mature cells that grow quickly and take over the bone marrow, causing both fibrosis and chronic inflammation. Approximately 60% of people with myelofibrosis have a mutation called "JAK2V617F". The V617F mutation causes Janus Associated Kinases (JAK) to become "constitutively active" resulting in the production of more blood cells. Other known mutations consist of MPL and CALR, which also affect the JAK signaling pathway [73, 74]. Prognosis is based on the Dynamic International Prognostic Scoring System-plus model, which uses 8 independent predictors of inferior survival to classify patients into low, intermediate 1, intermediate 2, and high-risk disease groups; with estimated median survivals of 15.4, 6.5, 2.9, and 1.3 years respectfully [75]. Treatment strategies may include observation alone, conventional or investigational (*e.g.*, JAK inhibitors, pomalidomide) drug therapy, allogeneic HCT with reduced or conventional intensity conditioning, splenectomy, or radiotherapy.

Therapies Used in T-cell Lymphomas

PRALATREXATE

Pharmacology/Pharmacokinetics/Pharmacodynamics

Pralatrexate (Folotyn®), an antifolate analog, was approved by the FDA in 2009 for the treatment of relapsed or refractory peripheral T-cell lymphoma. It inhibits DNA, RNA, and protein synthesis by selectively entering cells expressing reduced folate carrier (RFC-1). It is polyglutamylated by folylpolyglutamate synthetase (FPGS), which then competes for the DHFR-folate binding site to inhibit dihydrofolate reductase (DHFR). Pralatrexate is broken down into two isomers and excreted through the urine with approximately 34% in the form of unchanged drug. The half-life can range between 12-18 hours [76].

Pivotal Clinical Studies

In 2012, Horwitz SM and colleagues [77] showed that pralatrexate was well-tolerated in relapsed or refractory CTCL patients. The patients in this study had either MF, SS, or primary cutaneous anaplastic large cell lymphoma, which had progressed after 1 year of systemic therapy. Patients received 10-30 mg/m^2/week for 3-4 weeks for a median of 4 cycles. Response rates were 45% and the most common adverse events reported were leukopenia (3%, grade 4) and mucositis (17%, grade 3). This study concluded that pralatrexate at a dose of 15 mg/m^2/spell out week for 3 to 4 weeks shows high activity with acceptable toxicity in patients.

In 2011 the PROPEL study [78] was published, which included patients with relapsed/refractory PTCL. Patient in this study received pralatrexate intravenously at 30 mg/m^2/week for six weeks in 7-week cycles. Out of 109 patients, there was a 29% response rate which included 11% complete response and 18% partial response. Median duration of response was approximately 10 months. Median PFS and OS were 3.5 and 14.5 months, respectively. The most common grade 3/4 adverse events were thrombocytopenia (32%), mucositis (22%), neutropenia (22%), and anemia (18%).

ROMIDEPSIN

Pharmacology/Pharmacokinetics/Pharmacodynamics

Romidepsin (Istodax®), approved by the FDA in 2009, is a histone deacetylase inhibitor that catalyzes the acetyl group removal from protein lysine residues. It is indicated for the treatment of CTCL and PTCL in patients who have received at least one prior therapy. Inhibition of histone deacetylase results in accumulation of acetyl groups, leading to alterations in chromatin structure and transcription factor activation causing termination of cell growth and cell death. Romidepsin is metabolized hepatically primarily through CYP3A4 with a half-life around 3 hours [79].

Pivotal Clinical Studies

In a phase II study by Peikarz RL and colleagues [80], romidepsin was given to CTCL patients, subtypes MF or SS, who had received no more than two prior cytotoxic regimens. Complete response was observed in four out of 71 patients, and partial responses were observed in 20 patients for an overall response rate of 34% (95% CI, 23-46%). The median duration of response was 13.7 months. This study concluded that romidepsin has single-agent clinical activity with significant and durable responses in patients with CTCL.

In 2010 Whittaker SJ and colleagues [81] confirmed the efficacy of romidepsin in a study of 96 patients. Patients received romidepsin as an intravenous infusion at a dose of 14 mg/m^2 on days 1, 8, and 15, every 28 days. The study showed a response rate of 34%, which included 6 patients with a complete response. The median time to response was 2 months, with a duration of response of 15 months. A clinically meaningful improvement in pruritus was observed in 28 (43%) of 65 patients, including patients who did not achieve an objective response. Median duration of reduction in pruritus was 6 months. Drug-related adverse events consisted of gastrointestinal disturbances and asthenic conditions.

Peikarz RL and colleagues [82] published a phase 2 trial in 2011 which included both CTCL and PTCL patients. Forty-seven patients with PTCL of various subtypes including PTCL not otherwise specified, angioimmunoblastic, ALK-negative anaplastic large cell lymphoma, and enteropathy-associated T-cell lymphoma were enrolled. All patients had received prior therapy with a median of 3 previous treatments (range 1-11); 18 (38%) had undergone HCT. Common toxicities were nausea, fatigue, transient thrombocytopenia, and granulocytopenia. Complete responses were observed in 8 and partial responses in 9 of 45 patients, for an overall response rate of 38% (95% confidence interval 24-53%). The median duration of overall response was 8.9 months (range 2-74 months). Responses were observed in various subtypes, with 6 responses among the 18 patients with prior HCT. Romidepsin showed durable responses in patients with relapsed PTCL.

Romidepsin was also seen to be effective in relapsed/refractory AITL. Pro B and colleagues [83] showed induced durable responses. In 27 patients with AITL, most had advanced disease (96% had stage III/IV disease; 44% with bone marrow involvement; 52% with elevated lactate dehydrogenase) and were heavily pretreated (median, 2 [range, 1-8] prior therapies) and 37% were refractory to their last line of therapy. Single-agent romidepsin produced rapid, complete, and durable responses in some patients with relapsed/refractory AITL, with several responses ongoing for >3 years. Patients with long-term responses to romidepsin received maintenance dosing. These results support the use of romidepsin in relapsed/refractory AITL.

Bates S and investigators [84] confirmed the promising results in 84 patients with both CTCL and PTCL. Patients with PTCL receiving romidepsin as third-line therapy or later had a comparable response rate (32%) of similar duration as the total population (38%). Safety data show slightly greater hematological and constitutional toxicity in PTCL.

Dupuis J and colleagues [85] studied romidepsin with cyclophosphamide, doxorubicin, vincristine, and prednisone in previously untreated patients with peripheral T-cell lymphoma. This was a non-randomized trial that enrolled 37 patients with PTCL into a dose-escalation (phase 1b) and expansion (phase 2) study at 9 Lymphoma Study Association centers in France. Three of six patients initially treated at 10 mg/m^2 had a dose-limiting toxicity. Three patients were treated with 8 mg/m^2 of romidepsin, an additional three at 10 mg/m^2 (one dose-limiting toxicity), and six patients at 12 mg/m^2 (three dose-limiting toxicities). Romidepsin 12 mg/m^2 was the recommended dose for phase 2. Of the 37 patients treated, three had early cardiac events (two myocardial infarctions and one acute cardiac failure). Overall, the most frequent serious adverse events were febrile neutropenia, physical health deterioration, lung infection, and vomiting. Eighty-nine percent of patients had grade 3-4 neutropenia, and 29 patients (78%) had grade 3-4 thrombocytopenia. Authors concluded that romidepsin can potentially be combined with CHOP chemotherapy.

BELINOSTAT

Pharmacology/Pharmacokinetics/Pharmacodynamics

Belinostat (Beleodaq®), another histone deacetylase inhibitor, was approved in 2014 for the treatment of relapsed/refractory PTCL. It works by catalyzing acetyl group removal from protein lysine residues. Histone deacetylase results in accumulation of acetyl groups, leading to cell cycle arrest and apoptosis. Belinostat is primarily hepatically metabolized through UGT1A1 and approximately 40% of the drug is excreted through the urine. It is well distributed with a half-life of 1.1 hours [86].

Pivotal Clinical Studies

Pohlman B and colleagues [87] published a study in 2009 using belinostat in 53 patients with either PTCL and CTCL. A CR of 10% and a PR of 15% was reported, with an ORR of 25% in PTCLs. With respect to CTCLs, 14% of patients responded with a CR of 7%. Grade 3 or 4 hematologic toxicity was seen in less than 10% of patients.

The BELIEF study [88] was conducted utilizing belinostat in patients with relapsed/refractory PTCL. Belinostat 1,000 mg/m^2 administered intravenously over 30 minutes daily on days 1-5 of a 21-day regimen was given to 129 patients across 62 sites in North America, Europe, and Africa. Of the 120 evaluable patients, 13 achieved a complete response (11%). In responding patients, the median time to response was 5.6 weeks, with the earliest after 4.3 weeks and the latest at 50.4 weeks. The median duration of response, defined as the date of first response to the date of disease progression or death, was 8.4 months (95% confidence interval, 4.5-29.4). Notably, 9 patients (7.5%) were able to proceed to a stem cell transplant. With regard to toxicity, belinostat was well tolerated, with dose reductions of 25-50% occurring in 13% of patients. Progressive disease was the most common reason for discontinuation (64%), followed by death (11%), and patient request (8%). Significant myelosuppression was not a factor in this study, with less than 10% grade 3 or 4 thrombocytopenia or neutropenia.

Foss F and colleagues [89] published a multicenter study in patients with PTCL or CTCL who failed $\geq$ 1 prior systemic therapy and were treated with belinostat (1000 mg/m^2 intravenously for 5 days of a 21 day cycle). The ORRs were 25% (PTCL) and 14% (CTCL). Treatment-related adverse events occurred in 77% of patients and consisted of nausea (43%), vomiting (21%), infusion site pain (13%), and dizziness (11%). Treatment-related serious adverse events included Grade 5 ventricular fibrillation, grade 4 thrombocytopenia, grade 3 peripheral edema, apraxia, paralytic ileus, and pneumonitis; and grade 2 jugular vein thrombosis. Belinostat monotherapy was noted to be well tolerated and efficacious in patients with recurrent/refractory PTCL and CTCL.

Therapies Used in Multiple Myeloma

CARFILZOMIB

Pharmacology/Pharmacokinetics/Pharmacodynamics

Carfilzomib (Kyprolis®) was approved by the FDA in 2012 for relapsed/refractory MM. It works by inhibiting proteasomes, which are responsible for intracellular protein homeostasis. Specifically, it is a potent, selective, and irreversible inhibitor of chymotrypsin-like activity of the 20S proteasome, and leads to cell cycle arrest and apoptosis. Carfilzomib penetrates all tissues extensively except the brain. It is rapidly and extensively metabolized. There is a minimal metabolism through cytochrome P450-mediated mechanisms. The half-life elimination is less than 1 hour on day 1 of cycle 1 when doses are greater than or equal to 15 mg/m^2 [90].

Pivotal Clinical Studies

Shah JJ and colleagues [91] published an abstract at the American Society of Hematology meeting showing carfilzomib was well tolerated in combination with pomalidomide and dexamethasone. Treatment consisted of 28-day cycles of oral pomalidomide once daily on days 1-21, intravenous carfilzomib over 30 minutes on days 1, 2, 8, 9, 15, and 16, and oral or intravenous dexamethasone 40 mg on days 1, 8, 15, and 22. Carfilzomib was initiated at 20 mg/m^2 for Cycle 1, days 1-2 at all dose levels. This combination achieved a high response rate (ORR of 64%) in a heavily pre-treated lenalidomide-refractory population with prior bortezomib exposure, with a median of 6 lines of prior therapy.

Berdeja JG and investigators [92] assessed safety and efficacy of the combination of panobinostat and carfilzomib in patients with relapsed/refractory multiple myeloma. Forty-four patients were accrued into the trial with a overall response rate of 67%. At a median follow-up of 17 months, median PFS was 7.7 months, median time to progression (TTP) was also noted to be 7.7 months, and median OS had not been reached. Overall, carfilzomib was well tolerated. In conclusion, the combination of panobinostat and carfilzomib is feasible and effective in patients with relapsed/refractory multiple myeloma.

A multi-centered, open-label phase 2 trial determined the safety and efficacy of carfilzomib in combination with cyclophosphamide and dexamethasone in patients with newly diagnosed MM who were 65 years of age or greater or ineligible for autologous stem cell transplantation [93]. Fifty eight patients received carfilzomib, cyclophosphamide, and dexamethasone for up to nine 28-day cycles, followed by maintenance with carfilzomib until progression or intolerance. Ninety-five percent of patients achieved at least a partial response, 71% achieved at least a very good partial response, 49% achieved a near complete response, with 20% who achieved a stringent complete response. After a median follow-up of 18 months, the 2-year PFS and OS rates were 76% and 87%, respectively. The most frequent grade 3 to 5 toxicities were neutropenia (20%), anemia (11%), and cardiopulmonary adverse events (7%). Peripheral neuropathy was limited to grades 1 and 2 (9%). Fourteen percent of patients discontinued treatment because of adverse events and 21% of patients required carfilzomib dose reductions. Authors concluded that this combination showed high complete response rates and a tolerable safety profile.

POMALIDOMIDE

Pharmacology/Pharmacokinetics/Pharmacodynamics

Pomalidomide (Pomalyst®), approved by the FDA in 2013 for relapsed/refractory MM, works by inducing cell cycle arrest and apoptosis directly in multiple myeloma cells by enhancing T cell and natural killer cell-mediated cytotoxicity. It also inhibits production of the pro-inflammatory cytokines tumor necrosis factor-α (TNF-α), interleukins-1, 6, and 12, which further inhibits angiogenesis. Pomalidomide is rapidly absorbed on an empty stomach. It is metabolized hepatically by CYP1A2 and CYP3A4 with a half-life of 8-10 hours [94].

Pivotal Clinical Studies

Dispenzieri A and colleagues [95] analyzed pomalidomide and dexamethasone combination in 33 patients. The confirmed hematologic response rate was 48%, with a median time to response of 1.9 months. Organ improvement was documented in 5 patients. The median overall and PFS rates were 28 and 14 months, respectively; the 1-year overall and PFS rates were 76% and 59%, respectively. The most common grade 3-5 adverse events were neutropenia and fatigue.

Larocca A and investigators [96] performed a phase 1/2 trial to determine the maximum tolerated dose (MTD) of pomalidomide and to explore its efficacy when combined with cyclophosphamide-prednisone in relapsed/refractory myeloma patients. The median time-to-response was 1.83 months. After a median follow-up of 14.8 months, median PFS was 10.4 months and 1-year OS was 69%. At the MTD, grade 3 to 4 toxicities included anemia (9%), thrombocytopenia (11%), neutropenia (42%), neurologic events (7%), dermatologic events (7%), and thromboembolism (2%). Grade 3 to 5 infections occurred in 5 patients (9%). Five patients (9%) discontinued treatment for toxicity. New grade 3 to 4 adverse events were low during maintenance.

Leleu X and colleagues [97] showed that the combination of pomalidomide and low-dose dexamethasone can be safely administered to patients with end-stage relapsed/refractory multiple myeloma. However, shorter median PFS and OS were seen in these patients when characterized by adverse cytogenetics (deletion 17p and translocation [4, 14]). There was a striking difference in TTP, duration of response, and ORR according to the presence of del(17p) compared with t(4;14) (TTP, 7.3 *versus* 2.8 months; duration of response, 8.3 *versus* 2.4 months; and

ORR, 32% *versus* 15%, respectively). Overall survival was prolonged after pomalidomide and dexamethasone, particularly in t(4;14), given the short TTP, suggesting that patients were rescued at relapse with further lines of therapy. Pomalidomide and dexamethasone, a doublet immunomodulatory drug–based regimen, is active and well tolerated in adverse cytogenetic patients with early relapsed/refractory MM, particularly in those with del(17p), who are characterized by a high and rapid development of a refractoriness state and known for their poor prognosis.

A phase II randomized, multicenter, double-blind study, was published [98] in 2009 evaluating the safety and therapeutic activity of pomalidomide in patients with anemia associated with myelofibrosis. Four treatment arms were included: pomalidomide (2 mg per day) plus placebo, pomalidomide (2 mg per day) plus prednisone, pomalidomide (0.5 mg per day) plus prednisone, and prednisone plus placebo. Eighty-four patients in total were randomly assigned. Response in anemia was documented in 20 patients, including 15 who became transfusion independent. Response rates in the four treatment arms were 23% (95% CI, 5-41%), 16% (95% CI, 0-33%), 36% (95% CI, 16-56%), and 19% (95% CI, 2-36%). Response to pomalidomide with or without prednisone was durable (range, 3.2 to 16.9+ months) and significantly better in the absence of leukocytosis (37% *versus* 8%; P= 0.01); JAK2V617F or cytogenetic status did not affect response. Toxicities of grade 3 or higher were infrequent and included (in each treatment arm) neutropenia (9%; 16%; 5%; 5%, respectively), thrombocytopenia (14%; 16%; 9%; 5%, respectively), and thrombosis (9%; 5%; 0%; 0%, respectively).

Latest Therapies in Multiple Myeloma

Of importance to be mentioned, panobinostat (Farydak®) was granted accelerated approval by the FDA in February 2015 to be used in combination with bortezomib and dexamethasone for the treatment of patients with MM who have received at least 2 prior therapies, including bortezomib and an immunomodulatory agent. Panobinostat is a histone deacetylase inhibitor and has shown to have promising results in this patient population.

Therapies Used in Myelofibrosis

RUXOLITINIB

Pharmacology/Pharmacokinetics/Pharmacodynamics

Ruxolitinib (Jakafi®) was approved by the FDA in 2011. It is an oral medication indicated for the treatment of myelofibrosis and polycythemia vera. Ruxolitinib is a small molecule kinase inhibitor which selectively and potently inhibits JAKs,

JAK1 and JAK2. JAK1 and JAK2 mediate the signaling of cytokines and growth factors important for hematopoiesis and immune function. It modulates gene expression by interfering with the JAK signaling pathway, which involves recruitment, activation, and localization of signal transducers and activators of transcription to cytokine receptors and the nucleus. Ruxolitinib is rapidly absorbed and metabolized in the liver, primarily *via* CYP3A4. It forms active metabolites which are responsible for 20-50% of its activity. Time to peak is 1-2 hours and 74% of the drug is excreted unchanged in the urine [99].

Pivotal Clinical Studies

Cervantes F and colleagues [100] reported an analysis from a 3-year follow-up (median, 151 weeks) of the efficacy and safety of the Controlled Myelofibrosis Study With Oral Janus-associated Kinase Inhibitor Treatment-II (the COMFORT-II Trial), comparing ruxolitinib with the best available therapy in 219 patients with intermediate-2 and high-risk myelofibrosis. In the ruxolitinib arm, with continued therapy, spleen volume reductions of ≥ 35% by magnetic resonance imaging sustained for at least 144 weeks, with the probability of 50% (95% confidence interval, 36-63%) among patients achieving such degree of response. Anemia and thrombocytopenia were the main toxicities, but they were generally manageable, improved over time, and rarely led to treatment discontinuation (1% and 3.6% of patients, respectively). Additionally, patients randomized to ruxolitinib showed longer OS than those randomized to best available therapy (hazard ratio, 0.48; 95% CI, 0.28-0.85; log-rank test, P= 0.009).

Mead AJ and investigators [101] published the UK ROBUST trial, an open-label, phase II study evaluating the safety and efficacy of ruxolitinib in patients with myelofibrosis (N=48). Overall, 50% of patients and 57% of intermediate-1 risk patients, achieved treatment success; reductions in spleen length and symptoms were observed in all risk groups. The majority of patients (66.7%) experienced ≥50% reductions from baseline in spleen length at any time. Consistent with other studies of ruxolitinib, the most common hematological adverse events were anemia and thrombocytopenia. Results indicate that most patients with myelofibrosis, including intermediate-1 risk patients, may benefit from ruxolitinib treatment.

Verstovsek S and colleagues [102] revealed in the phase III COMFORT-I study, that ruxolitinib provided significant improvements in splenomegaly, key symptoms, and quality-of-life measures and was associated with an OS benefit relative to placebo in patients with intermediate-2 or high-risk myelofibrosis. At week 144, mean spleen volume reduction was 34% with ruxolitinib. Previously observed improvements in quality-of-life measures were sustained with longer-term ruxolitinib therapy. Ruxolitinib continued to be well tolerated; there was no pattern of worsening of grade ≥3 anemia or thrombocytopenia with longer-term ruxolitinib exposure.

Novel Uses of Ruxolitinib

As noted earlier, graft-*versus*-host disease (GVHD) is a severe complication of allogeneic HCT, accounting for 15-30% of deaths post-transplant. It is characterized by the production of high levels of pro-inflammatory cytokines. It is postulated that activated JAKs are required for T effector cell responses in various inflammatory disorders; thus, blockade could effectively reduce GVHD.

Spoerl S and colleagues treated six patients suffering from steroid-refractory GVHD with ruxolitinib after demonstrating that *in vivo* JAK 1/2 inhibition improved survival of mice developing acute GVHD and reduced histopathologic grading, serum levels of pro-inflammatory cytokines, and expansion of alloreactive luc-transgenic T cells. Patients were included if they had acute or chronic GVHD that was refractory to steroids given for at least one month and at least 2 other immunosuppressive approaches. Patients were treated with ruxolitinib at a starting dose of 5mg orally twice daily with a dose increase to 10mg twice daily if no side effects after three days of therapy. Four of the six patients had acute GVHD (gastrointestinal involvement in one; all others with skin involvement); two patients had chronic skin GVHD.

All patients were able to reduce their dose of steroids after ruxolitinib initiation. In addition, one hundred percent of patients responded with respect to clinical GVHD symptoms (time to response 1-1.5 weeks) and serum levels of pro-inflammatory cytokines. Treatment with ruxolitinib promoted FoxP3+ regulatory T cells, which are linked to immunological tolerance. Based on the pre-clinical and clinical data presented, JAK 1/2 inhibition may be introduced as a novel concept to mitigate this grave complication following allogeneic HCT [103].

Subsequently, the same group reported outcomes of 14 patients with GVHD refractory to steroids and at least two other lines of treatment who received ruxolitinib salvage treatment. Ten patients had acute GVHD and four patients had features consistent with cGVHD; various sites were involved including skin, gastrointestinal tract, and liver. Of 14 patients, 13 responded with respect to clinical GVHD symptoms and levels of pro-inflammatory cytokines (one patient discontinued therapy due to lack of response after one week). Steroids were reduced 1.5 weeks after ruxolitinib initiation. Two patients developed mild cytopenias during ruxolitinib treatment and did not require dose reduction or transfusion. These results further support therapeutic JAK 1/2 inhibition as salvage treatment in GVHD [104].

FUTURE DIRECTIONS

Multiple Myeloma

Like many of the disease states discussed in this chapter, the future of multiple myeloma is focused on both immunotherapeutic and targeted agents. Elotuzumab is a monoclonal antibody directed against Signaling Lymphocytic Activation Molecular F7 (SLAMF7). ELOQUENT-1, a phase III study compared elotuzumab in combination with lenalidomide and dexamethasone to lenalidomide and dexamethasone (Ld) alone for patients with relapsed/refractory multiple myeloma [107]. A large number of patients were enrolled with 321 in the elotuzumab arm and 325 in the Ld arm. Overall response was 79% for the elotuzumab arm *versus* 66% for the Ld arm, (P= 0.0002). Progression-free survival was 19.4 months and 14.9 months for the elotuzumab group and the Ld group, respectively (P= 0.0004). Grade 3 and 4 adverse events were similar between the two groups with the most frequently observed AEs being neutropenia and anemia.

Other investigational agents include those that inhibit spindle formation, specifically aurora Kinase A and the kinesin spindle protein, and the cyclin dependent kinase inhibitor, dinaciclib. There are several other agents active in the RAF/RAS/MEK/ERK and PI3K/AKT/mTOR pathways but as monotherapy in phase I and II studies these agents have not shown a clear benefit [108]. Likely, these agents may need to be studied in combination with proven active agents to see if there is a clinical advantage. Currently, two oral proteasome inhibitors are in early phase trials, ixazomib and oprozomib. With the advent of several new targeted agents and the continued development of others, the treatment of multiple myeloma will continue to be revolutionized improving patient's quality of life and survival.

Myelofibrosis

Telomerase has become a target for the treatment of cancer, as most cancers have a high level of telomerase activity and relatively short telomeres compared to normal cells. Imetelstat is a lipid-conjugated 13-mer oligonucleotide sequence that binds with high affinity to the RNA template of telomerase, which directly inhibiting telomerase activity. The tissue half-life of imetelstat is estimated to be 41 hours in humans. Imetelstat is the first telomerase inhibitor to advance to clinical development. Clinically relevant and significant inhibition of telomerase activity has been seen in various types of tissue in which telomerase activity is measurable, including normal bone marrow hematopoietic cells, malignant plasma cells, hair follicle cells, and peripheral blood mononuclear cells [105].

Thirty three high-risk or intermediate-2–risk myelofibrosis patients were given imetelstat, as a 2-hour intravenous infusion (starting dose, 9.4 mg/kg of body weight) every 1 to 3 weeks. A complete or partial remission occurred in 7 patients (21%), with a median duration of response of 18 months for complete responses and 10 months for partial responses. Bone marrow fibrosis was reversed in all 4 patients who had a complete response, and a molecular response occurred in 3 of the 4 patients. Response rates were 27% among patients with a JAK2 mutation *versus* 0% among those without a JAK2 mutation (P= 0.30) and 32% among patients without an ASXL1 mutation *versus* 0% among those with an ASXL1 mutation (P= 0.07). The rate of complete response was 38% among patients with a mutation in SF3B1 or U2AF1 *versus* 4% among patients without a mutation in these genes (P= 0.04). Responses did not correlate with baseline telomere length. Treatment-related adverse events included grade 4 thrombocytopenia (in 18% of patients), grade 4 neutropenia (in 12%), grade 3 anemia (in 30%), and grade 1 or 2 elevation in levels of total bilirubin (in 12%), alkaline phosphatase (in 21%), and aspartate aminotransferase (in 27%). Although imetelstat was found to be active in patients with myelofibrosis, it is important to note its potential to cause clinically significant myelosuppression. In conclusion, the current study suggests the potential value of telomerase-targeting treatment strategies in patients with myelofibrosis and identifies imetelstat as an active drug for this disease [106].

Figure adapted with permission from Lydon N. Attacking cancer at its foundation. Nature Medicine. 2009;15: 1153-57.

Figure adapted with permission from Parmar S, Patel K, Pinilla-Ibarz J. Ibrutinib (Imbruvica): A novel targeted therapy for chronic lymphocytic leukemia. P&T. 2014;39: 483-519.

Figure adapted with permission from Kapoor A, Rajput PS, Beniwal S, *et al.* Blinatumomab: A ray of hope for relapsed/refractory adult B-cell acute lymphoblastic leukemia. Clin Cancer Investig J. 2014;3: 577-8.

KEY CONCEPTS

Key Concepts in T-cell Lymphomas
• T-cell lymphoma is often split into cutaneous T-cell lymphoma and peripheral T-cell lymphoma subtypes.
• Initial treatment for CTCL consists of skin-directed therapies with milder systemic therapy for refractory, persistent, or progressive disease.
• PTCL may be treated with multi-agent chemotherapy regimens, or antifolates, histone deacetylase inhibitors, smonoclonal antibodies, nucleoside analogs, proteasome inhibitors, and signaling inhibitors.

Contd.....

Key Concepts in Multiple Myeloma
• Multiple myeloma is characterized by the progression of normal plasma cells to monoclonal gammopathy of undetermined significance.
• Treatment therapies are largely determined by stem cell transplant eligibility.
• Current and future treatments are focused on both immunotherapeutic and targeted agents including proteasome inhibitors, inhibition of spindle formation, and antibodies against Signaling lymphocytic Activation Molecular F7 (SLAMF7).
Key Concepts in Myelofibrosis
• Myelofibrosis is a chronic blood cancer that induces dysregulation of kinase signaling, clonal myeloproliferation, and abnormal cytokine expression.
• Treatment strategies include observation, investigational drug therapy, allogeneic stem cell transplant, splenectomy, or radiotherapy.
• Future treatment strategies include telomerase-targeting and inhibition.

CONCLUDING REMARKS

During the last decade, we have witnessed a complete transformation in how blood cancers are approached and managed. A plethora of novel therapeutic agents have resulted from a deeper understanding of the biology of specific hematologic malignancies. Data on biomarkers from clinical trials and subsequent laboratory evaluation have ensued gradual shifting from the use of non-specific chemotherapeutic agents toward an era of targeted therapy. These directed therapies reduce toxicity profiles and have demonstrated improved survival in many studies as mentioned throughout the chapter. Most exciting, this era of targeted treatments have allowed clinicians to expand on personalized medicine. In conclusion, the pace of drug discovery and fast-moving landscape in this specific field is extraordinary and ultimately offers new hopes for patients.

CONFLICT OF INTEREST

The authors confirm that they have no conflict of interest to declare for this publication.

ACKNOWLEDGEMENTS

Declared none.

REFERENCES

[1] Faderl S, Talpaz M, Estrov Z, Kantarjian HM. Chronic myelogenous leukemia: biology and therapy. Ann Intern Med 1999; 131(3): 207-19. [http://dx.doi.org/10.7326/0003-4819-131-3-199908030-00008] [PMID: 10428738]

[2] Siegel RL, Miller KD, Jemal A. Cancer statistics, 2015. CA Cancer J Clin 2015; 65(1): 5-29. [http://dx.doi.org/10.3322/caac.21254] [PMID: 25559415]

[3] Schiffer CA. BCR-ABL tyrosine kinase inhibitors for chronic myelogenous leukemia. N Engl J Med 2007; 357(3): 258-65.
[http://dx.doi.org/10.1056/NEJMct071828] [PMID: 17634461]

[4] Goldman JM, Melo JV. Chronic myeloid leukemia--advances in biology and new approaches to treatment. N Engl J Med 2003; 349(15): 1451-64.
[http://dx.doi.org/10.1056/NEJMra020777] [PMID: 14534339]

[5] Rao KV, Jabbour E. Current and future clinical strategies in the management of chronic myeloid leukemia. Pharmacotherapy 2010; 30: 77S-101S.
[http://dx.doi.org/10.1592/phco.30.pt2.77S]

[6] Parmar S, Patel K, Pinilla-Ibarz J. Ibrutinib (imbruvica): A novel targeted therapy for chronic lymphocytic leukemia. P&T 2014; 39(7): 483-519.
[PMID: 25083126]

[7] García-Escobar I, Sepúlveda J, Castellano D, Cortés-Funes H. Therapeutic management of chronic lymphocytic leukaemia: state of the art and future perspectives. Crit Rev Oncol Hematol 2011; 80(1): 100-13.
[http://dx.doi.org/10.1016/j.critrevonc.2010.10.006] [PMID: 21146422]

[8] Chronic lymphocytic leukemia [homepage on the Internet] American cancer society. Available from: http://www.cancer.org. , [[cited 27th September 2015]];

[9] Hallek M. Chronic lymphocytic leukemia: 2013 update on diagnosis, risk stratification and treatment. Am J Hematol 2013; 88(9): 803-16.
[http://dx.doi.org/10.1002/ajh.23491] [PMID: 23720127]

[10] Doan V, Wang A, Prescott H. Bosutinib for the treatment of chronic myeloid leukemia. Am J Health Syst Pharm 2015; 72(6): 439-47.
[http://dx.doi.org/10.2146/ajhp140221] [PMID: 25736937]

[11] Amsberg GK, Schafhausen P. Bosutinib in the management of chronic myelogenous leukemia. Biologics 2013; 7: 115-22.
[PMID: 23674887]

[12] Bosulif [package insert]. New York, NY: Pfizer labs 2013.

[13] Cortes JE, Kim DW, Kantarjian HM, *et al.* Bosutinib *versus* imatinib in newly diagnosed chronic-phase chronic myeloid leukemia: results from the BELA trial. J Clin Oncol 2012; 30(28): 3486-92.
[http://dx.doi.org/10.1200/JCO.2011.38.7522] [PMID: 22949154]

[14] Cortes JE, Kantarjian HM, Brümmendorf TH, *et al.* Safety and efficacy of bosutinib (SKI-606) in chronic phase Philadelphia chromosome-positive chronic myeloid leukemia patients with resistance or intolerance to imatinib. Blood 2011; 118(17): 4567-76.
[http://dx.doi.org/10.1182/blood-2011-05-355594] [PMID: 21865346]

[15] Khoury HJ, Cortes JE, Kantarjian HM, *et al.* Bosutinib is active in chronic phase chronic myeloid leukemia after imatinib and dasatinib and/or nilotinib therapy failure. Blood 2012; 119(15): 3403-12.
[http://dx.doi.org/10.1182/blood-2011-11-390120] [PMID: 22371878]

[16] Iclusig Cambridge, MA: Ariad pharmaceuticals, Inc; 2014. Cambridge, MA: Ariad pharmaceuticals, Inc. 2014.

[17] Shamroe CL, Comeau JM. Ponatinib: A new tyrosine kinase inhibitor for the treatment of chronic myeloid leukemia and Philadelphia chromosome-positive acute lymphoblastic leukemia. Ann Pharmacother 2013; 47(11): 1540-6.
[http://dx.doi.org/10.1177/1060028013501144] [PMID: 24265264]

[18] Cortes JE, Kim DW, Pinilla-Ibarz J, *et al.* PACE Investigators. A phase 2 trial of ponatinib in Philadelphia chromosome-positive leukemias. N Engl J Med 2013; 369(19): 1783-96.
[http://dx.doi.org/10.1056/NEJMoa1306494] [PMID: 24180494]

[19] Jain P, Kantarjian H, Jabbour E, *et al.* Ponatinib as first-line treatment for patients with chronic myeloid leukaemia in chronic phase: a phase 2 study. Lancet Haematol 2015; 2(9): e376-83. [http://dx.doi.org/10.1016/S2352-3026(15)00127-1] [PMID: 26436130]

[20] Synribo. North Wales: PA: Teva pharmaceuticals; 2012.

[21] Chen Y, Li S. Omacetaxine mepesuccinate in the treatment of intractable chronic myeloid leukemia. Onco Targets Ther 2014; 7: 177-86. [PMID: 24516334]

[22] Cortes J, Lipton JH, Rea D, *et al.* Omacetaxine 202 Study Group. Phase 2 study of subcutaneous omacetaxine mepesuccinate after TKI failure in patients with chronic-phase CML with T315I mutation. Blood 2012; 120(13): 2573-80. [http://dx.doi.org/10.1182/blood-2012-03-415307] [PMID: 22896000]

[23] Castillo J, Perez K. The role of ofatumumab in the treatment of chronic lymphocytic leukemia resistant to previous therapies. J Blood Med 2010; 1: 1-8. [http://dx.doi.org/10.2147/JBM.S7284] [PMID: 22282677]

[24] FDA approved drugs: of atumumab [homepage on the Internet]. U.S. Food and drug administration. Available from: http://www.fda.gov , 2015 [[cited 19th October]];

[25] Arzerra. Research Triangle Park, NC: Glaxo SmithKline. 2014.

[26] Hillmen P, Robak T, Janssens A, *et al.* COMPLEMENT 1 Study Investigators. Chlorambucil plus ofatumumab *versus* chlorambucil alone in previously untreated patients with chronic lymphocytic leukaemia (COMPLEMENT 1): a randomised, multicentre, open-label phase 3 trial. Lancet 2015; 385(9980): 1873-83. [http://dx.doi.org/10.1016/S0140-6736(15)60027-7] [PMID: 25882396]

[27] Pidala J, Kim J, Betts BC, *et al.* Ofatumumab in combination with glucocorticoids for primary therapy of chronic graft-*versus*-host disease: phase I trial results. Biol Blood Marrow Transplant 2015; 21(6): 1074-82. [http://dx.doi.org/10.1016/j.bbmt.2015.03.014] [PMID: 25805300]

[28] Basu B. Ofatumumab for rituximab-resistant nephrotic syndrome. N Engl J Med 2014; 370(13): 1268-70. [http://dx.doi.org/10.1056/NEJMc1308488] [PMID: 24670185]

[29] Hoy SM. Obinutuzumab: a review of its use in patients with chronic lymphocytic leukaemia. Drugs 2015; 75(3): 285-96. [http://dx.doi.org/10.1007/s40265-014-0340-3] [PMID: 25586272]

[30] Gazyva . South San Francisco, CA: Genentech 2013.

[31] Goede V, Fischer K, Busch R, *et al.* Obinutuzumab plus chlorambucil in patients with CLL and coexisting conditions. N Engl J Med 2014; 370(12): 1101-10. [http://dx.doi.org/10.1056/NEJMoa1313984] [PMID: 24401022]

[32] Cartron G, de Guibert S, Dilhuydy M-S, *et al.* Obinutuzumab (GA101) in relapsed/refractory CLL: Final data from the phase 1/2 GAUGUIN study. Blood 2014; 124(14) [http://dx.doi.org/10.1182/blood-2014-07-586610] [PMID: 25143487]

[33] Byrd JC, Brown JR, O'Brien S, *et al.* Ibrutinib *versus* ofatumumab in previously treated CLL. N Engl J Med 2014; 371: 213-23. [http://dx.doi.org/10.1056/NEJMoa1400376] [PMID: 24881631]

[34] O'Brien S, Jones JA, Coutre S, *et al.* Efficacy and safety of ibrutinib in patients with relapsed or refractory CLL or SLL with 17p deletion: Results from the phase II RESONATE-17 trial. Blood 2014; 124: 21.

[35] Dubovsky JA, Flynn R, Du J, *et al.* Ibrutinib treatment ameliorates murine chronic graft-*versus*-host disease. J Clin Invest 2014; 124(11): 4867-76.

[http://dx.doi.org/10.1172/JCI75328] [PMID: 25271622]

[36] Miklos DB, Arora M, Cutler CS, *et al.* A multicenter open-label phase 1b/2 study of ibrutinib in steroid dependent or refractory chronic graft-*versus*-host disease. J Clin Oncol 2015. (suppl; abstr 7024).

[37] Keating GM. Idelalisib: a review of its use in CLL and indolent NHL. Target Oncol 2015; 10: 141-51. [http://dx.doi.org/10.1007/s11523-015-0359-8] [PMID: 25637459]

[38] Furman RR, Sharman JP, Coutre SE, *et al.* Idelalisib and rituximab in relapsed CLL. N Engl J Med 2014; 370: 997-1007. [http://dx.doi.org/10.1056/NEJMoa1315226] [PMID: 24450857]

[39] Bar M, Radich J. Maintenance therapy with tyrosine kinase inhibitors after transplant in patients with chronic myeloid leukemia. J Natl Compr Canc Netw 2013; 11(3): 308-15. [PMID: 23486457]

[40] Baccarani M, Cortes J, Pane F, *et al.* European LeukemiaNet. Chronic myeloid leukemia: an update of concepts and management recommendations of European LeukemiaNet. J Clin Oncol 2009; 27(35): 6041-51. [http://dx.doi.org/10.1200/JCO.2009.25.0779] [PMID: 19884523]

[41] Kuznar W. Treatment for CLL will incorporate more targeted therapies in the near future. Oncology Pharmacist 2015; 8: 3.

[42] Hodgkin disease American cancer society. Available from: http://www.cancer.org , [[cited 3rd October 2015]];

[43] Non-hodgkin's lymphoma American cancer society [homepage on the Internet] Available from: www.cancer.org. Available from: http://www.cancer.org , [[cited 3rd October 2015]];

[44] Brentuximab. Bothell, WA: Seattle Genetics 2015.

[45] Younes A, Gopal AK, Smith SE, *et al.* Results of a pivotal phase II study of brentuximab vedotin for patients with relapsed or refractory Hodgkin's lymphoma. J Clin Oncol 2012; 30(18): 2183-9. [http://dx.doi.org/10.1200/JCO.2011.38.0410] [PMID: 22454421]

[46] Pro B, Advani R, Brice P, *et al.* Brentuximab vedotin (SGN-35) in patients with relapsed or refractory systemic anaplastic large-cell lymphoma: results of a phase II study. J Clin Oncol 2012; 30(18): 2190-6. [http://dx.doi.org/10.1200/JCO.2011.38.0402] [PMID: 22614995]

[47] Moskowitz C, Nadamanee A, Masszi T, *et al.* The Aethera Trial: Results of a Randomized, Double-Blind, Placebo-Controlled Phase 3 Study of Brentuximab Vedotin in the Treatment of Patients at Risk of Progression Following Autologous Stem Cell Transplant for Hodgkin Lymphoma ASH Abstract 2014; 21(S2): 2190-6. [http://dx.doi.org/http://dx.doi.org/10.1016/j.bbmt.2014.11.017]

[48] Ansell SM, Lesokhin AM, Borrello I, *et al.* PD-1 blockade with nivolumab in relapsed or refractory Hodgkin's lymphoma. N Engl J Med 2015; 372(4): 311-9. [http://dx.doi.org/10.1056/NEJMoa1411087] [PMID: 25482239]

[49] Lenalidomide. Summit, NJ: Celegene Corporation 2015.

[50] Goy A, Sinha R, Williams ME, *et al.* Single-agent lenalidomide in patients with mantle-cell lymphoma who relapsed or progressed after or were refractory to bortezomib: phase II MCL-001 (EMERGE) study. J Clin Oncol 2013; 31(29): 3688-95. [http://dx.doi.org/10.1200/JCO.2013.49.2835] [PMID: 24002500]

[51] Ibrutinib [package insert]. Horsham, PA: Janssen Biotech, Inc. 2015.

[52] Wang ML, Rule S, Martin P, *et al.* Targeting BTK with ibrutinib in relapsed or refractory mantle-cell lymphoma. N Engl J Med 2013; 369(6): 507-16. [http://dx.doi.org/10.1056/NEJMoa1306220] [PMID: 23782157]

[53] Acute lymphocytic leukemia [homepage on the Internet]. American cancer society. Available from: www.cancer.org , [cited 3rd October 2015];

[54] Blinatumomab. Thousand Oaks, CA:: Amgen Inc. 2014.

[55] Topp MS, Gökbuget N, Stein AS, *et al.* Safety and activity of blinatumomab for adult patients with relapsed or refractory B-precursor acute lymphoblastic leukaemia: a multicentre, single-arm, phase 2 study. Lancet Oncol 2015; 16(1): 57-66. [http://dx.doi.org/10.1016/S1470-2045(14)71170-2] [PMID: 25524800]

[56] Asparaginase Erwinia. Palo Alto, CA: Jazz Pharmaceuticals; 2014.

[57] Vincristine sulfate liposomal injection. San Francisco, CA: Talon Therapeutics, Inc. 2012.

[58] O'Brien S, Schiller G, Lister J, *et al.* High-dose vincristine sulfate liposome injection for advanced, relapsed, and refractory adult Philadelphia chromosome-negative acute lymphoblastic leukemia. J Clin Oncol 2013; 31(6): 676-83. [http://dx.doi.org/10.1200/JCO.2012.46.2309] [PMID: 23169518]

[59] DeAngelo DJ, Stelljes M, Martinelli G, *et al.* Efficacy and safety of inotuzumab ozogamicin vs standard of care in salvage 1 or 2 patients with acute lymphoblastic leukemia: an ongoing global phase 3 study. 20th Congress of the European Hematology Association (EHA). Vienna, Austria. 2015.

[60] Tasian SK, Gardner RA. CD19-redirected chimeric antigen receptor-modified T cells: a promising immunotherapy for children and adults with B-cell acute lymphoblastic leukemia (ALL). Ther Adv Hematol 2015; 6(5): 228-41. [http://dx.doi.org/10.1177/2040620715588916] [PMID: 26425336]

[61] Siegel R, Ma J, Zou Z, Jemal A. Cancer statistics, 2014. CA Cancer J Clin 2014; 64(1): 9-29. [http://dx.doi.org/10.3322/caac.21208] [PMID: 24399786]

[62] Fonseca R, Blood E, Rue M, *et al.* Clinical and biologic implications of recurrent genomic aberrations in myeloma. Blood 2003; 101(11): 4569-75. [http://dx.doi.org/10.1182/blood-2002-10-3017] [PMID: 12576322]

[63] Chng WJ, Santana-Dávila R, Van Wier SA, *et al.* Prognostic factors for hyperdiploid-myeloma: effects of chromosome 13 deletions and IgH translocations. Leukemia 2006; 20(5): 807-13. [http://dx.doi.org/10.1038/sj.leu.2404172] [PMID: 16511510]

[64] Fonseca R, Bergsagel PL, Drach J, *et al.* International Myeloma Working Group. International Myeloma Working Group molecular classification of multiple myeloma: spotlight review. Leukemia 2009; 23(12): 2210-21. [http://dx.doi.org/10.1038/leu.2009.174] [PMID: 19798094]

[65] Kyle RA, Therneau TM, Rajkumar SV, *et al.* A long-term study of prognosis in monoclonal gammopathy of undetermined significance. N Engl J Med 2002; 346(8): 564-9. [http://dx.doi.org/10.1056/NEJMoa01133202] [PMID: 11856795]

[66] Bird JM, Owen RG, D'Sa S, *et al.* Haemato-oncology Task Force of British Committee for Standards in Haematology (BCSH) and UK Myeloma Forum. Guidelines for the diagnosis and management of multiple myeloma 2011. Br J Haematol 2011; 154(1): 32-75. [http://dx.doi.org/10.1111/j.1365-2141.2011.08573.x] [PMID: 21569004]

[67] International Myeloma Working Group. Criteria for the classification of monoclonal gammopathies, multiple myeloma and related disorders: a report of the International Myeloma Working Group. Br J Haematol 2003; 121(5): 749-57. [http://dx.doi.org/10.1046/j.1365-2141.2003.04355.x] [PMID: 12780789]

[68] Kyle RA, Gertz MA, Witzig TE, *et al.* Review of 1027 patients with newly diagnosed multiple myeloma. Mayo Clin Proc 2003; 78(1): 21-33. [http://dx.doi.org/10.4065/78.1.21] [PMID: 12528874]

[69] Palumbo A, Anderson K. Multiple myeloma. N Engl J Med 2011; 364(11): 1046-60.

[http://dx.doi.org/10.1056/NEJMra1011442] [PMID: 21410373]

[70] Foss FM, Zinzani PL, Vose JM, Gascoyne RD, Rosen ST, Tobinai K. Peripheral T-cell lymphoma. Blood 2011; 117(25): 6756-67. [http://dx.doi.org/10.1182/blood-2010-05-231548] [PMID: 21493798]

[71] Campo E, Swerdlow SH, Harris NL, Pileri S, Stein H, Jaffe ES. The 2008 WHO classification of lymphoid neoplasms and beyond: evolving concepts and practical applications. Blood 2011; 117(19): 5019-32. [http://dx.doi.org/10.1182/blood-2011-01-293050] [PMID: 21300984]

[72] Kuter DJ, Bain B, Mufti G, Bagg A, Hasserjian RP. Bone marrow fibrosis: pathophysiology and clinical significance of increased bone marrow stromal fibres. Br J Haematol 2007; 139(3): 351-62. [http://dx.doi.org/10.1111/j.1365-2141.2007.06807.x] [PMID: 17910625]

[73] Tefferi A. Novel mutations and their functional and clinical relevance in myeloproliferative neoplasms: JAK2, MPL, TET2, ASXL1, CBL, IDH and IKZF1. Leukemia 2010; 24(6): 1128-38. [http://dx.doi.org/10.1038/leu.2010.69] [PMID: 20428194]

[74] Ernst T, Chase AJ, Score J, *et al.* Inactivating mutations of the histone methyltransferase gene EZH2 in myeloid disorders. Nat Genet 2010; 42(8): 722-6. [http://dx.doi.org/10.1038/ng.621] [PMID: 20601953]

[75] Gangat N, Caramazza D, Vaidya R, *et al.* DIPSS plus: a refined Dynamic International Prognostic Scoring System for primary myelofibrosis that incorporates prognostic information from karyotype, platelet count, and transfusion status. J Clin Oncol 2011; 29(4): 392-7. [http://dx.doi.org/10.1200/JCO.2010.32.2446] [PMID: 21149668]

[76] Folotyn. Westminister, CO: Allos Therapeutics, Inc. 2009.

[77] Horwitz SM, Kim YH, Foss F, *et al.* Identification of an active, well-tolerated dose of pralatrexate in patients with relapsed or refractory cutaneous T-cell lymphoma. Blood 2012; 119(18): 4115-22. [http://dx.doi.org/10.1182/blood-2011-11-390211] [PMID: 22394596]

[78] Owen A. Pralatrexate Is an Effective Treatment for Relapsed or Refractory Transformed Mycosis Fungoides: A Subgroup Efficacy Analysis From the PROPEL Study. Clin Oncol 2011; 29: 1182-9.

[79] Istodax [package insert]. Summit, NJ: Celgene Corporation, Inc. 2014.

[80] Piekarz RL, Frye R, Prince HM, *et al.* Phase 2 trial of romidepsin in patients with peripheral T-cell lymphoma. Blood 2011; 117(22): 5827-34. [http://dx.doi.org/10.1182/blood-2010-10-312603] [PMID: 21355097]

[81] Whittaker SJ, Demierre MF, Kim EJ, *et al.* Final results from a multicenter, international, pivotal study of romidepsin in refractory cutaneous T-cell lymphoma. J Clin Oncol 2010; 28(29): 4485-91. [http://dx.doi.org/10.1200/JCO.2010.28.9066] [PMID: 20697094]

[82] Piekarz RL, Frye R, Turner M, *et al.* Phase II multi-institutional trial of the histone deacetylase inhibitor romidepsin as monotherapy for patients with cutaneous T-cell lymphoma. J Clin Oncol 2009; 27(32): 5410-7. [http://dx.doi.org/10.1200/JCO.2008.21.6150] [PMID: 19826128]

[83] Pro B, Horwitz SM, Prince M, *et al.* Romidepsin Induces Durable Responses in Patients with Relapsed or Refractory Angioimmunoblastic T-Cell Lymphoma Blood 2014. (abstr 1742).

[84] Bates SE, Eisch R, Ling A, *et al.* Romidepsin in peripheral and cutaneous T-cell lymphoma: mechanistic implications from clinical and correlative data. Br J Haematol 2015; 170(1): 96-109. [http://dx.doi.org/10.1111/bjh.13400] [PMID: 25891346]

[85] Dupuis J, Morschhauser F, Ghesquières H, *et al.* Combination of romidepsin with cyclophosphamide, doxorubicin, vincristine, and prednisone in previously untreated patients with peripheral T-cell lymphoma: a non-randomised, phase 1b/2 study. Lancet Haematol 2015; 2(4): e160-5. [http://dx.doi.org/10.1016/S2352-3026(15)00023-X] [PMID: 26687958]

[86] Beleodaq. Irvine, CA: Spectrum Pharmaceuticals, Inc. 2014.

[87] Pohlman B, Advani R, Duvic M, *et al.* Final results of a phase II trial of belinostat (PXD101) in patients with recurrent or refractory peripheral or cutaneous T-cell lymphoma. Blood 2009; 114: 920.

[88] O'Connor OA, Horwitz S, Masszi T, *et al.* Belinostat in Patients With Relapsed or Refractory Peripheral T-Cell Lymphoma: Results of the Pivotal Phase II BELIEF (CLN-19) Study. J Clin Oncol 2015; 33(23): 2492-9.
[http://dx.doi.org/10.1200/JCO.2014.59.2782] [PMID: 26101246]

[89] Foss F, Advani R, Duvic M, *et al.* A Phase II trial of Belinostat (PXD101) in patients with relapsed or refractory peripheral or cutaneous T-cell lymphoma. Br J Haematol 2015; 168(6): 811-9.
[http://dx.doi.org/10.1111/bjh.13222] [PMID: 25404094]

[90] Kyprolis. South San Francisco, CA: Onyx Pharmaceuticals, Inc 2012.

[91] Shah JJ, Stadtmauer ED, Abonour R, *et al.* A Multi-Center Phase I/II Trial of Carfilzomib and Pomalidomide with Dexamethasone (Car-Pom-d) in Patients with Relapsed/Refractory Multiple Myeloma. ASH Annual Meeting. (Abstr 74).

[92] Berdeja JG, Hart LL, Mace JR, *et al.* Phase I/II study of the combination of panobinostat and carfilzomib in patients with relapsed/refractory multiple myeloma. Haematologica 2015; 100(5): 670-6.
[http://dx.doi.org/10.3324/haematol.2014.119735] [PMID: 25710456]

[93] Bringhen S, Petrucci MT, Larocca A, *et al.* Carfilzomib, cyclophosphamide, and dexamethasone in patients with newly diagnosed multiple myeloma: a multicenter, phase 2 study. Blood 2014; 124(1): 63-9.
[http://dx.doi.org/10.1182/blood-2014-03-563759] [PMID: 24855212]

[94] Pomalyst. Summit, NJ: Celgene Corporation 2013.

[95] Dispenzieri A, Buadi F, Laumann K, *et al.* Activity of pomalidomide in patients with immunoglobulin light-chain amyloidosis. Blood 2012; 119(23): 5397-404.
[http://dx.doi.org/10.1182/blood-2012-02-413161] [PMID: 22493299]

[96] Larocca A, Montefusco V, Bringhen S, *et al.* Pomalidomide, cyclophosphamide, and prednisone for relapsed/refractory multiple myeloma: a multicenter phase 1/2 open-label study. Blood 2013; 122(16): 2799-806.
[http://dx.doi.org/10.1182/blood-2013-03-488676] [PMID: 23954889]

[97] Leleu X, Karlin L, Macro M, *et al.* Intergroupe Francophone du Myélome (IFM). Pomalidomide plus low-dose dexamethasone in multiple myeloma with deletion 17p and/or translocation (4;14): IFM 2010-02 trial results. Blood 2015; 125(9): 1411-7.
[http://dx.doi.org/10.1182/blood-2014-11-612069] [PMID: 25575538]

[98] Tefferi A, Verstovsek S, Barosi G, *et al.* Pomalidomide is active in the treatment of anemia associated with myelofibrosis. J Clin Oncol 2009; 27(27): 4563-9.
[http://dx.doi.org/10.1200/JCO.2008.21.7356] [PMID: 19652059]

[99] Jakafi [package insert]. Wilmington, DE: Incyte Corporation 2011.

[100] Cervantes F, Vannucchi AM, Kiladjian JJ, *et al.* COMFORT-II investigators. Three-year efficacy, safety, and survival findings from COMFORT-II, a phase 3 study comparing ruxolitinib with best available therapy for myelofibrosis. Blood 2013; 122(25): 4047-53.
[http://dx.doi.org/10.1182/blood-2013-02-485888] [PMID: 24174625]

[101] Mead AJ, Milojkovic D, Knapper S, *et al.* Response to ruxolitinib in patients with intermediate-1-, intermediate-2-, and high-risk myelofibrosis: results of the UK ROBUST Trial. Br J Haematol 2015; 170(1): 29-39.
[http://dx.doi.org/10.1111/bjh.13379] [PMID: 25824940]

[102] Verstovsek S, Mesa RA, Gotlib J, *et al.* Three-year efficacy, overall survival, and safety of ruxolitinib

therapy in patients with myelofibrosis from the COMFORT-I study. Haematologica 2015; 100: 479-88.
[http://dx.doi.org/10.3324/haematol.2014.115840] [PMID: 25616577]

[103] Spoerl S, Mathew NR, Bscheider M, *et al.* Activity of therapeutic JAK 1/2 blockade in graft-*versus*-host disease. Blood 2014; 123(24): 3832-42.
[http://dx.doi.org/10.1182/blood-2013-12-543736] [PMID: 24711661]

[104] Spoerl S, Maas-Bauer K, Verbeek M, *et al.* Response to JAK 1/2 inhibition in patients with corticosteroid-refractory acute GVHD Blood 2014. (Abstr 722)

[105] Marian CO, Cho SK, McEllin BM, *et al.* The telomerase antagonist, imetelstat, efficiently targets glioblastoma tumor-initiating cells leading to decreased proliferation and tumor growth. Clin Cancer Res 2010; 16(1): 154-63.
[http://dx.doi.org/10.1158/1078-0432.CCR-09-2850] [PMID: 20048334]

[106] Tefferi A, Lasho TL, Begna KH, *et al.* A Pilot Study of the Telomerase Inhibitor Imetelstat for Myelofibrosis. N Engl J Med 2015; 373(10): 908-19.
[http://dx.doi.org/10.1056/NEJMoa1310523] [PMID: 26332545]

[107] Lonial S. ELOQUENT-2: A phase III, randomized, open-label study of lenalidomide (Len)/dexamethasone (dex) with/without elotuzumab (Elo) in patients (pts) with relapsed/refractory multiple myeloma (RRMM). ASCO Annual Meeting. Abstract #8508.

[108] Ocio EM, Mitsiades CS, Orlowski RZ, Anderson KC. Future agents and treatment directions in multiple myeloma. Expert Rev Hematol 2014; 7(1): 127-41.
[http://dx.doi.org/10.1586/17474086.2014.858595] [PMID: 24350987]

CHAPTER 2

Current Innovations in Management of Esophageal Carcinoma

Julie H. Rowe[2,5,*], Fathima Kamil[1,5], Melissa Yan[1,5], Curtis J. Wray[3,5] and Atilla Ertan[4,5]

[1] *Department of Internal Medicine*

[2] *Department of Internal Medicine, Division of Oncology*

[3] *Department of Surgery, Division of Minimally Invasive and Elective General Surgery*

[4] *Department of Internal Medicine, Division of Gastroenterology, Hepatology and Nutrition*

[5] *University of Texas Health Science Center-McGovern Medical School, Houston, Texas, USA*

Abstract: Esophageal cancer (EC) is the 8th most common cause of cancer worldwide and is endemic in certain parts of the world, especially in developing countries. The etiology of EC is multifactorial and includes tobacco and alcohol abuse, obesity, chronic gastroesophageal reflux disease (GERD), and Barrett's esophagus. In addition, there are hereditary cancer syndromes associated with an increased risk of ECs. Histologically, EC is classified as either squamous cell carcinoma (ESCC) or adenocarcinoma (EAC). The western hemisphere has seen a shift in decreasing incidence of ESCC *versus* increasing incidence of EAC. Human epidermal growth factor receptor 2 (Her2) gene and Her2 protein expression have been implicated in the pathogenesis of esophageal cancer. A multidisciplinary approach to EC is essential for workup, management, and treatment. Current therapeutic modalities include endoscopic treatments, such as endoscopic mucosal resection (EMR), endoscopic submucosal dissection (ESD), and ablation of early stage disease for both ESCC and EAC. For locally advanced disease, neoadjuvant chemotherapy and radiation followed by surgical resection are often used. However, the performance status of the patient as being "medically fit" *versus* "unfit" also plays an instrumental role in determining treatment. For metastatic EC, palliative chemotherapy remains the sole treatment. Most recently, there has been interest in moving beyond standard cytotoxic chemotherapy and to explore novel agents including immunotherapy, which could result in more promising outcomes in this malignancy.

Keywords: Endoscopy, Esophageal adenocarcinoma, Esophageal cancer, Immunotherapy, Squamous cell carcinoma, Targeted therapy.

* **Corresponding author Julie H. Rowe:** University of Texas Health Science Center-McGovern Medical School, Houston, Texas, USA; Tel: 713-500-5369, Fax: 713-512-7132; E-mail: julie.rowe@uth.tmc.edu

Atta-ur-Rahman and M. Iqbal Choudhary (Eds.)

EPIDEMIOLOGY

Esophageal cancer (EC) is the 8th most common cause of cancer worldwide and the 6th most common cause of cancer-related deaths. The incidence rates of EC vary regionally throughout the world with the highest rates seen in Southern and Eastern Africa and China [1]. In 2005, there were 497,700 new cases of EC, and the prevalence is expected to increase by approximately 140% by 2025 [2].

Worldwide, esophageal squamous cell carcinoma (ESCC) is the most common histological type of EC and predominates in Asian countries including China and Middle East and extends to southeastern Africa, often referred to as the "esophageal cancer belt" [3, 4]. However, focal areas in industrialized countries including northwestern France, Iceland, Scotland, Finland and eastern regions in the United States (US) including South Carolina and Washington D.C./Baltimore also have high rates of ESCC.

In the US and many Western countries, there has been a paradigm shift with increasing incidence of esophageal adenocarcinoma (EAC) and decreasing incidence of ESCC [1]; in which EAC has become the most prevalent form of EC. The annual incidence of EAC in the US increased sevenfold between 1974 (3.6 cases per million) and 2006 (25.6 per million) [4]. This epidemiological shift has been attributed to the rising incidence of gastroesophageal reflux disease (GERD) and obesity.

Age, Gender, and Race

Independent of histology, the incidence of EC increases with age and peaks in the seventh decade of life [5]. In the US and worldwide, the incidence of EC is higher in males than females. ESCC is higher in black males than white males; conversely, EAC occurs predominantly in white males. Interestingly, the rates of ESCC have steadily decreased in the US over the past 40 years, though ESCC is the most common histology among black men (refer to Fig. **1**) [4]. The incidence of EAC has increased dramatically within the last 3 decades and has become the major histologic type of EC in the US. The steep increase in incidence was largely seen in white males [6]. Based on a Surveillance, Epidemiology, and End Results (SEER) review, the incidence of EC is rising among white males and females and Hispanic males in the US. There is a steady decline in ESCC, most dramatically in black males but also seen in white males and females and black females [7]. Despite the rise of EAC in the western countries, ESCC is the most common histology worldwide with the peak incidence in regions of eastern Asia, eastern and southern Africa [8].

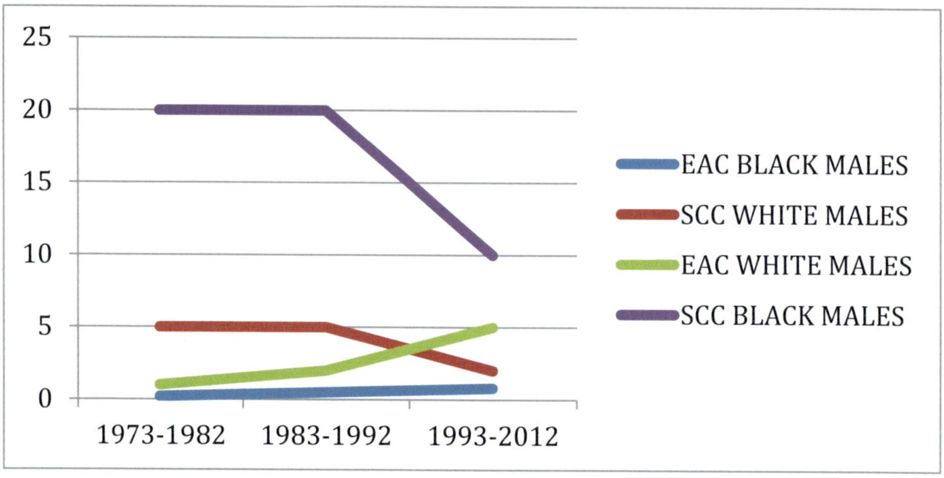

Fig. (1). Incidence of esophageal cancer in US males from 1973-2012. Data adapted from Holmes RS, Vaughan TL. Epidemiology and pathogenesis of esophageal cancer. InSeminars in radiation oncology 2007 Jan 31 (Vol. 17, No. 1, pp. 2-9). WB Saunders [6].

Risk Factors

Tobacco and alcohol are the 2 major independent risk factors and are synergistic in the pathogenesis of ESCC. Depending on the amount of tobacco use, smokers have a 5 to 10-fold increased risk of development of ESCC. The polynuclear aromatic hydrocarbons and nitrosamines contained in the tar fraction of tobacco are the propagators that initiate carcinogenesis [4, 9]. The duration of smoking history and the number of cigarettes inhaled per day have been directly correlated to the risk of EC. Other factors that cause chronic irritation and inflammation when combined with tobacco are synergistic in development of ESCC [5]. Similarly, the amount of alcohol consumed per week increases the relative risk of ESCC. The intensity and duration of alcohol used and type of alcoholic beverage have been implicated to affect the risks of ESCC. The pathogenesis of ESCC involving alcohol is less established but is thought to be attributed to local irritation of the esophageal mucosa from alcohol exposure, which can lead to increased susceptibility to carcinogenesis.

Several dietary factors have also been associated as a risk factor for ESCC. Consumption of large amounts of hot beverages and foods has been implicated to increase the risk of ESCC by causing thermal injury to the esophageal mucosa. Studies have shown an increased risk of ESCC with higher drinking temperature such as hot tea consumption as seen in northern Iran [4, 9]. Also, consumption of foods containing N-nitroso compounds increase the risk of ESCC as these compounds form potent electrophilic alkylating agents which subsequently reacts with DNA of target tissues to form altered bases, initiating carcinogenesis [10].

Chewing betal quid or areca nuts, which is common in certain regions of Asia, have been implicated in the development of ESCC. Vitamin and mineral deficiencies, such as molybdenum, B-carotene, vitamin A, vitamin E, selenium, and zinc have also been found to increase the risk of ESCC [11]. Chronic alcohol consumption can lead to nutritional deficiencies as described, which also plays a role in carcinogenesis [5]. In addition, dietary intake of fruits and vegetables contributes to the risk of ESCC. A meta-analysis revealed a significant association between high intake of fruits and vegetables and lower risk of ESCC [12]. Additionally, poor oral health and low socioeconomic status are considered risk factors [5]. The role of human papillomavirus (HPV) in ESCC is controversial with reports of 0-66%. HPV has been associated with other malignancies including cervical cancer and head and neck cancers, but its role in ESCC is less certain [13].

Chronic gastroesophageal reflux disease (GERD) is the strongest independent risk factor for the development of EAC. The refluxed acid and bile lead to esophageal mucosal inflammation and with chronic acid exposure, specialized intestinal metaplasia develops known as Barrett's esophagus (BE). The incidence of GERD in the general population has been estimated to be around 10-20%. Barrett's esophagus occurs around 3.5-7% in this affected population. BE is a precursor lesion of EAC and the presence of BE is associated with a 0.12% to 0.33% annual risk of developing EAC [30] (refer to *Barrett's esophagus* for further detail). There are several risk factors for GERD, including obesity, smoking, diet, hereditary factors, and pre-existing conditions. Obesity has been found to be an independent risk factor for EAC. Proposed mechanisms include increased intra-abdominal pressure and GERD promoting inflammation, adipocytes and inflammatory cells secreting cytokines, which may stimulate tumor growth and progression [5].

HEREDITARY CANCER SYNDROME

Over the past several years with the use of genetic testing and screening methods, familial ECs are becoming better delineated, though the incidence is quite low. Familial clustering is important in understanding the inheritance pattern of inherited cancer syndromes. For familial esophageal cancer, the pattern of inheritance is suggested to be autosomal dominant. Gathering family history of affected members is instrumental in this type of cancer. Interestingly, a study that compared risk factors between familial esophageal cancer patients *versus* (*vs*) sporadic esophageal cancer patients did not find any differences in gender, ethnicity, or tobacco and/or alcohol consumption. However, in familial EC patients, younger age of diagnosis and lower body mass index (BMI) appeared to be more common; though there is still conflicting data [15].

Genetic Mutations

Certain genetic changes have been linked to esophageal cancer. Genetic mutations associated with ESCC are not as well defined as compared to EAC. However, genome-wide association studies (GWAS) have identified common disease alleles associated with ESCC. Single nucleotide polymorphisms in TP53, MDM21, CASP8, and COX2 are risk factors for ESCC. Specifically, certain single-nucleotide changes in the following have been implicated with ESCC: 1) rs4135113, which regulates non-synonymous coding in base excision repair; 2) rs1800450, which regulates monosaccharide binding; and 3) rs3769823, which regulate CASP8 [16]. In addition, chromosomal losses of 4q, 5q, 9p, and 18q, chromosomal gains of 8q, 17q, and 20q, and genetic amplifications of 7, 8, and 17q are frequently implicated. Wu *et al.* [17] described two (2q22 and 13q33) of nine new ESCC susceptibility loci that have significant association with gene-alcohol interaction. One of nine loci, 4q23, includes ADH cluster, which has similar gene-alcohol interaction. Variants in ADH gene and/or ALDH2 have been implicated with ESCC in recent GWAS studies in European and Japanese populations with ESCC. Another study had demonstrated a four-fold increased risk for ESCC in those with both ADH1B and ALDH2 risk alleles and who drank alcohol compared to non-drinkers [18]. These studies emphasize the potential interaction of genetic changes with alcohol consumption [5].

Cyclin D1 (CCND1) G870A polymorphism has been implicated as a risk factor for other malignancies and has also been studied as a risk factor for EAC. Earlier studies by Casson *et al.* [19] in 2005 demonstrated CCND1 G870A as risk factor for EAC; however, a recent study done by Liu *et al.* [20] provided contradictory conclusions. The methods of the two groups were different. Casson used polymerase chain reaction (PCR)-restriction fragment length polymorphism, while Liu applied 5'-nuclease assay, which is considered to be the gold standard in genotyping in current-day standards. Additionally, the control populations used in both studies were different. Another study demonstrated increased risk of EC among Asians who were homozygous for this allele [21]. In conclusion, the role of CCND1 G870A polymorphism as a potential risk factor is still not well delineated and needs further studies [5]. Orloff *et al.* has described potential germline mutations in macrophage scavenger receptor 1 (MSR1), activating signal co-integrator 1 complex subunit 1 (ASCC1), and collagen triple helix repeat containing 1 (CTHRC1) associated with BE and EAC [15].

Bloom Syndrome

Bloom syndrome is an autosomal recessive genetic disorder caused by a mutation in the BLM gene at chromosome 15q26.1, which codes for the DNA repair enzyme RecQL3 helicase [22, 23]. Many different mutations have been identified and include missense, nonsense, frame-shift, exon skipping, and exonic deletions. Bloom syndrome is more common in Ashkenazi Jews and a founder mutation designated BLM^{ash}, a 6 base pair (bp) deletion/7bp insertion, has been identified in this population. This syndrome is characterized by a constellation of features including proportionate small stature with mild microcephaly, photosensitivity and telangiectasia generally on the face and dorsa of the hands and forearms, and characteristic facies: malar hypoplasia, nasal prominence, small mandible, and dolichocephalic skull [23]. The absence of RecQL3 helicase leads to improper DNA repair mechanisms and high sister chromatid exchange rates occur. The resulting genetic instability increases frequency of malignancy at all ages, with acute leukemia, lymphoid neoplasms, and Wilms tumor predominating before the age of 25; after age 20, solid tumor cancers including ESCC are more frequent [22, 23].

Familial Barrett's Esophagus

The spectrum of Familial Barrett's Esophagus (FBE) includes EAC. This aggregation suggests a biological relationship between BE and EAC, which may be caused by common environmental exposures in family members, genetic predisposition to disease, or both. A positive family history of BE should raise suspicion of this disease and consider upper endoscopy evaluation. Current evidence demonstrates possible autosomal dominant inheritance and EAC diagnosed at a significantly earlier age when compared to non-familial EAC; however, it is still not well understood if other risk factors are implicated in FBE inheritance [15, 24].

Fanconi Anemia

Fanconi anemia (FA) is an autosomal recessive or X-linked disorder associated with congenital abnormalities (such as short stature, microcephaly, thumb abnormalities, and café-au-lait spots), pancytopenia, and a predisposition to leukemia and solid tumors. Multiple genes appear to be responsible for FA and thirteen complementation groups (FA-A through FA-N) and their corresponding genes have been identified [23]. The gene responsible for FA-A, which occurs in approximately 66% of patients with FA, is FANCA and is located on chromosome 16q24.3. Many of the FA genes interact in a nuclear complex that is involved with the mono-ubiquitination of FANCD2, which interacts with multiple proteins involved with genomic stability, including BRCA1, FANCD1/BRCA2, FANCN/PALB2 and RAD51 [25]. The genomic instability results in increased frequency of malignancy, particularly acute myeloid leukemia, ESCC, squamous cell carcinoma of the head/neck and vulva, and hepatocellular carcinoma.

Tylosis Esophageal Cancer

Tylosis, which is also known as Palmoplantar Keratosis or Howel Evans syndrome, is an autosomal dominant familial cancer syndrome involving a missense mutation in RHBDF2 that encodes the inactive rhomboid protease, which functions in growth-factor signaling in esophageal cancer. This syndrome is characterized by a constellation of features including hyperkeratosis of the palms or soles, oral precursor lesions, and high lifetime risk of esophageal cancer. The cutaneous features, including focal non-epidermolytic palmoplantar keratoderma and oral leukokeratosis usually manifest by the onset of puberty (refer to Fig. **2**). More than 90% of affected patients will be diagnosed with ESCC by the age of 65 [26].

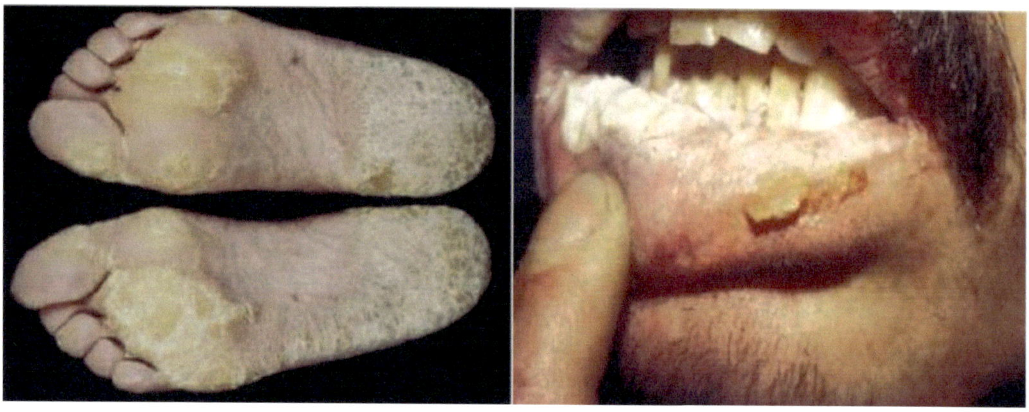

Fig. (2). Cutaneous manifestations of Tylosis Esophageal Cancer—focal non-epidermolytic palmoplantar keratoderma (left) and oral leukokeratosis (right) [26].

RHBDF2, also known as RHBDL6 or iRhom2, belongs to transmembrane protein family rhomboids, which function in preparation of proteins such as epidermal growth factor (EGF) and mitochondrial remodeling. Currently, the exact role of RHBDF2 is not well known; however, it has been found that RHBDF2 regulates epidermal growth factor receptor (EGFR) expression through ER-associated degradation of EGF. The EGFR pathway is involved in tumorigenesis of many cancers, including esophageal. Blaydon *et al.* [26] had elucidated how constitutive EGFR signaling results in a hyper-proliferative state, which leads to precancerous lesions transforming into malignancy. Further discussion on the role of EGFR inhibitors in esophageal cancer will be reviewed in *Targeted Therapies in Esophageal Cancer.*

PATHOLOGY

Anatomy

The esophagus is a muscular tube that extends from the upper sphincter to the lower sphincter and divided into three regions: cervical, thoracic, and abdominal. Structurally, the esophageal wall is composed of four layers: innermost mucosa, submucosa, muscularis propria, and adventitia. Unlike the remainder of the GI tract, the esophagus has no serosa. The z-line is the transition from esophageal to gastric mucosa and differentiates between two areas of different colored mucosa. The middle third of esophagus consists of a mixture of smooth and skeletal muscle. The esophagus has two high-pressure zones consisting of the upper esophageal sphincter (UES) and the lower esophageal sphincter (LES). The UES is composed of 3 muscles including the cricopharyngeus, thyropharyngeus, and cranial cervical esophagus and the thyroid and cricoid cartilage, and the hyoid bone and controlled by a variety of reflexes. The LES is composed of an intrinsic and extrinsic component. The esophageal muscle fibers and neuro-hormonal influence comprises the intrinsic component; the diaphragm muscle makes up the extrinsic component. Malfunction of either component results in GERD [27].

The mucous membrane is a non-keratinized squamous epithelium that covers the entire inner surface of the esophagus, except for the LES. The submucosa contains connective tissue as well as lymphocytes, plasma cells, nerve cells called Messner's plexus, and mucous glands. The esophageal glands are important in esophageal clearance and tissue resistance to acid. The muscularis propria is responsible for motor function. The upper third portion of the esophagus is predominantly striated muscles, the distal third is mostly smooth muscle, and the transition zone is a mixture of both striated and smooth muscle. The adventitia covers the esophagus and connects it with the surrounding structures [27].

Based on the 7th edition of the American Joint Committee on Cancer (AJCC) Cancer Staging Manual, the esophagus is divided into 4 divisions based on the distance from the incisors. The cervical esophagus begins at the lower border of the cricoid cartilage and ends at the suprasternal notch, which is approximately 18 centimeters (cm) from the incisors. The upper thoracic is 20-25 cm from the incisors, mid-thoracic from 25-30 cm, and lower thoracic & intra-abdominal from 30-40 cm, respectively. Clinically, physicians including cardiothoracic surgeons and radiologists divide the esophagus into 3 divisions. The upper third extends from the cricopharyngeus to the superior portion of the aortic arch; middle third, from the superior portion of the aortic arch to the inferior pulmonary vein; and the distal third, from the inferior pulmonary vein to the GEJ (refer Fig. **3**) [28, 29].

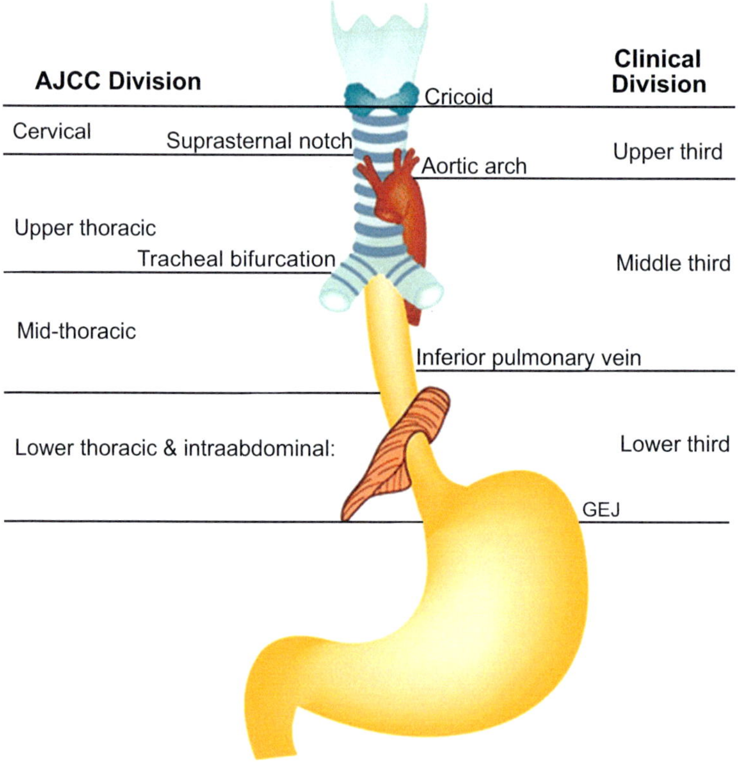

Fig. (3). The anatomic divisions of the esophagus based on AJCC Cancer Staging Manual. Adapted from Rice TW, Blackstone EH, Rusch VW. of the AJCC Cancer Staging Manual: esophagus and esophagogastric junction. Annals of surgical oncology. 2010 Jul 1; 17(7):1721-4 and Kim TJ, Kim HY, Lee KW, *et al.* Multimodality assessment of esophageal cancer: preoperative staging and monitoring of response to therapy 1. Radiographics. 2009 Mar; 29(2):403-21.

Siewert Classification and EGJ

Esophagogastric junction (EGJ) tumors are defined as being within 5 cm proximal and distal of the anatomic cardia. Siewert *et al.* classified EGJ adenocarcinoma into three types based on the anatomic location of the tumor mass. Type I tumors are defined as adenocarcinoma of the distal esophagus with the tumor center located within 1 to 5 cm above the anatomic EGJ. These tumors usually arise from areas of intestinal metaplasia in Barrett's esophagus as a consequence of chronic gastroesophageal reflux. Type II tumors are defined as the true carcinoma of the cardia with the tumor center within 1 cm above and 2 cm below the EGJ. Type III is defined as the subcardial carcinoma with the tumor center between 2 to 5 cm below the EGJ, infiltrating the EGJ and the distal esophagus from below.

The routes of tumor spread of EC can result from direct extension of tumor, lymphatic spread, and hematogenous metastasis. The esophagus lacks a serosal wall, which makes local extension to surrounding structures within mediastinum easier. Complications due to direct extension can result in tracheoesophageal or bronchoesophageal fistulas. There are 2 lymphatic drainage systems of the esophagus within the mucosa and muscular layer. Due to bidirectional flow in the tracheal bifurcation, lymph node metastasis can be found in the upper thorax and lower abdomen region. Common hematogenous sites of spread involve the liver, lung, bone, and adrenal glands [29].

Precursor Lesions

The precursor lesions for ESCC and EAC differ. The multistep process starts from normal squamous epithelium to low-grade dysplasia (LGD) to high-grade dysplasia (HGD) and finally invasive carcinoma (see Fig. **4**). LGD involves less than 50% of the thickness of the epithelium with dysplastic cells; HGD involves more than 50% of the epithelium. Chromoendoscopy, the use of dye stains or an image that changes the color visualized at endoscopy to enhance visualization of potential neoplastic lesions, can be used to help distinguish LGD, HGD, and cancer [30]. The pathologic classification of ESCC includes a description of the mitotic activity, nuclear atypia, and degree of squamous differentiated as defined as well differentiated, moderately differentiated, poorly differentiated, and undifferentiated [16]. The precursor lesions for EAC are described below.

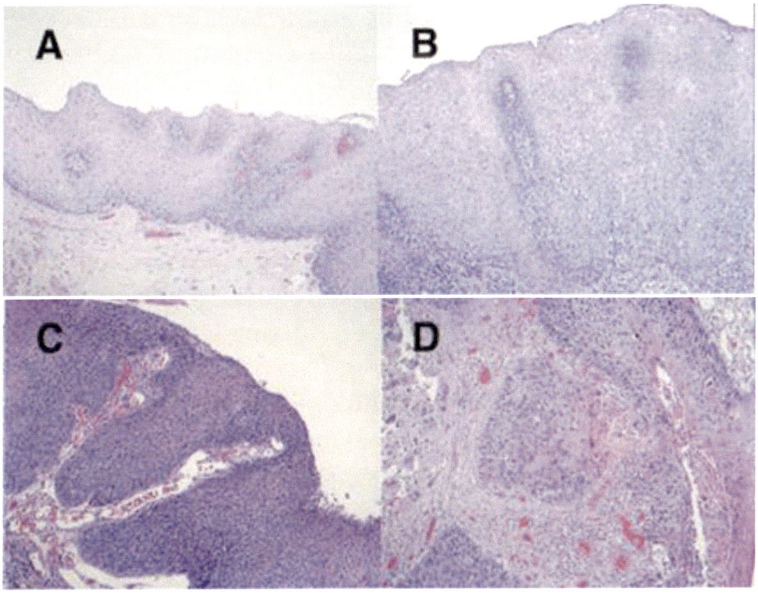

Fig. (4). Neoplastic progression in the esophageal squamous epithelium. **A.** Normal squamous epithelium. **B.** Low grade squamous dysplasia. **C.** High grade squamous dysplasia. **D.** Squamous cell carcinoma. Photographs are courtesy of Mamoun Younes MD, FCAP, AGAF.

Barrett's Esophagus

Barrett's esophagus (BE) has a predilection for white males and occurs 2-3 times more in males than females. Other risk factors include obesity, especially associated with intra-abdominal fat distribution, and cigarette smoking as previously discussed in risk factors of EC. Interestingly, the incidence of BE is less common in African Americans and rare in Asian Americans. In a US Radiofrequency patient registry of 5521 patients, women had shorter and less aggressive histology. The usual tendency toward BE in men was absent in African American and Asians [31]. One study suggested that the prevalence of Barrett's metaplasia (BM) in Hispanics is similar to whites [7].

BE is further defined based on the distance between the GEJ and the most proximal extent of BM and divided into long-segment which is defined as > 3 cm or short segment which is < 3 cm. Long segment BE is commonly associated with chronic heartburn, presence of a hiatal hernia, and severe reflux esophagitis. Patients with short segment BE often do not complain of reflux symptoms and are more often asymptomatic. However, the prevalence of short-segment is more common. Long-segment BE is at higher risk of malignancy as the higher risk of adenocarcinoma varies on the length of BM; however fewer than 5% diagnosed with EC have a prior diagnosis of BM [30].

BE is characterized by a metaplasia, a transformational process in which normal squamous epithelium is replaced by specialized columnar epithelium, with the inciting factor attributed to chronic GERD. Due to chronic exposure to gastroesophageal reflux, damaged esophageal squamous cells are replaced by columnar cells with two proposed mechanisms: transdifferentiation and transcommitment. Transdifferentiation is characterized by expression of important transcription factors leading to metaplasia, whereas transcommitment is the process in which esophageal stem cells differentiate into columnar cells, instead of normal squamous cells. Recent animal studies have demonstrated that BM may develop from stem cells derived from the circulating bone marrow stem cells or embryonic cells migrating from different areas of the gastric cardia or gastroesophageal junction [30]. The morphologic grading of dysplasia in BM can be subjective to observer variation. Surveillance programs for patients with BM include periodic endoscopy with biopsy; the follow-up interval of the visit depends on the grade of dysplasia. There have been efforts to identify molecular markers that can be used to predict malignant transformation of BM to EC. A study of 120 patients with BM, which were evaluated for p53 protein, Glut1 expression by immunohistochemistry, DNA ploidy, and dysplasia, suggested a potential mechanism in which oxidative DNA damage leads to G1/G2 arrest of the cell cycle, which can lead to p53 mutation and subsequently DNA aneuploidy (refer to Fig. **5**) [32]. Further studies on p53 as a potential marker for neoplastic progression have demonstrated a sensitivity of 100%, specificity of 93%, and positive predictive value of 0.56. P53 accumulation in LGD could be an early molecular marker for development of HGD and EC [33]. Kaye *et al.* showed improved reliability of p53 immunostaining as compared to routine hematoxylin and eosin evaluation and use of p53 immunostaining as an adjunct tool to assist in distinguishing LGD and HGD [34].

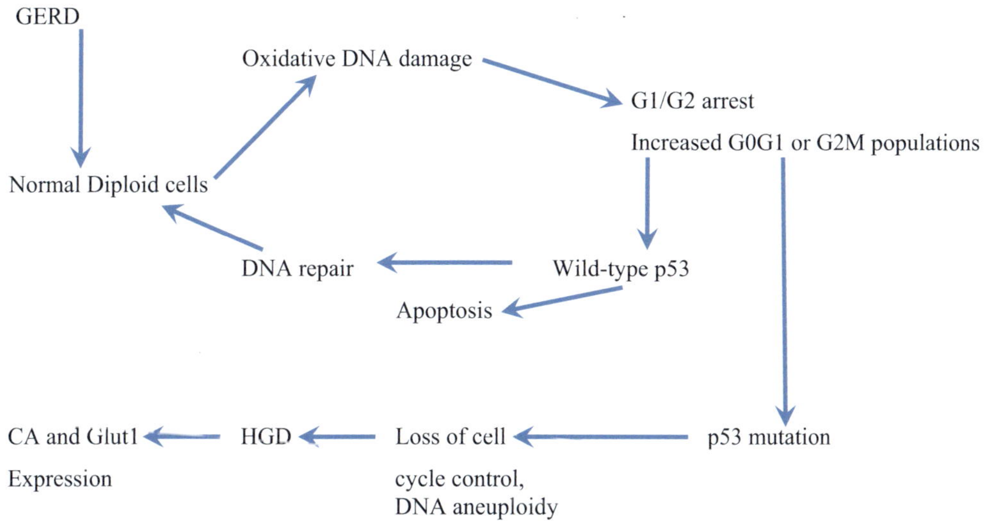

Fig. (5). Malignant progression of Barrett's Esophagus. Adapted from Younes M, Lechago J, Chakraborty S, *et al.* Relationship between dysplasia, p53 protein accumulation, DNA ploidy, and Glut1 overexpression in Barrett metaplasia. Scandinavian journal of gastroenterology. 2000 Jan 1; 35(2):131-7.

Dysplasia is the most useful biomarker for transformation into EC. The progression of HGD is around 6% per year. Due to this increased risk, current guidelines by the American Gastroenterological Association (AGA) and the American Society for Gastrointestinal Endoscopy (ASGE) recommend endoscopic eradication therapy including endoscopic mucosal resection (EMR) and/or radiofrequency ablation (RFA) for HGD. Management of LGD is controversial based on inconsistencies of its natural history and disagreements among pathologists, which highlights the complexity of pathologic evaluation of dysplasia [30]. Biopsies that are indefinite for dysplasia (IND) have evidence of crypt dysplasia but the surface epithelium is not involved, denuded, or replaced by squamous epithelium, which could be attributed to regenerative changes or inflammation, especially in the setting or proton pump inhibitors (PPIs) or endoscopic therapies [35]. Several studies have evaluated the clinical implications of IND and the rate of progression into HGD and EC [35, 36]. A study of over

2200 patients found IND in 83 patients and LGD in 79 patients. The combined incidence of HGD and EC in IND and LGD was about 0.86% per year and 1.53% per year, respectively, which implies similar biological behavior. Interestingly, the regression rates of IND after first follow-up endoscopy was around 80%, suggesting that surveillance of IND and LGD can be applied similarly [36].

Dysplasia in BE is classified in a five-tiered system and is based on the Riddell classification initially developed for dysplasia in inflammatory bowel disease [37, 38]. Based on histological criteria, it is classified into the following categories: negative for dysplasia, IND, LGD, HGD, and intramucosal carcinoma (see Fig. **6**).

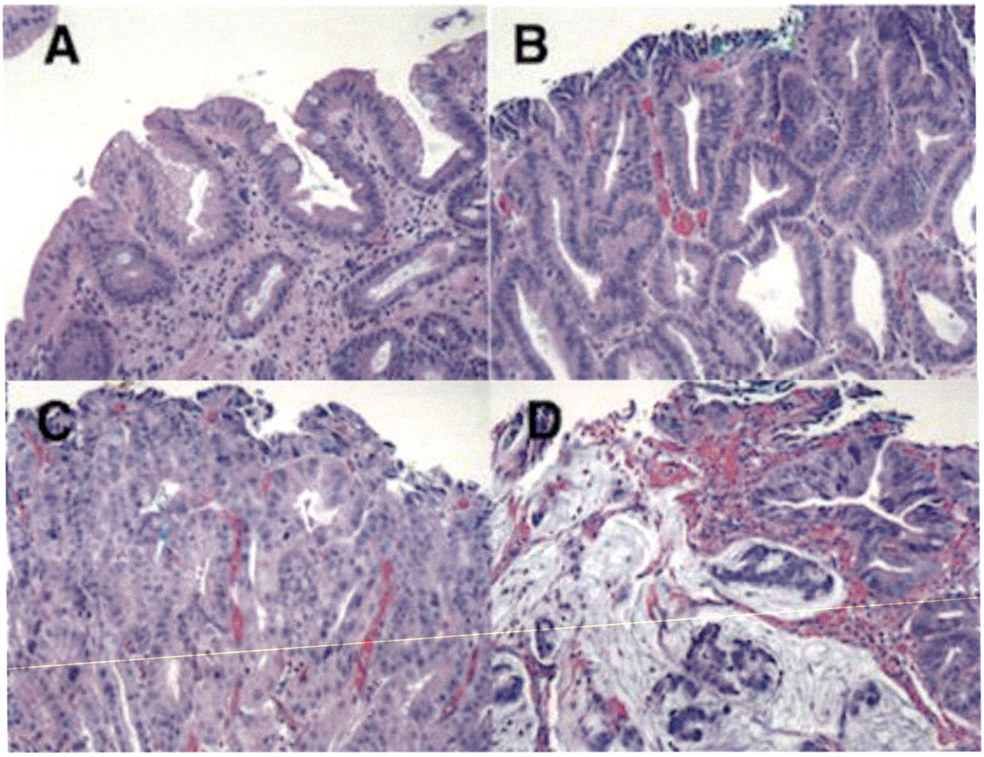

Fig. (6). Neoplastic progression in Barrett's esophagus (Barrett's metaplasia, BM): **A.** BM negative for dysplasia. **B.** BM with low-grade dysplasia. **C.** BM with high-grade dysplasia. **D.** Adenocarcinoma. Photographs are courtesy of Mamoun Younes MD, FCAP, AGAF.

Studies have supported that non-dysplastic BE may be a precursor to neoplasia and typically shows a variable degree of regenerative changes with evidence of crypt budding, atrophy, branching, increased mitotic activity, dystrophic goblet cells, mucin depletion, and nuclear hyper-chromaticity. At the severe end of the regeneration spectrum, the degree of cytologic atypia may overlap with true dysplasia. A diagnosis of IND is made when the definite distinction between regeneration and dysplasia cannot be made with certainty and when the diagnosis is difficult due to technical issues. The diagnosis of LGD or HGD is based on the severity of architectural and cytologic changes. LGD shows relatively preserved crypt architecture and cytologically atypical nuclear limited to the basal half of the cell cytoplasm. The nuclear are typically hyperchromatic, elongated, chromatin clumping, and an irregular contour. With neoplastic progression, HGD is defined by the presence of increased crypt complexity, crowding, irregularity, and branching in addition for increased nuclear stratification, loss of cell polarity, pleomorphism, and mitotic activity. Intramucosal carcinoma is defined as neoplastic epithelium that has penetrated through the basement membrane into the lamina propria [37, 38].

Table 1. Summary of guidelines for surveillance for Barrett's Esophagus.

Disease Stage	*British Society of Gastroenterology*	*American College of Gastroenterology*	*American Society of Gastrointestinal Endoscopy*	*American Gastroenterology Association*
Non-Dysplastic Barrett's Esophagus (BE)	■ If <3 cm with intestinal metaplasia, surveillance endoscopy every 3-5 years. ■ If >3 cm, surveillance endoscopy 2-3 years.	Surveillance endoscopy every 3-5 years.	■ Options include no surveillance endoscopy *vs* surveillance endoscopy every 3-5 years with 4-quadrant biopsies every 2 cm.	Surveillance endoscopy every 3-5 years.
Barrett's Esophagus, indeterminate for dysplasia	■ Second GI pathology review including p53 immunostain evaluation. ■ Optimization of acid suppressive therapy (AST). ■ If no definite dysplasia, then surveillance endoscopy as for non-dysplastic BE.	■ Second GI pathology review. ■ Repeat endoscopy after optimization with AST for 3-6 months. - If indeterminate for dysplasia again, then repeat endoscopy in 12 months.	■ Second GI pathology review. ■ Increase AST. ■ Repeat endoscopy and biopsy. ■ Consideration of endoscopic ablation.	--

(Table 1) contd.....

Disease Stage	*British Society of Gastroenterology*	*American College of Gastroenterology*	*American Society of Gastrointestinal Endoscopy*	*American Gastroenterology Association*
Low-Grade Dysplasia (LGD)	■ P53 immunostain ■ Repeat endoscopy in 6 months - If LGD again, then second GI pathology review and offer endoscopic therapy. - If endoscopic therapy declined, then repeat surveillance every 6 months.	■ Second GI pathology review. ■ Endoscopic therapy preferred or surveillance every 12 months. ■ Follow-up every year until no dysplasia seen on 2 consecutive endoscopies.	■ Confirm pathology. ■ Repeat endoscopy in 6 months to confirm LGD. ■ Surveillance endoscopy every year with 4 quadrant biopsies every 1-2 cm. ■ Consideration of endoscopic ablation or resection.	■ Confirm pathology. ■ Repeat endoscopy in 6 months to confirm LGD. ■ Surveillance endoscopy every year with 4 quadrant biopsies every 1-2cm. ■ Consideration endoscopic therapies.
High-Grade Dysplasia (HGD) or intramucosal carcinoma	■ Endoscopic therapy preferred (*i.e.* endoscopic mucosal resection [EMR]) over esophagectomy or endoscopic surveillance. ■ EMR recommended as most accurate staging intervention and therapy of choice if visible irregularities.	■ Second GI pathology review. ■ EMR recommended if visible irregularities.	■ Confirm pathology. ■ Consideration of endoscopic ablation or resection. ■ EUS for staging. ■ Surveillance endoscopy every 3 months in select patients with 4 quadrant biopsies every 1 cm.	■ Confirm pathology. ■ If mucosal irregularity, recommend EMR. ■ Endoscopic therapy preferred over esophagectomy or endoscopic surveillance. ■ If no treatment is elected, surveillance every 3 months.

Summary of Guidelines on Surveillance of Barrett's Esophagus based on four gastroenterological societies. Adapted from Pophali P, Halland M. Barrett's oesophagus: diagnosis and management. BMJ. 2016 May 11; 353:i2373.

Screening and Surveillance of Barrett's Esophagus

Patients with chronic or severe GERD and at least 2 or more risk factors including age over 50 years, male, white race, obesity, or smoking history are screened for BE. Screening is considered in patients with a first-degree relative who have BE. Surveillance every 3-5 years is recommended for patients with BE without dysplasia. For LGD and HGD, endoscopic eradication therapy is recommended. Subsequent surveillance with repeat endoscopy should be 6-12 months for LGD and 3 months for HGD. If patients declined endoscopic eradication therapy, surveillance should continue every 6-12 months [39]. Several studies have demonstrated that a substantial number of patients with BE are asymptomatic [40].

Treatment of GERD and Barrett's Esophagus

Lifestyle modifications and medical therapy including acid suppressive medications such as histamine- 2 blockers (H2Bs) and proton pump inhibitors (PPIs) are the first-line treatment for GERD [41]. Successful treatment of GERD is attributed to PPIs; however, around 30-40% of patients are not adequately treated [42]. Long-term medical treatment with acid-suppressive medications have been linked to osteoporosis, vitamin and mineral malabsorption including B12 and iron deficiency, increased infection risk, cardiovascular events, chronic kidney disease, and dementia based on observational studies [43 - 45]. However, therapies to reduce gastric exposure including acid suppression therapy (AST) with H2B or PPI or anti-reflux surgery failed to change the malignant progression of BE into EC. Moreover, p53 protein accumulation was not altered when patients were treated with AST [46].

Endoscopic eradication therapy for BE include ablative therapies with RFA, photodynamic therapy (PDT), cryotherapy, and argon plasma coagulation (APC) *vs* minimally invasive procedures with endoscopic mucosal resection (EMR) and endoscopic submucosal dissection (ESD). RFA is the preferred endoscopic ablative therapy for flat lesions or intramucosal carcinoma and applies high frequency energy to areas of interest. PDT uses photosensitizers which have high affinity for cancerous tissue and when light-activated, results in tissue destruction. Esophageal strictures are common complications for RFA and PDT [35]. A comparison of efficacy, safety, and cost analysis between RFA and PDT demonstrated higher rates of histologic response, decreased costs, and no serious safety concerns with RFA [47]. A multicenter RFA registry demonstrated less than 1% of BE patients died from EC. BE segment length and high baseline pathologic grade were associated with increased risk of EC [48]. Similarly, BM recurrence were associated with the following risk factors including increasing BE segment length, older age, non-Caucasian race [44]. EMR and ESD will be discussed more *Management of Early Stage Esophageal Cancer.*

Other Rare Histologies

Squamous cell carcinoma and adenocarcinoma are the most common histologies of EC. The World Health Organization (WHO) had proposed a histologic classification for EC including ESCC, EAC, and other types including mucoepidermoid carcinoma, adenoid cystic carcinoma, and adenosquamous and variants of squamous cell carcinoma such as verrucous and spindle cell and high-grade neuroendocrine carcinomas. These histologies are rare compared to ESCC and EAC (refer to Table **2**).

Table 2. WHO Classification of Carcinoma in Esophagus.

Squamous cell carcinoma
Verrucous (squamous) carcinoma
Spindle cell (squamous) carcinoma
Adenocarcinoma
Adenosquamous carcinoma
Mucoepidermoid carcinoma
High grade neuroendocrine carcinoma - Large cell neuroendocrine carcinoma - Small cell neuroendocrine carcinoma
Undifferentiated carcinoma
Others

Other rare histologies that have also been described are primary malignant melanoma of the esophagus (PMME) [50], esophageal lymphoma [51], and basaloid ESCC [52]. These rare histologies account for 0.1-5% of primary neoplasms of the esophagus [50 - 52]. PMME typically present with nodal metastasis, which is an indicator of poor prognosis [50]. The clinical course of esophageal lymphoma varies based on the subtype, which are typically B-cell type [51]. For basaloid ESCC, there does not appear to be any significant differences in staging or survival rates with ESCC [52].

SIGNALING PATHWAYS IN ESOPHAGEAL CANCER

BE is the precursor to development of EC. There is a multistep molecular pathogenesis involving tumor proto-oncogenes, tumor suppressor genes, mismatch repair genes, and mitotic checkpoints, and epigenetic changes from BE to EC. Along with inactivation of p16, loss of p53 and aneuploidy, recent studies has also shown that epigenetic changes have been implicated in the progression of HGD to EAC. However, it is still unknown which primary driver mutation(s) result in EC [56].

The molecular profiles of EC have been further elucidated based on the histologic subtypes-ESCC and EAC. There is a higher mutational burden for EC compared to other solid tumors. Agrawal *et al.* performed whole exome sequencing (WES) on 23 EC (12 ESCC, 11 EAC) from the US population and demonstrated different mutations between the 2 types. Further, when compared to EC in a Chinese population, there were disparities noted as well. For example, inactivating mutations in NOTCH-1 were identified in 21% and 0% in ESCC and EAC, respectively, whereas in Chinese ESCC, only 2% demonstrated this inactivating mutation [54]. In ESCC, genes that regulated cell cycle including TP53, CDKN2A, RB1, NFE2L2, CHEK1, and CHEK2 are commonly mutated. TP53 is a key player in development of ESCC [14]. Similarly, in EAC, these cell-cycle gene regulators, especially p53, are implicated in transition from BE to EAC [53]. Other studies have shown that PIK3CA, PTEN, CHEK2 mutations and somatic mutations in Wnt and cell cycle pathways were found in ESCC. KRAS mutations, HER2 amplification, and mutations in SWI/SNF family of chromatin remodeling factors including ARID1A, SMARCA4, and ARID2 were demonstrated in EAC [54].

Epidermal growth factor receptor (EGFR), HER2, HER3, and HER4 comprise the HER family of transmembrane receptor tyrosine kinases that functions in epithelial cell growth, survival, proliferation, and differentiation. The structures of these dimeric receptors include a glycosylated extracellular ligand-binding domain, a hydrophobic transmembrane domain, and an intracellular domain that contains the tyrosine kinase activity. In EC, EGFR is commonly overexpressed, ranging from 50 to 80%, whereas HER2 expression is more variable, ranging from 0 to 65% [55]. When comparing ESCC to EAC, HER-2-Neu overexpression is more common in EAC than ESCC. However, amplification of HER-2-Neu and EGFR overexpression is associated with poor prognosis in both ESCC and EAC. EGFR overexpression is more common in ESCC, ranging from 60-80% and similarly associated with a dismal prognosis. Amplification and mutations in EGFR are not as frequent in ESCC at 10-25% and 0-2%, respectively. Activating mutations in exon 18 and 21 of the EGFR gene occur in about 15% of BE and EAC. Around 15% of EAC demonstrate co-amplification of HER-2-neu and EGFR [14, 53]. Epidermal growth factor (EGF) and transforming growth factor-α (TGFα) stimulate cell proliferation through ligand activation with EGFR. EGF and TGFα are elevated BE and EAC [53].

The vascular endothelial growth factors (VEGF) have been implicated in early progression of BE and EAC. Studies have shown an incremental increase of VEGF-A expression from non-dysplastic BE to dysplasia to EAC. The prognostic value of VEGF overexpression remains unclear [53]. In EAC, 30-40% demonstrates overexpression of VEGF and VEGF receptors (VEGFR) [54].

Other pathways involved in EAC include insulin-like growth factor pathway and tumor necrosis factor receptor (TNF) which promote cell growth, survival, and angiogenesis. Transforming growth factor β (TGFβ) signaling is often mediated by mutations in downstream transcription factors like SMAD4 and is active in EAC and other epithelial cancers. This pathway is involved in epithelial to mesenchymal transition (EMT) in cancer cells and stimulates invasion and metastasis. Downstream signaling through RAS/RAF/MAPK and PI3-

kinase/AKT pathways is integral in cell growth, proliferation, differentiation, and motility. Modulation of these pathways have been found to contribute to progression of BE to EAC [53].

As discussed earlier, there are not only differences between the histologic types of EC but disparities noted among different ethnicities. Several genome-wide association studies in Asian populations have revealed two functional SNPs in alcohol dehydrogenase 1B (ADH1B) and aldehyde dehydrogenase 2 family (ALDH2), as well as 3 additional SNPs, associated with ESCC risk. Also it was found that there are gene-environmental interactions with alcohol drinking and smoking. Epidemiologic studies on Asian populations have shown genes that regulate alcohol and folate metabolism, DNA repair, cell cycle control, apoptosis, and carcinogen detoxification are involved in genetic susceptibility in ESCC carcinogenesis. However, there is limited information in ESCC in Western populations. Similarly, there is limited amount of data in the genetic susceptibility in EAC; however, some studies have shown variants of genes encoding phase I and II enzymes, DNA repair genes, and cell cycle control, and SNPs in VEGF are linked to EAC [8].

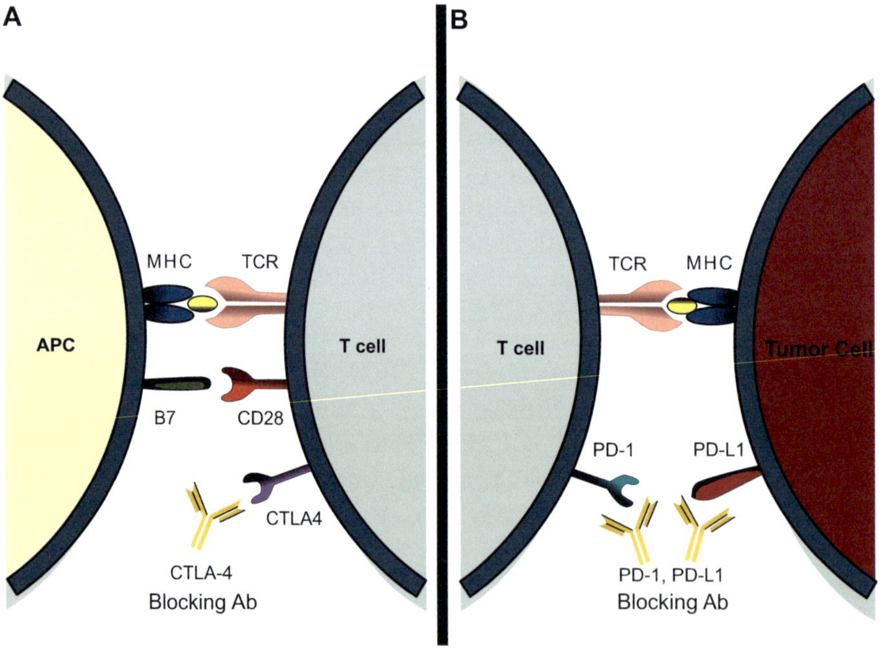

Fig. (7). Checkpoint blockade. **A**) CTLA-4 interactions with antigen-presenting cell through MHC/TCR and B7/CD28. **B**) PD-1 interaction with PL-1 on tumor cells. Raufi AG, Klempner SJ. Immunotherapy for advanced gastric and esophageal cancer: preclinical rationale and ongoing clinical investigations. Journal of gastrointestinal oncology. 2015 Oct; 6(5):561.

Another exciting area of interest in oncology is the role of immune checkpoint pathway in regulating human adaptive immune response to cancer. Tumor cells thwart this pathway through immune tolerance which are mediated by cytotoxic T-lymphocyte antigen 4 (CTLA-4) and programmed cell death protein 1 receptor (PD-1), which are T-cell receptors important in checkpoint modulation. The effects of CTLA-4 differs based on the type of T-cell which results in downregulation of CD4+ helper T-cell activity and upregulation of CD4+ T-regulatory cells. PD-1 interacts with programmed death ligand 1 and 2 (PD-L1 and PD-L2); refer to Fig. (**7**) [56].

Ohigashi *et al.* demonstrated that around 44% of ESCC express PD-L1 or PD-L2 [16]. Early translational and Phase I trials are investigating the role of checkpoint inhibition in EC [56].

SCREENING

The goal of screening for cancer is to capture a premalignant state and potentially alter the natural history. There is no routine screening for EC in the general population in the US. Patients with risk factors for chronic or severe GERD as described in *Screening and Surveillance of Barrett's Esophagus* are screened for BE. Patients with history of oral and/or oropharyngeal squamous cell carcinoma are at risk for concomitant ESCC and should be screened. Also patients with tylosis should be considered for screening for ESCC.

The modality of screening is *via* conventional upper endoscopy with biopsy. Other techniques including unsedated small-caliber endoscopy, transnasal or capsule endoscopy has been evaluated [40]. On endoscopy, superficial ESCC could present with subtle findings including color changes of the mucosa. Lugol's chromoendoscopy uses an iodine-containing solution, which stains normal epithelium. The pink color sign demonstrates cancerous lesions on Lugol's chromoendoscopy and can distinguish ESCC or HGD from LGD. The use of chromoendoscopy can also detect squamous dysplasia, which is the precursor lesion to ESCC. The sensitivity and specificity is 92% and 94%, respectively. Also, narrow-band imaging (NBI) system which uses narrow band illumination of wavelengths to enhance visualization during endoscopy with sensitivity of 97.2%, specificity of 42.1%, and 88.9% accuracy [16].

In Asian countries such as Northern and rural areas of China, cost-benefit studies have shown that endoscopy in high risk areas, which is defined as an incidence of EC more than 30 cases per 100,000 inhabitants per year, is cost-effective. However, other areas in the world with high EC incidence do not support this [57].

PREVENTION

Risk factors including alcohol, smoking, obesity, low intake of fruits and vegetables are modifiable and can be altered by lifestyle changes. Potential chemoprevention has been evaluated with PPIs, nonsteroidal anti-inflammatory drugs (NSAIDs), and aspirin. Existing data has shown that acid suppression could lead to regression of dysplasia. Further evaluation on the pathogenesis of GERD on the cellular level shows activation of the arachidonic acid pathway in the esophagus. Animal studies have shown that administration of NSAIDs has decreased EAC development. Moreover, a meta-analysis revealed that there is a protective association between aspirin/NSAIDs and esophageal cancer of both histological types [40].

STAGING AND WORKUP OF ESOPHAGEAL CANCER

Clinical Presentation

Dysphagia is the most common presenting symptom of EC and is initially experienced with solid foods that can progress to include liquids. The dysphagia and change in diet subsequently can cause malnutrition and significant weight loss. Early symptoms of EC can be subtle and nonspecific and patients may experience transient "sticking" of certain foods or retrosternal discomfort that may precede frank dysphagia. Chronic gastrointestinal blood loss from the tumor itself is common and may present as iron-deficiency anemia. Hoarseness may occur if the recurrent laryngeal nerve is invaded.

Diagnostic Evaluation

Esophageal malignancies are diagnosed *via* upper endoscopy with mucosal biopsies. The sensitivity for mucosal biopsies to detect EC reaches 100% when 6 or more samples are obtained. Barium swallow studies can be considered as the initial tool for diagnosis and characterize the tumor and aid in surgical planning. However, this modality is falling out of favor due to accuracy of endoscopy in tumor assessment [58]. Completing staging of esophageal cancer involves endoscopic ultrasound (EUS) and fine needle aspiration (FNA) in conjunction with cross-sectional imaging with CT. The 7th edition of the AJCC Cancer Staging Manual was updated in 2010 and revised based on worldwide analysis of 4,627 esophagectomy patients from 13 institutions including 5 countries and 3 continents (Asia, Europe, and North America). Please refer to Table **3 - 6** for the Tumor-Node-Metastasis (TNM) Classification of EC and EGJ Cancer. Regional lymph nodes are defined as any peri-esophageal lymph node from cervical nodes to celiac nodes. Recent changes to the TNM staging have identified the importance of histopathologic cell type, histologic grade, and tumor location and differences in survival between ESCC and EAC, especially in early-stage cancers. Therefore, ESCC and EAC have separate TNM Anatomic Staging/Prognostic groups; refer to Table **4** and **5**, respectively [28].

Table 3. TNM Classification of Esophageal Carcinoma and Esophagogastric Junction, American Joint Committee on Cancer (AJCC), 7th Edition, 2010.

Primary Tumor (T)	
TX	Primary tumor cannot be assessed.
T0	No evidence of primary tumor
Tis	High-grade dysplasia
T1	Tumor invades lamina propria, muscularis mucosae, or submucosa
	T1a Tumor invades lamina propria or muscularis mucosae T1b Tumor invades submucosa
T2	Tumor invades muscularis propria
T3	Tumor invades adventitia
T4	Tumor invades adjacent structures
	T4a Resectable tumor invading pleura, pericardium, or diaphragm T4b Unresectable tumor invading other adjacent structures (such as aorta, vertebral body, trachea).
Regional Lymph Nodes (N)	
NX	Regional lymph nodes cannot be assessed
N0	No regional lymph node metastasis
N1	Metastasis in 1-2 regional lymph nodes
N2	Metastasis in 3-6 regional lymph nodes
N3	Metastasis in 7 or more regional lymph nodes
Distant Metastasis (M)	
M0	No distant metastasis
M1	Distant metastasis

Table 4. Anatomic Staging/Prognostic Groups for Esophageal Squamous Cell Carcinoma.

STAGE	T	N	M	Grade	Tumor Location
Stage 0	Tis (HGD)	N0	M0	1, X	Any
Stage IA	T1	N0	M0	1, X	Any
Stage IB	T1	N0	M0	2-3	Any
	T2-3	N0	M0	1, X	Lower, X
Stage IIA	T2-3	N0	M0	1, X	Upper, middle
	T2-3	N0	M0	2-3	Lower, X

(Table 4) contd.....

STAGE	T	N	M	Grade	Tumor Location
Stage IIB	T2-3	N0	MO	2-3	Upper, middle
	T1-2	N1	M0	Any	Any
Stage IIIA	T1-2	N2	M0	Any	Any
	T3	N1	M0	Any	Any
	T4a	N0	M0	Any	Any
Stage IIIB	T3	N2	M0	Any	Any
Stage IIIC	T4a	N1-2	M0	Any	Any
	T4b	Any	M0	Any	Any
	Any	N3	M0	Any	Any
Stage IV	Any	Any	M1	Any	Any

Table 5. Anatomic Staging/Prognostic Groups for Esophageal Adenocarcinoma.

STAGE	T	N	M	Grade
Stage 0	Tis (HGD)	N0	M0	1, X
	T1	N0	M0	1-2, X
Stage IB	T1	N0	M0	3
	T2	N0	M0	1-2, X
Stage IIA	T2	N0	M0	3
Stage IIB	T3	N0	MO	Any
	T1-2	N1	M0	Any
Stage IIIA	T1-2	N2	M0	Any
	T3	N1	M0	Any
	T4a	N0	M0	Any
Stage IIIB	T3	N2	M0	Any
Stage IIIC	T4a	N1-2	M0	Any
	T4b	Any	M0	Any
	Any	N3	M0	Any
Stage IV	Any	Any	M1	Any

Table 6. Histologic Grade (G).

GX	Grade cannot be assessed --stage grouping as G1
G1	Well-differentiated
G2	Moderately differentiated

(Table 6) contd.....

G3	Poorly differentiated
G4	Undifferentiated --stage grouping as G3 squamous

The T stage describes the depth of tumor invasion and is primarily evaluated with EUS [14]. The accuracy of EUS for delineating T stage is 75-82% for T1, 64-82% for T2, 89-94% for T3, and 88-100% for T4. Though the accuracy of CT for T stage is lower than EUS, it can accurately define T4 disease through evaluation of the fat planes between the tumor and surrounding structures or displacement or indentation of other mediastinal structures. The sensitivity and specificity of CT for detecting mediastinal invasion is 88-100% and 85-100%, respectively. The depth of tumor invasion is important in determining the use of multimodality treatment.

Regional nodal spread, N stage, can be identified by EUS and CT imaging and the lymph nodes stations are depicted in Fig. (**8**). The status of regional and non-regional lymph nodes is important prognostically. Table **7** describes the location of regional lymph nodes based on tumor site. For example, for a patient with a tumor in the distal thoracic esophagus, a celiac axis lymph node metastasis is considered a non-regional lymph node and classified as M1a disease, whereas a gastric lymph node is regional lymph node metastasis are classified as N1 disease [29].

The endosonographic characteristics of malignant lymph nodes include size > 10mm, round and smooth features, proximity to the primary tumor, and hypoechogenicity. The accuracy of EUS for nodal staging based solely on these imaging characteristics approaches 80%. FNA of lymph nodes increases nodal staging accuracy to 92% to 98% by using pathologic staging. A recent meta-analysis compared sensitivity and specificity of N stage between EUS and CT; EUS has a sensitivity and specificity of 80% and 70%, *vs* CT with 50% and 83%, respectively [16]. Limitations of EUS are that the accuracy of EUS is operator dependent and evaluation of stenotic tumors can be difficult due to incomplete visualization of the tumor and the surrounding lymph nodes. Lymph nodes greater than 1 cm is considered enlarged with sensitivity and specificity of 30-60% and 60-80%, respectively. Despite CT findings of lymph node enlargement, pathologic confirmation is needed to confirm metastatic involvement [29].

For detection of metastatic disease, CT and positron emission tomography (PET) with 2-[fluorine 18] fluoro-2-deoxy-D-glucose (FDG) scans are utilized. The sensitivity of CT imaging detecting metastasis is up to 90%. The sensitivity of PET scans in detecting distant metastasis is 97% *vs* 67% for distant lymph node metastasis [16, 29]. Due to its high negative predictive value, PET scans are often used for initial staging for locally advanced esophageal cancer to rule out distant metastasis [58]. PET scans are also useful in treatment response to neoadjuvant chemotherapy as studies have shown that decrease in FDG-uptake as measured by standard uptake value (SUV) correlated with patient survival and pathologic response to therapy. The timing on when to obtain post-therapy PET scans or clinical implications of "responders" *vs* "non-responders" as defined by decrease SUV-uptake is not well defined [16, 29]. To improve diagnostic yield, staging laparoscopy can be considered in locally advanced (T3/T4) tumors of the EGJ. Studies have shown that the sensitivity and specificity ranges from 64-90% and 60-96%, respectively. However, the disadvantages of this procedure are due to the invasiveness and the lack of reproducibility of this accuracy at other centers. If considering staging laparoscopy for initial staging workup, should be performed by well-experienced surgeons [58].

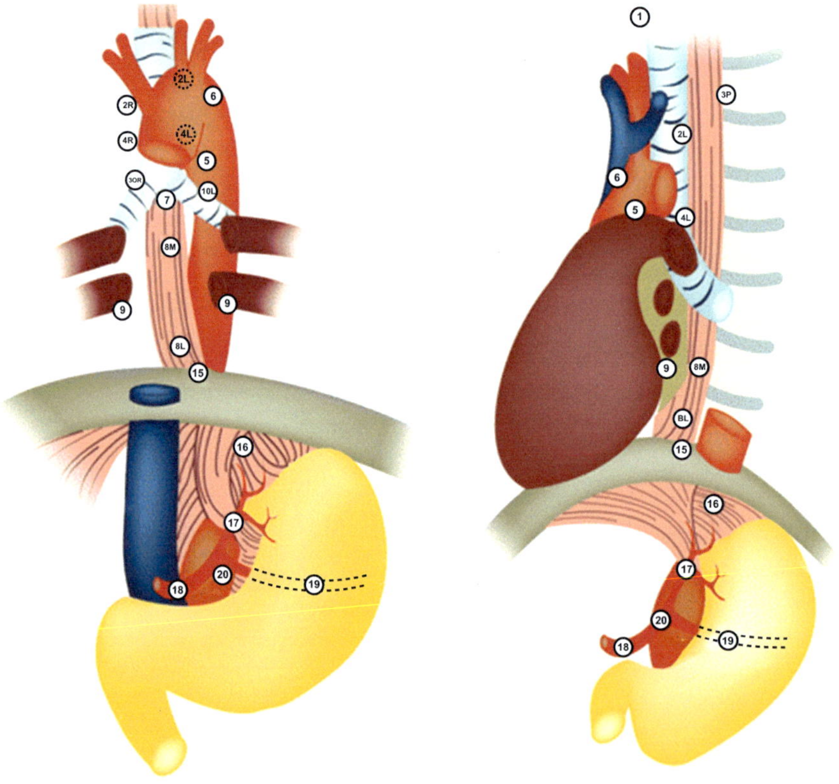

Fig. (8). Lymph node stations of esophageal cancer: *1* = supraclavicular, *2L* = left paratracheal, *2R* = right paratracheal, *3P* = posterior mediastinal, *4L* = left tracheobronchial angle, *4R* = right tracheobronchial angle, *5* = aortopulmonary, = anterior mediastinal, *7* = subcarinal, *8L* = lower paraesophageal, *8M* = middle paraesophageal, *9* = inferior pulmonary ligament, *10L* = left hilar, *10R* = right hilar, *6 15* = diaphragmatic, *16* = paracardial, *17* = left gastric, *18* = common hepatic, *19* = splenic, *20* = celiac. Adapted from Kim TJ, Kim HY, Lee KW, *et al.* Multimodality assessment of esophageal cancer: preoperative staging and monitoring of response to therapy 1. Radiographics. 2009 Mar;29(2):403-21.

Table 7. Regional lymph nodes of EC.

Cervical esophagus	Scalene, Internal jugular, Upper and Lower cervical, Periesophageal, Supraclavicular
Intrathoracic (upper, middle, and lower)	Upper periesophageal, Subcarinal, Lower periesophageal
GEJ	Lower esophageal (below the azygos vein), Diaphragmatic, Pericardial, Left gastric, Celiac

PATHOLOGY EVALUATION

Based on the College of American Pathologists (CAP), there are certain standards and guidelines when describing pathologic specimens for cancer. For biopsy specimens, a description of the extent of invasion, histologic type, grade, and presence or absence of BE must be included. If the sample is indeterminate for BE or evidence of low grade or high-grade dysplasia, a second pathologist who specializes in GI malignancies should review pathology as discussed in *Barrett's Esophagus*. Please refer to *Summary of Guidelines for Surveillance for Barrett's Esophagus*. For endoscopic resection, in addition to the descriptors as described above for biopsy specimens, further interpretation should provide the depth of tumor invasion, vascular invasion, and mucosal and deep margins. For esophagectomy specimens, the location of the tumor in the esophagus and the midpoint of the tumor in relation to the macroscopic EGJ and if the tumor crosses the EGJ should be noted. Tumors involving the EGJ are classified under the staging of EC. Histologic type should also be described (please refer to Table **2**, WHO Classification of Carcinoma of the Esophagus). Margins for the esophagectomy specimens include proximal, distal, and radial margins. R0 resection is when no margins are involved with cancer, R1 is microscopic evidence of cancer, and R2 is macroscopic evidence of cancer. The number of lymph nodes evaluated and the number of lymph nodes involved with cancer should be included. Other findings including the presence of BE or any non-malignant pathologic findings are also described [59]. Further discussion about treatment response evaluation from chemotherapy or chemoradiation (CRT) will be discussed in *Assessment of Treatment Response*.

HER-2-Neu Evaluation

Studies of HER-2-neu overexpression in EC and EGJ have varied widely from 9-60% and 2-45%, respectively [60]. These variations may be attributed to multiple factors such as methodological and scoring differences. Assessment of overexpression of HER-2-neu through immunohistochemical (IHC) and fluorescence *in situ* hybridization (FISH) is routinely done on pathologic specimens. IHC status is based on the pattern of membranous immunoreactivity on tumor cells and the scoring system is based on the intensity of the reactivity (refer to Table **8**). The drawbacks of IHC include problems with reproducibility and interpretation of the IHC assays, which can lead to false-positive or false-negative results. FISH is a gene amplification testing of the HER-2 gene and is typically used to for discordant results when IHC is 2+ (refer to Table **9**) [61].

Table 8. Immunohistochemical Criteria for HER-2-neu Expression.

Score	*Surgical Specimen Expression Pattern*	*Biopsy Specimen Expression Pattern*	*HER-2-neu Overexpression Assessment*
0	**No** reactivity or membranous reactivity in <10% cancer cells	**No** reactivity or membranous reactivity in any cancer cell	Negative
1+	**Faint or barely** perceptible membranous reactivity in **>10% of cancer cells**; cells are reactive only in part of their membrane	Cancer cell cluster with a **faint or barely** perceptible membranous reactivity irrespective of percentage of cancer cells positive	Negative
2+	**Weak to moderate** complete, basolateral or lateral membranous reactivity in **>10% of cancer cells**	Cancer cell cluster with a **weak to moderate** complete, basolateral, or lateral membranous reactivity irrespective of percentage of cancer cells positive	Equivocal
3+	**Strong** complete, basolateral or lateral membranous reactivity in **>10% of cancer cells**	Cluster of 5 or more cancer cells with **strong** complete, basolateral, or lateral membranous reactivity irrespective of percentage of cancer cells positive	Positive

Table 9. HER-2-neu Gene Amplifications with FISH.

Score	*Result of HER2:CEP17 (centromeric probe 17)*
Negative	< 1.8
Equivocal	1.8-2.2
Positive	> 2.2

ASSESSMENT OF TREATMENT RESPONSE

The response to treatment can be assessed by using the modified Ryan scheme (refer to Table **10**), which describes the extent of tumor regression and has been found to have good interobserver reproducibility.

Wu *et al.* demonstrated that disease-free-survival (DFS) and overall survival (OS) could be predicted by pathologic evaluation of any residual carcinoma after preoperative CRT [62]. Wu *et al.* also compared a 4-tiered *vs* 3-tiered classification (see Table **11**) and demonstrated better interobserver agreement among pathologists with the 3-tiered classification. Moreover, the extent of residual carcinoma as defined by the 3-tiered classification provided significant prognostic value and better-predicted OS [63].

Table 10. Modified Ryan Scheme for Tumor Regression Score.

Description	*Tumor Regression Score*
COMPLETE RESPONSE- No viable cancer cells	0
NEAR COMPLETE RESPONSE - Single cells or rare small groups of cancer cells	1
PARTIAL RESPONSE -Residual cancer with evident tumor regression, but more than single cells or rare small groups of cancer cells	2
POOR OR NO RESPONSE - Extensive residual cancer with no evident of tumor regression	3

Table 11. 4-Tiered *vs* 3-Tiered Classification for Post-Therapy Pathologic Stage.

3-Tier	*4-Tier*
P0 = 0% residual carcinoma	No residual carcinoma
P1 = 1%-50% residual carcinoma	1%-10% residual carcinoma
P2 = >50% residual carcinoma	11%-50% residual carcinoma
--	>50% residual carcinoma

These studies have demonstrated prognostic information is better provided with pathologic evaluation for residual carcinoma. The pre-treatment clinical stage is not predictive of outcome [62, 63].

Role of PET Scans in Treatment Response

As discussed earlier, the role of PET scans in providing prognostic information after preoperative CRT has been explored. Studies are still unclear about survival benefit of surgical resection after CRT and local failure rates are high if surgical resection is not pursued. A study evaluated FDG-PET response in patients who underwent preoperative CRT and defined complete response (PET-CR) as SUV ≤ 3. PET-CR after CRT was predictive of improved OS and freedom from local-failure; however, this was not demonstrated in patients treated with trimodality treatment [64]. Studies are underway to evaluate the role of PET scan after preoperative treatment and its possible clinical implications in patients who are non-responsive to therapy. Pathologic evaluation remains the best tool in treatment response; however, there are emerging techniques to not only assess treatment response but to also provide prognostic information.

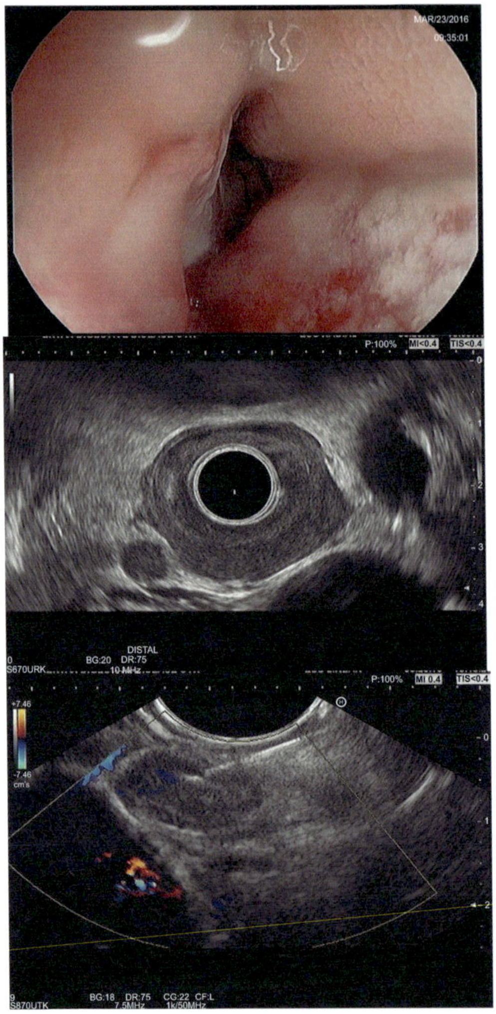

Fig. (9). T3N1 Esophageal Cancer. **A.** Ulcerated esophageal mucosa. **B.** T3 esophageal cancer invading muscularis propria along with enlarge periesophageal mediastinal lymph node. **C.** EUS FNA of mediastinal lymphadenopathy. Photographs are courtesy of Nirav Thosani MD, MHA.

Role of Micro-RNAs in Treatment Response

Micro-RNAs are small fragments of non-coding DNA that help regulate cell pathways. Altered expression of micro-RNAs may play a role in cancer carcinogenesis and chemoresistance [65]. One type of micro-RNA, miR-21, has been well studied as a proto-oncogenic marker of chemoresistance in other types of cancers [66, 67] with studies investigating its role in EC. In one study, the pre-treatment levels of miR-21 in a small group of patients with ESCC undergoing neoadjuvant chemotherapy were obtained and their subsequent histopathologic response was noted [68]. The study showed that patients with a higher pretreatment miR-21 level had a significantly lower histopathologic response. Analysis also concluded that high levels of miR-21 were an independent risk factor for chemoresistance.

Another study evaluated the signaling pathways in patients with chemoresistant adenocarcinoma. The authors analyzed 4 pairs of cell lines from patients with EAC and corresponding 5-FU resistant variants with overexpression of miR-21. DKK2 was identified as the target gene influenced by miR-21. Knockout of miR-21 in chemoresistant cell lines showed decreased tumor growth, increased apoptosis and chemosensitivity with inactivation of pathways mediated by DKK2 [69].

Other micro-RNAs such as miR-367, miR-100 and miR-26b have also been studied in EC [70 - 72]. Several more studies on the cell signaling pathways associated with micro-RNAs are ongoing, which may help personalize chemotherapeutic regimen based on the tumor molecular profile.

MANAGEMENT OF EARLY STAGE ESOPHAGEAL CANCER

This section describes the management of early stage EC where the goal of endoscopic therapy is curative. Patients who fall into this category are those with tumor classification pTis, pT1a, and selected superficial pT1b without lymphovascular invasion (LVI). Early stage EC can be managed endoscopically or surgically. The localized treatments for ESCC differs from EAC so will be discussed separately.

Endoscopic Procedures

Endoscopic therapy of early stage EC can be divided broadly into resection and ablation techniques. Endoscopic mucosal resection (EMR) or endoscopic submucosal dissection (ESD) are endoscopic techniques that permit targeted removal of superficial tissue, where EMR involves snare resection of dysplastic lesions and ESD uses endoscopic tools to dissect lesions from the submucosa. EMR has been widely accepted as an effective and minimally invasive treatment for patients with superficial early stage ESCC, nodular IS and T1a lesions, and flat BE with HGD. ESD can be used in similar situations but is preferred to EMR for large areas of dysplasia (>2 cm) or T1b malignancies. A retrospective study by Takahashi *et al.* reviewed ESD *vs* EMR for the treatment of early ESCC and reported higher en-bloc resection (100% *vs* 53.5%, $P < 0.05$) and lower local recurrence rates (0.9% *vs* 9.8%, P<0.05) with ESD [73]. Potential complications of EMR include bleeding, perforation, and stricture formation.

Ablative techniques include RFA, cryoablation, photodynamic therapy (PDT), and argon plasma coagulation (APC), which can be used independently or in combination with endoscopic resection. Some of these techniques were discussed in *Treatment of GERD and Barrett's Esophagus.* Supplementing endoscopic resection with the use of ablation therapy eliminates all flat neoplastic or dysplastic disease and all precursor disease such as BE. In patients with early stage EC treated with EMR or ESD, the remaining BE generally contains residual dysplasia and carcinoma recurrence can occur in 19% to 30% of cases [74]. Therefore, the goal in endoscopic management is to eradicate all BE in the treatment process using ablative techniques. Several studies have evaluated the long-term outcomes after combination endoscopic treatment for HGD or pTis. For example, Pech *et al.* evaluated outcomes of 1000 patients who underwent endoscopic treatment of intramucosal carcinomas by combination therapy of EMR followed by ablative therapy including APC or RFA [75]. A complete remission rate of 96% was achieved with combination therapy, and this rate remained largely stable even over a long-term follow-up period of approximately 5 years. Major complications from endoscopic therapy, including bleeding and perforation, occurred in 1.5% of patients in contrast to the higher morbidity and mortality rates associated with surgical esophageal resection. Similarly, a retrospective study by Zehetner *et al.* compared outcomes of endoscopic therapy and esophagectomy for HGD or intramucosal adenocarcinoma [76]. Endoscopic therapy was performed in 40 patients, which consisted of 102 endoscopic resections and 79 mucosal ablations, and esophagectomy in 61 patients. Compared with esophagectomy, endoscopic therapy was associated with significantly lower morbidity (39% *vs* 0%, P <0.001) and had similar survival (94% at 3 years in both groups).

Over the past 10 years, the use of endoscopic therapies has increased by over 15% as it has been shown to be an effective treatment options for patients with early stage EC. While traditional therapy had been an esophagectomy, the reduced morbidity, similar oncologic outcome, and ability to preserve the esophagus with endoscopic therapy led to a paradigm shift in the treatment of these patients [77]. Berry *et al.* analyzed 1458 patients with T1N0M0 EC using the SEER database from 1998 to 2008 and demonstrated that the OS rates were similar after treatment with surgery or endoscopic therapy; however, patients treated with endoscopic therapy had better cancer-specific survival. The patient and tumor characteristics were similar. However, the limitations of this study include that lack of data on the comorbidities of these patients. Patients who typically undergo local endoscopic therapies tend to have more comorbidities that make them "less fit" to undergo surgical resection. This study does provide support that endoscopic therapies may be a suitable alternative for patients with early stage (T1a) EC; however, this treatment strategy should be investigated in a clinical trial [78].

Treatment options for a subset of early stage EAC with T1b N0 include ER followed by ablation or esophagectomy. Although mortality rates of esophagectomy ranges from 0-4% at high-quality centers, the impact of increased morbidity and worsened quality life after surgery is a significant issue. In patients who are unfit for esophagectomy, alternative therapies including endoscopic therapies, chemoradiation, or surveillance are considered after primary treatment with ER. A retrospective cohort study of 69 patients with T1b EAC undergoing endoscopic resection was stratified by extent of ER and pathologic parameters. Low risk was defined as evidence of submucosal (SM) invasion <500 nanometers (nm), good to moderately differentiated (G1-G2), and no LVI; high risk was defined by deep SM invasion >500 nm, and/or presence of LVI and/or poor tumor differentiation (refer to Fig. **10**). Of the 14 low risk submucosal EAC, none developed metastatic disease. Notably, the high risk submucosal EAC had a lower rate of metastatic disease compared to prior studies, which highlights the possibility that these patients can be considered for alternative therapies as above. However, more studies should investigate this role [79].

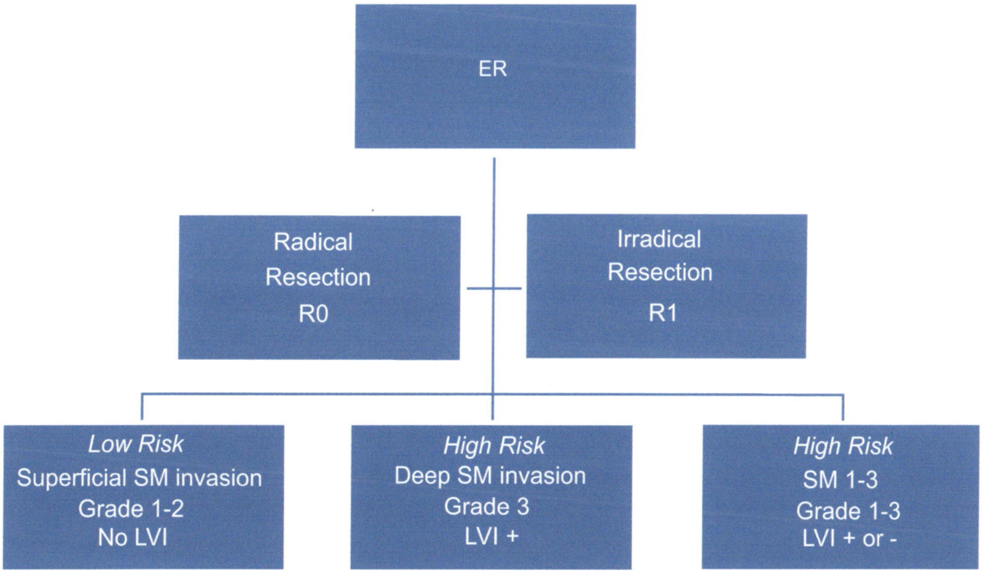

Fig. (10). Classification of T1b EAC based on endoscopic resection specimens. Adapted from Schölvinck D, Künzli H, Meijer S, Seldenrijk K, van Berge Henegouwen M, Bergman J, Weusten B. Management of patients with T1b esophageal adenocarcinoma: a retrospective cohort study on patient management and risk of metastatic disease. Surgical endoscopy. 2016 Jun 29:1-2.

The initial assessment of EC is dependent on the overall stage of disease but is also dependent on the functional status of the patient. Discussion of EC management of will be divided up into surgically resectable and unresectable. Patients who are surgical candidates but are not medically fit due to comorbidities are typically treated as unresectable.

MANAGEMENT OF SURGICALLY RESECTABLE ESOPHAGEAL CANCER

This section describes the management of resectable local disease where the goal of treatment is curative. Patients who fall in this category are those with TNM stages T1b to T4a disease with or without positive lymph nodes (any N).

Criteria for Surgery

Surgery is classically the first line curative therapy for patients with resectable esophageal cancer. Historically, surgery was utilized as monotherapy for these patients but this has been challenged in several studies in the past few decades (see *Trimodality Therapy* below).

Criteria for resection include patients with Tis-T4a disease. Patient with distant metastases, advanced age, and other comorbidities are best treated with either chemotherapy or chemoradiation (see *How to Approach a Non-resectable Esophageal Cancer Patient*). Currently, surgery can be offered as first line therapy or in combination with chemotherapy or chemoradiation, also termed trimodality therapy (TMT).

Patients with Tis or T1a disease are candidates for endoscopic resection or surgical esophagectomy, while resection in patients with T1bN0 disease should be managed by surgery alone. As described in the previous section (see *Management of Early Stage Esophageal Cancer*), these patients do not need to receive chemoradiation as part of therapy. Patients with more advanced disease including T1b-T3 tumors are resectable even with regional lymph node metastasis. Tumors invading into pleura, pericardium or diaphragm (T4a) are also resectable. Esophageal cancer patients should be considered for multimodality treatment with esophagectomy, chemotherapy and possibly radiation (see *Combined Trimodality Therapy*). Unresectable tumors are T4b involving heart, trachea, great vessels, or adjacent abdominal organs (liver, pancreas, spleen). Patients with bulky, multilevel lymphadenopathy should be classified as unresectable.

Surgical Techniques

Several surgical techniques are available in the surgical management of EC. The two main approaches include a transthoracic esophagogastrectomy (TTE) or a transhiatal esophagogastrectomy (THE) as described below:

- Transthoracic (Ivor Lewis) Esophagogastrectomy (TTE): Initially described by Ivor Lewis in 1948, TTE involves a laparotomy and right thoracotomy with thoracic esophagogastric anastomosis. This allows the surgeon to visualize the thoracic esophagus to perform a thoracic lymphadenectomy. This is usually performed for tumors in the middle to distal third of the esophagus. The McKeown esophagectomy involves a laparotomy, right thoracotomy and left cervical anastomosis. This three-field procedure allows for resection of proximal, middle and distal tumors.
- Transhiatal Esophagogastrectomy (THE): This is done through abdominal and left lateral neck incisions without a thoracotomy. The thoracic esophagus is dissected and a cervical anastomosis is created with a gastric pull-up approach. This can be used for transcervical, transthoracic and EGJ tumors.

Comparison Between TTE and THE

There have been several studies comparing TTE to THE. A transthoracic technique allows better locoregional control with a higher chance of curative resection and DFS [80]. However, this approach is thought to have a higher rate of postoperative complications due to the wide excisional approach. A randomized control trial assigned 220 patients to either TTE or THE concluded that patients with TTE had higher perioperative morbidity [81]. THE was associated with a longer median duration of surgery, more pulmonary complications, longer intensive care unit stay and more chylous leakage but there was no significant difference in in-hospital mortality. However, the study also concluded that patients who underwent THE had a non-significant higher rate of 5 year OS (39% *vs* 29%).

While TTE was commonly recommended for lesions in the distal third of the esophagus, another study supported its use in resection of cancers in the mid esophagus. They evaluated patients with cancers in the mid-esophagus who had undergone either TTE or THE and concluded that there were no differences in postoperative complications and OS [82]. Another study evaluated 1085 patients who had undergone either TTE or THE and concluded that while TTE had a higher rate of postoperative blood transfusions, return to the operating room and infections, there was no differences in operative mortality and 30-day mortality. There may be an early survival advantage in patients with THE as demonstrated in a study that evaluated the surgical outcomes of 868 patients. They noted a lower operative mortality rate in THE compared to TTE (6.7% *vs* 13.1%) but there was no significant difference in 5-year survival after adjusting for tumor stage, and patient and provider factors [83].

Minimally Invasive Esophagectomy

While esophagectomy has traditionally been performed as open operation, there is a current trend towards minimally invasive approaches. A review of 220 minimally invasive esophagectomies [84] noted a favorable operative mortality of 1.4% compared to reported mortalities of 2.5-12% in patients who undergo open esophagectomy [85 - 87]. However 81% of this cohort had previously received induction chemotherapy. A follow up Phase II multicenter trial, the E2202 study, evaluated the feasibility of minimally invasive esophagectomy in 95 patients and noted a 30-day mortality of 2.1% and an estimated 3-year survival of 58.4% [88]. The complications of this technique included anastomotic leak (8.6%), acute respiratory distress syndrome (5.7%), pneumonitis (3.8%), and atrial fibrillation (2.9%). In 2012, European investigators published results from the TIME trial (Traditional Invasive *vs* Minimally invasive Esophagectomy) as surgical treatment for EC [89]. A total of 115 patients were randomized to either open esophagectomy (Ivor Lewis) or minimally invasive esophagectomy (right thoracoscopy and laparoscopy) and 93% of patients in both arms of the study received neoadjuvant chemoradiation. The primary outcome was postoperative respiratory complications. There was a significant reduction in postoperative pulmonary infection, length of stay, and improved quality of life scores in the minimally invasive esophagectomy group.

Lymph Node Dissection

The extent of lymph node dissection and the number of lymph nodes removed has been found to be an independent predictor of survival after esophagectomy. Furthermore, the number of involved lymph nodes can predict systemic disease; the probability of systemic disease is near 100% if there are more than 8 lymph nodes involved [90]. Several large retrospective studies have shown improved survival with more extensive lymph node dissection. Results from SEER review evaluated 4882 patients who had removal of zero lymph nodes, 1-11 lymph nodes, 12-20 lymph nodes, and 30 or more lymph nodes. The authors demonstrated that patients who had more than 12 lymph nodes removed had a significant reduction of mortality. However, the group with more than 30 lymph nodes removed had the lowest reduction in mortality and the authors recommended removal of at least 30 lymph nodes in patients [91]. Similarly, Yuan *et al.* evaluated the survival rates of patients who underwent removal of < 29 lymph nodes and > 29 lymph nodes and concluded that the latter group had a significantly higher survival and that removal of > 29 lymph node was an independent predictor of survival [92]. However, this study did not stratify outcomes based on stage. A study that compared aggressive lymph node dissection (>15 LN) in patients with stage N0-N1 *vs* stage N2-N3 concluded that aggressive lymph node dissection influenced survival in N0-N1 disease but not in N2-N3 disease [93].

According to the 2016 NCCN guidelines, recommendations for patients who have not received preoperative treatment are to have at least 15 lymph nodes removed. In patients who have received preoperative treatment, it is unknown how many lymph nodes should be removed [94].

Timing of Surgery

The 2016 NCCN guidelines and the American Thoracic Surgery guidelines do not specify an optimum time for surgery after neoadjuvant therapy. A general consensus of 8 weeks has been used in most studies [94]. Previous data have shown no relationship between timing of surgery and clinical outcome [95, 96]. On the other hand, some studies have shown better outcomes with earlier surgeries [97, 98].

Since most studies included smaller patient populations with both ESCC and EAC, a recent study that evaluated a larger population with only EAC was designed. It retrospectively evaluated 4284 patients with EAC who underwent neoadjuvant CRT followed by surgery [99]. The median interval between completion of radiation and surgery was 7.1 weeks and the overall 30-day mortality and 90-day mortality were 2.9% and 7.8%, respectively. The authors noted that a post-radiation interval greater than 9 weeks was associated with increased perioperative 30- and 90-day mortality and lower OS but also showed an increased incidence of complete pathologic primary tumor and nodal response. Longer periods of follow up are needed before an optimal interval time can be recommended.

Postoperative Complications

Post-operatively, patients are started on enteral feeds until a barium swallow confirms no anastomotic leak. The postoperative mortality depends on the surgeon and facility and can range from 2.5 to 10% with better rates noted at higher volume surgical institutions [100 - 103]. The most common systemic complications include pneumonia and atrial fibrillation and the most common procedure related complications were anastomotic leak, recurrent laryngeal nerve injury, and hiatal hernias [104]. The incidence of anastomotic leak is about 10.6% and can be associated with longer hospital stay and in-hospital mortality [105].

THE DEVELOPMENT OF CHEMORADIOTHERAPY

Historically, locally advanced EC was treated by radiation alone. The 5-year survival rates in these patients were 2% [106] and the 2-year survival rate in another study was between 15-20% [107]. In current practice, radiation is rarely used as monotherapy unless in the palliative setting.

Definitive Chemoradiation

The landmark trial, RTOG 85-01, was one of the first major studies that randomized 123 patients with locally advanced EC to either combined CRT with cisplatin and 5-FU or to radiotherapy alone. Ninety percent of the patients were ESCC. Results showed superiority of the combination therapy compared to radiation alone; the median survival time and 5-year survival were 14.1 months and 27% in the CRT arm and 9.3 months and 0% in the radiation-only arm, respectively. This study led to the development of combined CRT (also termed *bimodality treatment*, BMT) as definitive treatment and standard of care in locally advanced disease [108].

A follow up study, US Intergroup Study 0123 (INT-0123) trial randomized 236 nonsurgical patients with stage T1-T4 to high dose radiotherapy (64.8 Gy) with concurrent chemotherapy (cisplatin/5-FU) or standard dose radiotherapy (50.4 Gy) with concurrent chemotherapy. The study concluded that there were no differences in survival, locoregional failure or persistence in disease in the two arms, which concluded that higher dose of radiotherapy, did not provide any benefit [109]. The optimal radiation dose in combined preoperative CRT is usually a total of 41.4 to 50.4 Gy in daily fractions of 1.8 to 2 Gy. Postoperative radiotherapy is similar and aims for a total of 45 to 50.4 Gy. Patients who are not surgical candidates who undergo definitive CRT should be given higher doses of radiation with a total dose of 50 to 50.4 Gy. Higher doses above 60 Gy are not recommended and can lead to a higher incidence of adverse effects.

Other chemotherapeutic agents have been explored for definitive CRT. A retrospective study of 179 locally advanced EC patients who underwent BMT with paclitaxel and carboplatin demonstrated a median OS of 19 months. Follow up endoscopies showed remission in 53%, and the 1- and 2-year survival rates were 70% and 47%, respectively. However, 56% of patients developed severe acute toxicities including febrile neutropenia, infections, and cytopenias [110].

Discussion about the role of definitive CRT in ESCC is further discussed under Preoperative Chemoradiotherapy in *Combined Trimodality Treatment*.

Current and Novel Radiotherapy Techniques

Radiotherapy destroys cells by ionizing damage to DNA, leading to breaks in the DNA chain. The most common way of delivering radiation is from an outside source, termed external beam radiation therapy (EBRT). Conformal 3D radiation uses X-ray beams that enter and exit the body and 'conforms' the radiation to the tumor. It uses high resolution imaging to identify the tumor margins and directs radiation to the lesion as well as surrounding margins. However, this approach exposes lung and cardiac tissue to radiation leading to early and late complications, described under Radiation and Radiation esophagitis in *Supportive care.*

Newer radiotherapy techniques such as Intensity Modulated Radiotherapy (IMRT) have been studied in combination with chemotherapy in EC and it is thought that they have a favorable side effect profile compared to EBRT. IMRT uses beams at different angles and varying intensities to concentrate radiation at the tumor with lower doses of radiation on the surrounding tissue. Another technique, Image Guided Radiotherapy (IGRT) uses real time imaging during radiotherapy to continually ensure targeted delivery. Particle therapy is another novel form of radiotherapy that is relatively new and delivers either high-energy protons or electrons to tumor cells. Proton therapy treatment plans are thought to have a lower side effect profile by relative sparing of the heart and lung as described in a study that compared 3D RT, IMRT, and proton therapy in EC [111]. A review of the literature on proton beam therapy (PBT) in EC concluded that PBT has significantly lower dose toxicity compared to traditional photon radiation [112]. The best choice of radiotherapy is still debated and a randomized clinical trial comparing proton beam therapy to IMRT in EC (both resectable and unresectable) is currently ongoing [113].

Choice of Chemotherapeutic Agent

Cisplatin and 5-Fluorouracil (5-FU) were the first drugs studied in EC and remain first line therapy in the treatment of several solid tumors. Cisplatin is a platinum based drug that binds to DNA of actively proliferating tumor cells, leading to DNA crosslinking and eventual cell apoptosis. Other drugs in this class include carboplatin and oxaliplatin. The most common side effects are nephrotoxicity, neurotoxicity, ototoxicity, in addition to nausea and vomiting.

5-FU belongs to a class of drugs called fluoropyrimidines. Other drugs in this class include oral prodrugs, Capecitabine and Tegafur, which are converted to 5-FU in the body. While unavailable in the US, S1 and UFT are also members of this class and are oral combinations of Tegafur with other synergistic agents. Fluoropyrimidines, once converted to 5-FU, inhibit thymidylate synthase, which blocks the synthesis of thymine. Thymine is a key nucleoside component of DNA and its depletion in actively replicating tumor cells leads to cell death. Folinic acid, also known as leucovorin, is usually given with 5-FU as it has a synergistic effect in inhibiting thymidylate synthase. The most common adverse effects of the fluoropyrimidine drug class are myelosuppression, diarrhea, and cardiotoxicity as well hand-foot syndrome. Of note, fluoropyrimidines are metabolized by an enzyme dihydropyrimidine dehydrogenase and patients deficient in this enzyme by genetic variations in the dihydropyrimidine dehydrogenase (DPYD) gene are at higher risk for adverse effects including increased risk of developing severe and potentially fatal neutropenia, mucositis, and diarrhea [114]. Screening for this polymorphism prior to initiating treatment is controversial and not routinely performed [115].

Table 12. Chemotherapeutic Agents Used in EC and Classified by Mechanisms of Action.

Chemotherapeutic Agents
Antimetabolites
- Fluoropyrimidine (either 5-FU or Capecitabine)
Alkylating agents
- Cisplatin
- Oxaliplatin
- Carboplatin
Topoisomerase II Inhibitor
- Epirubicin
- Doxorubicin
Antimicrotubule agents (Taxanes derivatives)
- Paclitaxel
- Docetaxel

While cisplatin and 5-FU were traditionally used as the first line drugs in BMT, several studies began exploring other agents such as taxanes and anthracyclines. Taxanes, such as docetaxel and paclitaxel, are anti-microtubule agents, which interfere in spindle formation in mitosis, thus reducing tumor cell growth. The most common side effect is sensory neuropathy, which can either resolve or persist after completion of chemotherapy. Anthracyclines, such as doxorubicin and epirubicin, work by intercalating with DNA strands to form complexes that trigger cell death. The most serious side effect of anthracyclines is dose dependent cardiotoxicity and most oncologists will monitor cardiac function by serial echocardiography during treatment [116].

A Phase III trial, REAL-2, played a critical role in establishing the non-inferiority of oral capecitabine to infusional 5-FU [117]. It assigned 1002 patients with advanced esophageal-gastric cancer (30% were EC) to one of four arms; epirubicin, cisplatin and either capecitabine or infusional FU or epirubicin, oxaliplatin and either capecitabine or infusional FU. The trial showed no significant differences in response rates or OS among the four groups and the authors concluded that the substitution of capecitabine for infusional FU did not change outcomes.

COMBINED TRIMODALITY TREATMENTS

Preoperative Chemoradiotherapy

There have been several clinical trials that compared CRT and surgery to surgery alone in patients with localized disease. The Dutch CROSS trial randomly assigned 363 patients with resectable disease (T2-T3) to preoperative or also termed as neoadjuvant CRT with carboplatin and paclitaxel followed by surgery (TMT) or to surgery alone [118]. This pivotal trial was the largest Phase III of EC and EGJ cancers with 75% of EAC and 23% ESCC. The complete resection (R0) rate [see *Assessment of Response*] was higher in the chemotherapy group (92% *vs* 69%). After median follow up of 84.1 months, the median survival and recurrence rates were 49 months and 35% in the TMT and 24 months and 58% in the surgery group, respectively. Moreover, the 3- and 5-year survival rate was higher in the TMT group compared to surgery group; 58% *vs* 44% and 47% *vs* 33%, respectively.

In contrast, the FFCD 9901 study randomized 195 patients with T1-T2 disease to TMT with cisplatin and 5FU or to surgery alone [119]]. The authors concluded that there was no significant difference in 3-year survival (47.5% in TMT *vs* 53% in surgery). However, the TMT group had higher postoperative mortality (11.1% *vs* 3.4%). Notably, a majority of the patients had lower T stage disease than the CROSS trial; about 19% of the patients had Stage I disease and around 53% and 28% had Stage IIA and IIB, respectively. In contrast, a great majority of both groups of patients in the CROSS trial had T3 disease (84% and 78%).

Other combinations with 5-FU and cisplatin have been explored including a Phase II trial of 40 patients with T3 disease who received cisplatin and paclitaxel, which was compared to historical cohort of patients treated with cisplatin and 5-FU. Both groups underwent standard radiotherapy and surgery as part of their treatment. The study concluded that while the paclitaxel group had higher toxicity, there was no difference in survival, locoregional control, and development of distant metastasis [120]. Another Phase II study demonstrated similar results which did not support paclitaxel and cisplatin as another first line chemotherapy for locally advanced EC [121].

A meta-analysis of 12 randomized controlled trials including the CROSS and FFCD 9901 trials concluded a survival benefit of 8.7% at two years in TMT with neoadjuvant CRT followed by surgery *vs* surgery alone [122]. These landmark trials demonstrated the survival benefit for patients with locally advanced resectable disease treated with a combination of preoperative CRT followed by surgical resection, also termed neoadjuvant CRT.

Furthermore, two robust meta-analyses provided support of improved survival with neoadjuvant chemotherapy or CRT [122, 123]. One meta-analysis included 17 trials with 4188 patients and found the hazard ratio (HR) for all-cause mortality for neoadjuvant CRT and chemotherapy was 0·78 and 0·87, respectively [122]. The Cochrane meta-analysis, which included 13 randomized studies with 2122 patients who received preoperative chemotherapy, also demonstrated improved OS with HR of 0.88 and significantly higher rate of complete (R0) resection [123]. There is significant evidence that supports neoadjuvant therapy and Phase II studies that have favored neoadjuvant CRT over chemotherapy; however, there has been no randomized study that directly compared neoadjuvant chemotherapy *vs* neoadjuvant CRT.

Despite evidence showing survival benefit with TMT, there is still debate on the role of surgery in patients who have responded to CRT. Stahl *et al.* conducted a Phase III trial of locally advanced (T3-4, N0-1) ESCC patients who were randomized to: arm A) induction chemotherapy followed by CRT and surgery *vs* arm B) induction chemotherapy followed CRT. The arm A induction chemotherapy included three courses of bolus 5-FU, leucovorin, etoposide, and cisplatin on days 1 to 3 every 3 weeks, followed by concurrent CRT with cisplatin and etoposide and 40 Gy of irradiation. Treatment of arm B consisted of the same induction chemotherapy and the same combined CRT up to 65 Gy. The 2-year progression-free survival (PFS) survival was better in the surgery arm at 62%; however, the OS was similar in both arms. The trial closed due to poor accrual. However, the results of the trial lend support for possible consideration of surveillance for patients who have responded to CRT in lieu of surgery due to comparable OS [123]. A subsequent French trial demonstrated similar results with 5-FU and cisplatin [125]. The majority of patients in these trials were ESCC. Also, in locally advanced ESCC patients who are non-surgical candidates, definitive CRT is a suitable option as discussed in *Definitive Chemoradiation*. The data in non-surgical management in EAC is more limited. Two retrospective analyses suggest better locoregional control in patients who have undergone surgical resection [126, 127]. Further clinical trials investigating this should be pursued.

Postoperative Treatment

Patients with locally advanced EGJ adenocarcinoma who undergo surgery without neoadjuvant CRT may be candidates for postoperative CRT. The benefit of postoperative chemotherapy was noted in the INT-0116 trial, which randomized 556 patients with resected T1-T4 EGJ and gastric adenocarcinoma to CRT with 5-FU and leucovorin or to observation alone. The 3-year survival rates and median survival were significantly higher in the postoperative CRT arm compared to the observation group; 50% *vs* 41% and 36 months *vs* 27 months, respectively. This study had advanced tumors with around 70% with T3 or T4 tumors and 85% with node positive disease. Limitations of this study included that the type of surgical resection was not uniform and patients were eligible for the study only after the recovery from surgery, which provide arguments that the population included the "fit" patients. This landmark trial established postoperative CRT as standard of care for EGJ adenocarcinomas [128]. At the 10-year follow-up, the OS and relapse-free survival (RFS) benefit was demonstrated in the treated arm (HR for OS is 1.32 (95% CI, 1.10 to 1.60; P = .0046, refer to Fig. **11**) [129]. The role of adjuvant CRT in thoracic EC is not well established; though there are sparse data that supports adjuvant CRT. Similarly, adjuvant chemotherapy after resection in patients who have not received preoperative chemotherapy or CRT can be considered and demonstrates potential benefit but also has not been studied in a randomized trial setting.

Another study evaluated the role of postoperative CRT in 50 patients with poorer prognosis (Stage T3, N1, M1a disease) and noted acceptable toxicities with projected 4-year OS of 51%, distant metastatic control of 56%, and locoregional control of 86% [130].

The role of further treatment in adjuvant chemotherapy after TMT is still not well studied. A study of 145 patients received TMT and 62 of 145 patients received postoperative chemotherapy after TMT [131]. About 34% of the patients had complete pathologic response and 66% had evidence of residual disease. Patients with macroscopic residual disease who underwent postoperative chemotherapy (predominantly with docetaxel) had a higher 5-year OS (38.7% *vs* 13.9%) and cause-specific survival advantage (42.8% *vs* 18.8%). This survival benefit was absent in patients with complete pathologic response or microscopic residual disease. The authors therefore advocated for postoperative chemotherapy in patients with residual macroscopic disease (R2 resection) who had undergone neoadjuvant chemotherapy and resection. Soon after this trial was published, a similar retrospective study was done on a larger scale where 3592 patients who had undergone neoadjuvant CRT and surgery were given adjuvant chemotherapy (AC) [132]. EAC made up around 85% of the cohort with 9.9% receiving AC.

ESCC made up the remaining 15% with 6.4% receiving AC. The authors noted no difference in risk of death in patients with no residual disease (R0 resection) or residual non-nodal disease who had received AC. However, patients with residual nodal disease who had received AC had a 30% lower risk of death. This emphasizes the point that patients with residual nodal metastases are most likely to have micrometastatic systemic disease and may benefit for AC as demonstrated by results.

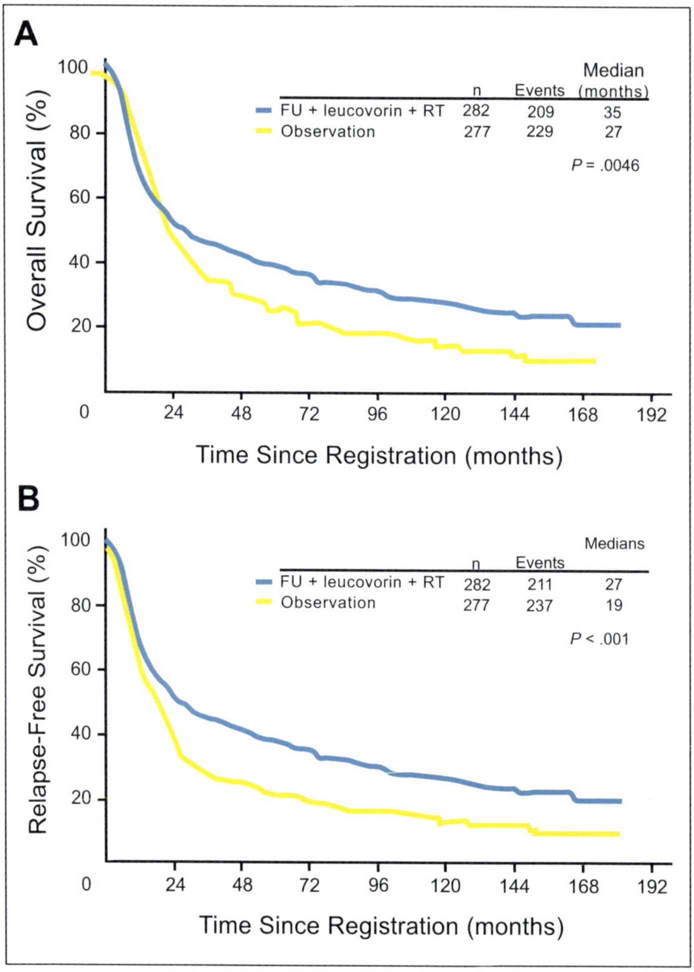

Fig. (11). Kaplan Meier curves for (**A**) Overall survival by arm; (**B**) relapse-free survival by arm.

The prognostic value of residual nodal disease even with complete pathologic response (defined as absence of malignant cells at the primary lesion, ypT0) after neoadjuvant chemotherapy has been well described in the literature. One study described the survival of complete pathologic responders with residual nodal disease as similar as or worse than non-complete responders [133]. In a study of 487 patients who underwent neoadjuvant chemotherapy and surgery, the OS of patients with complete pathologic response was 92.2 months in those with no residual nodal disease and 14 months in those with residual nodal disease. Patients with non-complete pathologic response but without residual nodal disease had a longer OS as well (29.6 and 27.5 months for pathologic Stage II and III, respectively) compared to complete responders with residual nodal disease. This along with the previous studies provides support for postoperative chemotherapy especially if there is residual disease noted. However, further randomized controlled trials should further investigate this role.

PERIOPERATIVE CHEMOTHERAPY

Perioperative chemotherapy (chemotherapy before and after surgery) was evaluated in the MAGIC trial where 503 patients with resectable gastric (74%), esophageal (11%) and EGJ adenocarcinomas (11%) were randomized to surgery alone or to surgery with perioperative chemotherapy 1 [134]. Three cycles of epirubicin, cisplatin and 5-FU (ECF) were given preoperatively and postoperatively. The authors noted a lower locoregional failure and development of distant metastases in the perioperative group compared to the surgery alone group; 14% *vs* 21% and 24% *vs* 37% respectively. Most importantly, the perioperative chemotherapy group had a higher likelihood of OS (HR for death 0.75) and a better 5-year survival (36% *vs* 26%). The MAGIC trial established perioperative chemotherapy in locally advanced EC patients as a potential treatment option. Another study, the FNCLCC/FFCD multicenter phase III trial compared perioperative chemotherapy to surgery in 224 patients with resectable gastroesophageal adenocarcinoma. The study showed that patients in the perioperative group had a significantly better 5-year OS (38% *vs* 24%) and a longer DFS (34% *vs* 19%) [135]. However, there have been other negative trials that did not demonstrate survival benefit.

In summary, there are several options for management of surgically resectable EC including TMT or perioperative chemotherapy. Studies have concluded that TMT is superior to surgery alone as discussed above. TMT options can include either preoperative CRT or in EGJ adenocarcinoma, postoperative CRT. In GEJ adenocarcinoma, perioperative chemotherapy is considered an optimal plan of care. There are no randomized clinical trials comparing these approaches, and management should involve a multidisciplinary approach of cardiothoracic and surgical oncologists, medical and radiation oncologists, gastroenterologists, and nutritionists. There is currently a large randomized multicenter clinical trial (ESOPEC) ongoing that is comparing neoadjuvant CRT to perioperative chemotherapy in patients with localized EAC (Stage T1-T2). As the first randomized clinical trial of this nature, it is hoped that this trial will help guide oncologists to determine which route of TMT to offer to patients [136].

The following table lists the combination of chemotherapeutic drugs used in combined modality treatment of EC.

Table 13. Systemic Therapy for Resectable Esophageal Cancer.

PREOPERATIVE CHEMORADIATION
Preferred Regimens: - Paclitaxel and Carboplatin **(CATEGORY 1)** - Fluoropyrimidine (either 5-FU or Capecitabine) and Cisplatin **(CATEGORY 1)** - Fluoropyrimidine (either 5-FU or Capecitabine) and Oxaliplatin **(CATEGORY 1)** Other Regimens: - Irinotecan and Cisplatin **(CATEGORY 2B)** - Fluoropyrimidine (either 5-FU or Capecitabine) and Paclitaxel **(CATEGORY 2B)**
PERI-OPERATIVE CHEMOTHERAPY
- Fluoropyrimidine (either 5-FU or Capecitabine) and Cisplatin **(CATEGORY 1)** - ECF and ECF modifications **(CATEGORY 3)** - Epirubicin, Cisplatin, and 5-FU (ECF) - Epirubicin, Oxaliplatin and 5-FU (EOF) - Epirubicin, Cisplatin and Capecitabine (ECX) - Epirubicin, Oxaliplatin and Capecitabine (EOX) ***Only for adenocarcinoma of the thoracic esophagus or esophagogastric junction* ***3 cycles preoperative and 3 cycles post-operative*
PREOPERATIVE CHEMOTHERAPY
- Fluoropyrimidine (either 5-FU or Capecitabine) and Cisplatin **(CATEGORY 2B)** ***Only for adenocarcinoma of the thoracic esophagus or esophagogastric junction*
POSTOPERATIVE CHEMORADIATION
- Fluoropyrimidine (either infusional 5-FU or Capecitabine) before and after fluoropyrimidine-based chemoradiation

Adapted from National Comprehensive Cancer Network (NCCN) Guidelines for Esophageal and Esophagogastric Junction Cancer, version 2.2016. Category 1: Based upon high-level evidence, there is uniform NCCN consensus that the intervention is appropriate. Category 2A: Based upon lower-level evidence, there is uniform NCCN consensus that the intervention is appropriate. Category 2B: Based upon lower-level evidence, there is NCCN consensus that the intervention is appropriate. Category 3: Based upon any level of evidence, there is major NCCN disagreement that the intervention is appropriate.

HOW TO APPROACH A NON-RESECTABLE ESOPHAGEAL CANCER PATIENT

This section refers to patients who are found to have locally advanced ESCC or EAC who are not considered surgical candidates due to presence of T4b disease, or not medically fit given comorbidities and advanced age and in addition, applies to potentially resectable patients who refuse surgery. These patients also do not have distant metastases. Patients with distant metastases (any M) will be discussed in *Management of Metastatic Disease.* T4 can be further sub-classified into T4a or T4b. As described earlier, T4b disease involves local invasion of the tumor into adjacent structures such as the aorta, trachea, paravertebral tissues or bone or the presence of a tracheoesophageal fistula, which is considered unresectable. However, invasion of the pleural, pericardial or diaphragmatic tissues is still considered resectable and these patients would be classified as T4a.

The prognosis of patients with locally advanced disease is poor, as disease tends to recur after definitive treatment. The median survival of 206 patients with locally advanced cancer (equally split between ESCC and EAC) treated with definitive platinum based CRT was 20.6 months [137] and the 1-, 3- and 5-year survival rates were 43.6%, 32.9% and 19.5%, respectively. Longer disease length and greater tumor burden were associated with a worse outcome. Another study analyzed 184 patients with inoperable EC treated with carboplatin and paclitaxel and noted a 41% loco-regional recurrence rate after a follow up of 22 months [138]. The 1-, 3-, and 5-year survival rates were 65%, 28% and 21%, respectively.

Therefore, the goal of treatment for patients with inoperable disease would be palliative, rather than curative and to improve PFS.

Definitive Treatment

Radiation

Historically, patients with unresectable EC or nonsurgical candidates with EC were treated with EBRT alone. As described earlier, the 5-year survival rates in one study was 2% [139] and the 2-year survival rate in another study was between 15-20% [140]. The OS in one study with 127 patients treated with different doses of radiotherapy was 7.4 months [141]. However, radiotherapy did improve dysphagia with a 70% response rate noted in that same patient population. Radiation therapy can therefore be considered for palliation of dysphagia in medically unfit or comfort care patients, see Radiation and Radiation Esophagitis under *Supportive Care*. The most serious complication of radiation is the development of tracheoesophageal fistula, which limits further radiation.

Chemoradiation

As described earlier, the RTOG 85-01 trial showed survival benefit in patients with CRT compared to radiation alone in patients with locally advanced EC, which led to the development of BMT as definitive treatment and standard of care in locally advanced disease.

Chemotherapeutic Agent Options

Once CRT had been established as standard of care, several studies began comparing different chemotherapeutic regimens to the well-studied cisplatin/5-FU. As mentioned earlier, the REAL- 2 trial established the noninferiority of capecitabine to 5-FU as well as the non-inferiority of oxaliplatin to cisplatin. Therefore, the standard cisplatin/5-FU regimen is often modified to cisplatin/capecitabine, oxaliplatin/5-FU or oxaliplatin/capecitabine. All four regimens can be used as first-line treatment in patients with locally advanced EC. Notably, the 2 arms treated with EOX *vs* ECF had a median survival of 11.2 *vs.* 9.9 months, which has led some oncologists to prefer EOX over ECF [117].

Other alternative first-line regimens have been evaluated. A study of 50 patients with locally advanced and metastatic EC underwent treatment with carboplatin and paclitaxel in the first-line setting [142]. Concurrent radiation was given and patients who were surgical candidates underwent esophagectomy. The results showed a median survival of 32 months; 44 months for localized disease treated with surgery, >44 months for localized disease treated with definitive CRT and 12 months for metastatic disease. Another study retrospectively compared carboplatin/paclitaxel to cisplatin/irinotecan in patients with locally advanced EC [143]. Results showed that carboplatin/paclitaxel was superior in terms of 3-year OS (56% *vs* 19.7%). Other combinations such as irinotecan and cisplatin and 5-FU and paclitaxel can also be considered in combination with radiation therapy [144, 145]. Another study worth mentioning is the PRODIGE5/ACCORD17 trial, which randomized patients with locally advanced cancer to Leucovorin, 5-FU, Oxaliplatin (FOLFOX) or standard cisplatin/5-FU in addition to radiotherapy [146]. There was no significant difference in treatment related adverse events or median PFS (9.7 months in FOLFOX and 9.4 months in cisplatin/5-FU). As a result, FOLFOX was suggested as an alternative therapy for patients with locally advanced inoperable cancer.

Table **14** below summarizes the preferred first line agents for definitive chemotherapy in patients with unresectable disease.

Table 14. Systemic therapy for definitive chemoradiation.

Preferred Regimen:
- Fluoropyrimidine (either 5-FU or Capecitabine) and Cisplatin **(CATEGORY 1)**
- Fluoropyrimidine (either 5-FU or Capecitabine) and Oxaliplatin **(CATEGORY 1)**
- Paclitaxel and Carboplatin

(Table 14) contd.....

Other Regimens: - Irinotecan and Cisplatin **(CATEGORY 2B)** - Fluoropyrimidine (either 5-FU or Capecitabine) and Paclitaxel **(CATEGORY 2B)** - Cisplatin and Docetaxel or Paclitaxel

Adapted from National Comprehensive Cancer Network (NCCN) Guidelines for Esophageal and Esophagogastric Junction Cancer, version 2.2016. Category 1: Based upon high-level evidence, there is uniform NCCN consensus that the intervention is appropriate. Category 2A: Based upon lower-level evidence, there is uniform NCCN consensus that the intervention is appropriate. Category 2B: Based upon lower-level evidence, there is NCCN consensus that the intervention is appropriate. Category 3: Based upon any level of evidence, there is major NCCN disagreement that the intervention is appropriate.

Resectability after CRT can be considered depending on response and potential for resection. There have been no clinical trials comparing the use of post chemoradiotherapy surgical intervention in patients with T4 disease; however, surgery can be considered on a case-by-case evaluation.

SURVEILLANCE AND FOLLOW UP

Even after curative treatment, the recurrence of EC in these patients is significantly high (between 40-60%) and approximately 90% of patients will eventually die from their disease [147]. Therefore, aggressive surveillance after treatment plays a crucial role in early detection of recurrence since intervention can potentially increase survival. There is a paucity of data about the best surveillance algorithm and this has been acknowledged by the NCCN [94]. Currently, options include a combination of lab work, CT scans, PET scans, tumor markers, and surveillance endoscopies in addition to regular clinic visits for history and physicals.

Role of Surveillance

The need for an endoscopy driven surveillance strategy compared to an imaging based surveillance strategy depends on whether esophagectomy was part of the primary treatment plan. Patients who undergo endoscopic resection/ablation or BMT have a higher rate of local recurrence compared to patients who undergo surgery [148]. Kazuki *et al.* evaluated recurrence patterns in 275 patients with esophageal cancer who underwent BMT alone. Disease recurred in about 66.7% of patients; of these 23.2% were locoregional recurrence only and 43.5% were distant metastasis with or without local recurrence. In patients with local recurrence, 36% (8% of the original cohort) underwent salvage surgery with improved survival. In these patients, the median survival was 58.6 months compared to 9.5 months in those who did not undergo surgery. This study therefore argued for aggressive endoscopic surveillance of patients with BMT as it identifies patients with local recurrence early with the potential for salvage surgery and improved survival.

Kazuki *et al.* also evaluated relapse patterns of 518 patients who underwent TMT [149]. Recurrence was seen in about 41.5% of the cohort, of which only 5% were locoregional recurrence and 36% were distant metastasis with or without local recurrence. Of the patients with local recurrence (27 out of the 518 patients), the median survival was around 17 months. Of these 27 patients, 12 underwent salvage chemotherapy and only 10 patients survived more than 2 years. The authors concluded that only 2% of the original cohort benefited from endoscopic surveillance and salvage therapy, raising questions about the benefit of endoscopic surveillance in patients with TMT.

Lou *et al.* retrospectively analyzed 1187 patients who underwent an esophagectomy for their disease [150]. Of this cohort, 63% had received neoadjuvant CRT before surgery (TMT). During follow-up, there were 595 deaths (52%) and 435 recurrences (38%). About 75% of the recurrences were in the first 2 years as seen below in Fig. (**12**).

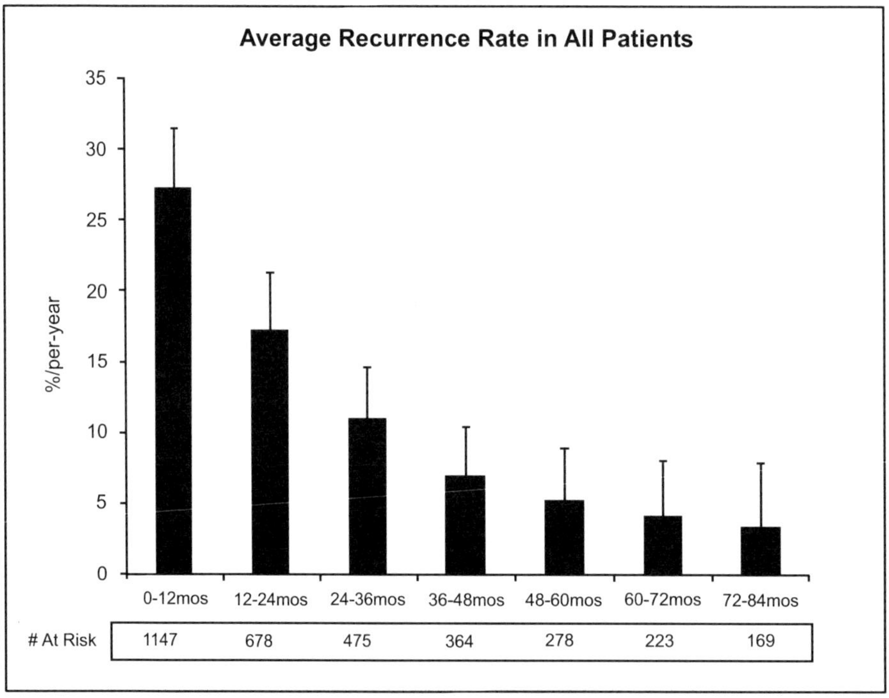

Fig. (12). Average recurrence rate in patients who underwent esophagectomy [150].

This study also looked at the modality through which recurrence was diagnosed. About half the recurrences were detected after the patient complained of symptoms, primarily dysphagia. The other half of recurrences were detected by routine CT scans and only 1% were detected by surveillance upper endoscopy.

These groups of patients that were non-clinically diagnosed had an increased survival than patients who presented with concerning histories and physicals. The otherwise asymptomatic patients who were diagnosed with recurrence based on surveillance endoscopy (done every 6 months for 2 years and annually after that in this study population) were only 6 patients out of the cohort. Of these 6 patients, only one patient underwent additional salvage surgery with curative intent. Therefore, the authors conclude that routine endoscopy has little benefit for surveillance in patients after curative esophagectomy.

They also further analyzed the pattern of recurrence in patients with TMT *vs* surgery alone. They noted that patients with TMT had a higher rate of recurrence in the first year (83%) with a sharp decline in recurrence rates after. In contrast, patients with esophagectomy alone had a lower rate of recurrence in the first year (63%) with a slower decline in recurrence rates after. This difference is likely secondary to the stage of disease in these two patient categories. TMT was likely to be offered to patients with advanced disease while surgery was offered to patients with early stage disease with better prognosis.

This pattern was previously noted in a similar study done in 2010, which retrospectively analyzed 590 patients [151]. Of this population, about 40% had disease recurrence. In this study as well, patients who underwent TMT had a shorter interval to recurrence (8 months) compared to patients who underwent surgery alone (12 months).

Recurrence was detected by history and physical in 17%, CT scan in 60%, PET scan 18% and elevated CEA in 5%. Though, it should be noted that CEA are not always routinely ordered for surveillance. By CT scan, the most common site of recurrence was the liver, followed by the lymph nodes and lung. In the patients suspected of having a recurrence based on elevated CEA, the median increase in CEA was 51.

Around 70% of the patients were treated for their recurrence and median survival was about 9 months in this subset compared with 3 months in those untreated as seen in Fig. (**13**). This increased survival benefit therefore confirms the need for frequent follow up.

The authors concluded that aggressive follow up was beneficial as more than 90% of recurrences occurred within 2 years after TMT and within 3 years after surgery alone. Beyond this, about 2-3% of recurrences were diagnosed each year. This is in accordance with previous studies and therefore aggressive surveillance should only be continued for about 3 years and surveillance after that may be annual or as clinically needed.

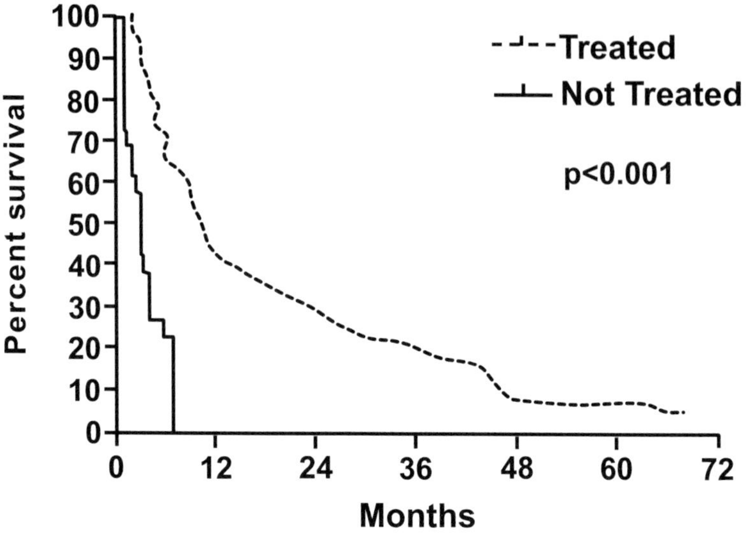

Fig. (13). Survival after recurrence in patients either treated or not treated for their recurrence [151].

Surveillance Strategy

Based on the available data, the NCCN has put forward guidelines for follow up and surveillance [94]. They recommend office visits with history and physical every 3-6 months for 1 to 3 years and then every 6 months for the next 2 years and then annually. Lab work such as a complete blood count and chemistries can be obtained at these visits. The need for and frequency of imaging and upper GI endoscopy are dependent on the stage and are as follows per NCCN guidelines:

Stage 1:

- Tis treated with ER/ablation: EGD every 6 months for 1-2 years, then annually for 3 more years. Imaging studies are not recommended.
- Tis treated with esophagectomy: EGD based on symptoms. Routine imaging is not recommended.
- T1a treated with ER/ablation: EGD every 3 months for first year, every 4-6 months for the second year and then annually for 3 more years
- T1a treated with esophagectomy: EGD based on symptoms. Routine imaging is not recommended.
- T1b treated with ER/ablation, N0: EGD every 3 months for first year, every 4-6 months for second year and annually for 3 more years. Imaging (CT or PET-CT) every 6-12 months for 2 years or annually for a total of 3 years.
- T1b, any N treated with esophagectomy: Imaging (CT or PET CT) every 6-12 months for up to 3 years. EGD should be done based on symptoms or on

radiographic findings

- T1b, any N treated with BMT (non-surgical candidate): EGD every 6-12 months for the first 2 years and then annually for 3 more years. Imaging every 6-9 months for the first 2 years and then annually up to 5 years
- T1b, any N treated with BMT (candidate for salvage esophagectomy): EGD every 6-12 months for the first 2 years and then annually for 3 more years. Imaging every 6-9 months for the first 2 years and then annually up to 5 years

Stage 2 or 3:

- BMT: Endoscopy every 3-4 months for 2 years and then every 6 months for the third year and then as warranted. Imaging studies were complementary.
- TMT: Imaging studies (CT or PET) every 4-6 months in the first year and then every 6-9 months in the second and third year and then as warranted. Endoscopy was not recommended.

MANAGEMENT OF METASTATIC DISEASE:

Despite advances in chemotherapy and immunotherapy, the 5-year survival rate for EC remains dismally low at 14% and over 50% of patients present with metastatic disease at diagnosis [152]. Management of metastatic EC as well as unresectable disease is largely supportive. The goals of treatment are to palliate symptoms, to improve quality of life, and to prolong survival.

A meta-analysis of 35 trials by Wagner *et al.* concluded that palliative chemotherapy prolongs survival in patients with advanced gastric adenocarcinoma [153]. As with other gastric adenocarcinoma trials, many have applied this data to patients with advanced EAC.

Current Strategies with First-Line Chemotherapy

Historically, metastatic esophageal and gastric carcinoma was treated with single drugs such as platinum-based agents or taxanes with good response rates [154, 155]. Combination of chemotherapeutic agents led to significantly higher response rates (RR) but only modest improvements in survival [153, 156 - 158].

Currently, multidrug regimens such as a combination of fluoropyrimidines (5-FU or capecitabine) and a platinum agent (cisplatin or oxaliplatin) are considered first line therapy for metastatic or locally advanced esophageal cancer. For more medically fit patients, three drug regimens such as ECF (epirubicin, cisplatin, and fluoropyrimidine) or combinations as discussed in the REAL-2 trial [159] or DCF (docetaxel, cisplatin and a fluoropyrimidine) as first line for metastatic or unresectable disease [160, 161]. The landmark TAX-325 trial demonstrated better

RR, time to progression (TTP), and 2-year survival with the addition of docetaxel to cisplatin and 5-FU combination; however, there was an increase of adverse effects including grade 3-4 diarrhea and neutropenia [161]. Due to the increased association of toxicity, modifications of DCF with was studied in a Phase II trial and demonstrated less toxicity with improved median OS in the modified DCF arm. The DCF arm was closed early because of toxicity [162]. For more information on the adverse effects of chemotherapy, please refer to *Choice of Chemotherapeutic Agents*.

Table **15** provides the list of the preferred combination of agents that can be considered in first-line therapy in locally advanced or metastatic disease.

Table 15. Systemic Therapy for Locally Advanced or Metastatic Esophageal Cancer.

Preferred Regimens: **Two drug:** - Fluoropyrimidine (either 5-FU or Capecitabine) and Cisplatin **(CATEGORY 1)** - Fluoropyrimidine (either 5-FU or Capecitabine) and Oxaliplatin
Three drug: DCF modifications - Docetaxel, Cisplatin and 5-FU (DCF) - Docetaxel, Oxaliplatin and 5-FU (DOX) - Docetaxel, Carboplatin and 5-FU **(CATEGORY 2B)** ECF modifications **(CATEGORY 1)** - Epirubicin, Cisplatin, and 5FU (ECF) - Epirubicin, Oxaliplatin and 5-FU (EOX) - Epirubicin, Cisplatin and Capecitabine (ECX) - Epirubicin, Oxaliplatin and Capecitabine (EOX)
Other regimens: - Paclitaxel with Carboplatin or Cisplatin - Docetaxel with Cisplatin - 5-FU and Irinotecan **(CATEGORY 1)**
Single agents: - 5-FU or Capecitabine - Docetaxel - Paclitaxel
Targeted Agents: - Trastuzumab can be added to all chemotherapeutic regimens in eligible candidates [see *Targeted Therapies in Esophageal Cancer*].

Adapted from National Comprehensive Cancer Network (NCCN) Guidelines for Esophageal and Esophagogastric Junction Cancer, version 2.2016. Category 1: Based upon high-level evidence, there is uniform NCCN consensus that the intervention is appropriate. Category 2A: Based upon lower-level evidence, there is uniform NCCN consensus that the intervention is appropriate. Category 2B: Based upon lower-level evidence, there is NCCN consensus that the intervention is appropriate. Category 3: Based upon any level of evidence, there is major NCCN disagreement that the intervention is appropriate.

Other combination therapies that have been recently evaluated include irinotecan-based regimens. A Phase II study investigated the use of irinotecan and cisplatin in 27 patients with metastatic ESCC and noted a median PFS of 4.5 months and OS of 8.8 months with manageable toxicities [163]. In a Phase III trial, irinotecan and 5-FU (IF) were compared to cisplatin and fluorouracil (CF) and concluded to be non-inferior in regards to PFS and TTP. IF was considered better tolerated, and patients experienced less adverse effects including severe neutropenia, thrombocytopenia, and stomatitis [164]. A subsequent study evaluated epirubicin, cisplatin, capecitabine (ECX) *vs* 5-FU, irinotecan, and leucovorin (FOLFIRI) in first-line treatment of EAC and GEJ adenocarcinoma and found that time to treatment failure was significantly longer in the FOLFIRI arm (FOLFIRI 5.1 months *vs* ECF 4.2 months) but no difference in median PFS, OS, or RR. This established FOLFIRI as another regimen that could be considered first line. Grade 3 to 4 toxicity and hematologic adverse events were significantly higher in ECX arm compared to FOLFIRI arm [165].

Clinical trials are currently ongoing with other chemotherapeutic regimens. One trial is evaluating FOLFIRINOX (5-FU, oxaliplatin, irinotecan, and leucovorin) in advanced esophageal or gastric cancers with trastuzumab given to patients with Her-2-neu positive disease [166].

Monotherapy

For patients who are medically unfit with a poor performance score, single agent therapy with either a fluoropyrimidine or a taxane can be considered. There have been several studies that investigated the use of single agent chemotherapy in patients with primary or recurrent metastatic disease. Taxanes have been studied as monotherapy in patients with metastatic EC who failed first line platinum based chemotherapy and a median survival of 10.4 months was noted [167]. Similarly, single agent docetaxel in metastatic EC (both treated and untreated) showed a survival rate of 8.1 months [168]. The most common side effect with taxanes was neutropenia. Single agent fluoropyrimidines can also be considered with median survival of 10.4 months and 9.5 months in previously treated and untreated cancer, respectively [169].

Second Line Therapy

In patients with recurrent cancer that is either unresectable or metastatic, single agent taxanes or single agent irinotecan or ramucirumab (see *Targeted Therapy in Esophageal Cancer*) either alone or in combination with a taxane can be used. A meta-analysis confirmed that second-line therapy in patients with metastatic gastric and esophageal adenocarcinoma previously treated with platinum and fluoropyrimidine therapy had significantly improved OS compared to supportive care [170]. However, the choice of second line therapy is dependent a number of factors including prior therapy, functional status, and toxicities experienced from prior treatment.

Table **16** is adapted from the NCCN and lists the second line chemotherapeutic options for locally advanced or metastatic disease.

Radiation

Unless contraindicated, palliative radiotherapy can be added to drug regimens in metastatic disease (refer to Table **14** and **15**) with several trials showing significant improvement in dysphagia and quality of life [171, 172] and in one trial, improved survival compared to stenting alone [171].

Table 16. Second Line Systemic Therapy for Locally Advanced or Metastatic Esophageal Cancer.

Preferred Regimens:
Ramucirumab and Paclitaxel **(CATEGORY 1 for EGJ adenocarcinoma, CATEGORY 2A for esophageal adenocarcinoma)**
Docetaxel (**CATEGORY 1)**
Paclitaxel (**CATEGORY 1)**
Irinotecan (**CATEGORY 1)**
Docetaxel (**CATEGORY 1)**
Ramucirumab **(CATEGORY 1 for EGJ adenocarcinoma, CATEGORY 2A for esophageal adenocarcinoma)**
Other Regimens:
Irinotecan and Cisplatin
Fluoropyrimidine (Capecitabine or 5-FU) and Irinotecan **(CATEGORY 2B)**
Docetaxel and Irinotecan **(CATEGORY 2B)**

Adapted from National Comprehensive Cancer Network (NCCN) Guidelines for Esophageal and Esophagogastric Junction Cancer, version 2.2016. Category 1: Based upon high-level evidence, there is uniform NCCN consensus that the intervention is appropriate. Category 2A: Based upon lower-level evidence, there is uniform NCCN consensus that the intervention is appropriate. Category 2B: Based upon lower-level evidence, there is NCCN consensus that the intervention is appropriate. Category 3: Based upon any level of evidence, there is major NCCN disagreement that the intervention is appropriate.

TARGETED THERAPIES IN ESOPHAGEAL CANCER

In almost all types of cancers, the approach to treatment has transformed towards molecular profiling and the use of targeted therapy. EC is no different and several studies have analyzed the expression of growth factor receptors, markers of angiogenesis, and cell cycle control in EC tumor biology. Antibodies against these antigens have been used in clinical trials and the most notable ones are listed below.

Trastuzumab

Currently, trastuzumab is the only targeted agent used for first-line treatment of Her2-neu positive metastatic EC. Trastuzumab is a human monoclonal antibody against the Her2-neu antigen, a proto-oncogene that promotes cell growth and invasiveness [173]. Her2-neu is part of a four member group of growth receptors ranging from Her1 to Her4 and antibodies to these growth factor receptors are a major component of targeted therapy in various cancers [174]. As Fig. (**14**) demonstrates, trastuzumab binds to Her2-neu and blocks dimerization, ultimately leading to tumor cell apoptosis, decreased transcription of growth factors, and overall tumor shrinkage [174].

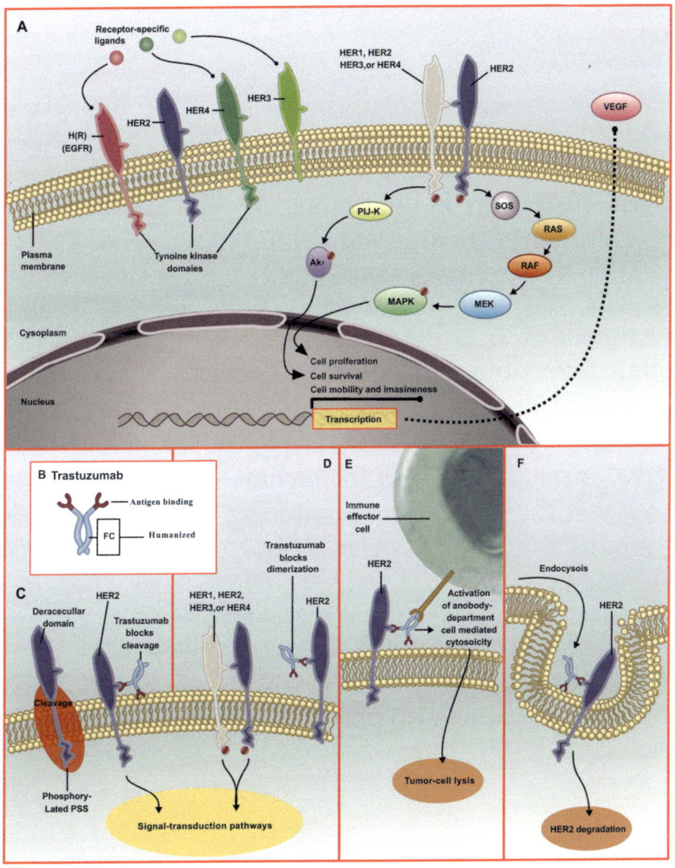

Fig. (14). Mechanism of action of Trastuzumab [174].

Ross *et al.* analyzed several patient populations and concluded that Her2-neu overexpression was seen in an average of 23% of patients with ESCC and 22% of patients with EAC [175]. As described in *Signaling Pathways in Esophageal*

Cancer, there is much heterogeneity in studies with reports of HER2 expression ranging from 0 to 65% [55]. Some studies have analyzed the role of Her2-neu in the transition of BE to EAC and noted a correlation between Her2-neu amplification and presence of dysplasia [175].

The first clinical trial that demonstrated the benefit of adding trastuzumab to cisplatin and fluoropyrimidine, either 5-FU or capecitabine was the Trastuzumab for Gastric Cancer, ToGA, trial [176]. This was a phase III randomized study that randomized 594 patients with Her2-neu positive (either positive by IHC or FISH) advanced gastric adenocarcinoma to either trastuzumab and chemotherapy or to chemotherapy alone. Results showed a significantly higher response rate (47% *vs* 35%) and modestly improved survival (13.8 months *vs* 11.1 months) in the trastuzumab group.

Based on this trial, the NCCN guidelines recommend that all patients with metastatic or locally advanced EAC who are candidates for trastuzumab therapy should undergo tumor analysis for Her2-neu and trastuzumab be added if Her2-neu is overexpressed [94]. This is determined by IHC classification and FISH analysis as described earlier in *HER-2-Neu Evaluation.*

The most notable side effect of trastuzumab is cardiotoxicity and obtaining a baseline echocardiogram is vital before starting therapy. The cardiotoxicity of trastuzumab is often reversible and not dose-dependent. Patients ineligible for trastuzumab include patients with depressed ejection fractions, valvular disease, chronic angina, and arrhythmias on medications or history of congestive heart failure or myocardial infarctions. Once trastuzumab is started, patients will need to have serial echocardiograms for monitoring of ejection fraction. Dose reductions and modifications are utilized by on patient's symptoms and echocardiographic results.

Trastuzumab is currently being investigated in patients with locally advanced disease. An ongoing phase III randomized controlled trial is investigating the addition of Trastuzumab to trimodality therapy in patients with Stage 1-3 disease with Her2 amplified EAC [177].

Ramucirumab

As described earlier, ramucirumab is recommended by the NCCN as second line therapy for metastatic or unresectable GEJ or EAC. Ramucirumab is a monoclonal human antibody that binds to VEGF-2, a potent mitogen that stimulates angiogenesis and cell growth. Secreted in response to hypoxia and cytokines by proliferating cells, VEGF binds to receptors on endothelial cells and leads to transcription of factors involved in cell proliferation, vascular permeability, and is thought to correlate to tumor invasiveness and metastasis [178]. The signaling pathways involved are illustrated below in Fig. (**15**).

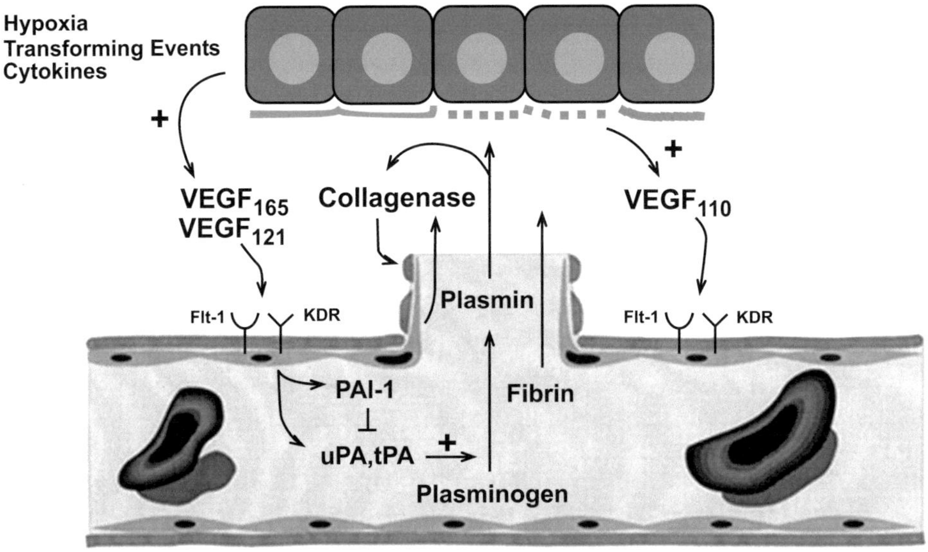

Fig. (15). Role of VEGF in carcinogenesis [178].

The addition of ramucirumab to first line therapy with FOLFOX failed to show any improvement in survival [179]. However, two Phase III trials (REGARD and RAINBOW) have shown benefit of ramucirumab as second line therapy. The REGARD trial randomized 355 patients with previously treated advanced gastric or GEJ adenocarcinoma to either ramucirumab or placebo [180]. A modest survival benefit was noted in the ramucirumab arm (5.2 months *vs* 3.8 months). That same year, the RAINBOW trial randomized 665 patients with advanced gastric or GEJ adenocarcinoma who had also failed first line chemotherapy to two arms: ramucirumab and paclitaxel *vs* paclitaxel alone [181]. As with the REGARD trial, a survival benefit was seen in the ramucirumab group (9.6 months *vs* 7.4 months). The first line chemotherapy that was used in both trials was platinum and fluoropyrimidine therapy with the addition of anthracyclines in the RAINBOW trial.

Based on the results of these trials, ramucirumab was approved as second line therapy, either alone or in combination with paclitaxel for patients who had disease progression after first line platinum or fluoropyrimidine therapy. The side effect profile of ramucirumab includes hypertension, headache and proteinuria. Rare side effects include gastrointestinal perforation and life threatening gastrointestinal hemorrhage, after which the medication should be permanently discontinued. Ramucirumab should also be discontinued if the patient develops complications secondary to poor wound healing.

FUTURE AND NOVEL THERAPEUTIC AGENTS

Other targeted therapies that have been studied with no significant survival benefit include lapatinib, gefitinib, bevacizumab, and cetuximab. Lapatinib, an EGFR type I and II inhibitor, and bevacizumab, a monoclonal antibody to VEGF, have each been evaluated in first line therapy with disappointing results [182, 183]. The Phase III GATSBY trial of ado-trastuzumab emtansine (T-DM1) *vs* taxane monotherapy did not demonstrate any survival advantage in the second line setting [54]. A Phase II Study conducted by the US cooperative group examined the role of cetuximab, a monoclonal antibody that blocks the ligand-binding site of EGFR, in previously treated esophageal or gastroesophageal junction cancers and found no significant differences with the addition of agent. EGFR expression is common in both ESCC and EAC as described earlier [184].

Despite evidence demonstrating the role of EGFR in EC carcinogenesis, the success of targeted agents against EGFR as previously described has been disappointing. It highlights the possibility that select populations may benefit from these therapies; however, this is not well studied in EC. In advanced colon cancer (CRC), extended RAS testing is obtained in order target populations who will benefit from EGFR-directed therapies. The presence of RAS mutations in advanced CRC has shown resistance against these agents [185]. The significance of RAS mutations was evaluated in the Phase 3 REAL3 study in which the study arm received up to eight 21-day cycles of EOX and a humanized monoclonal antibody to EGFR, panitumumab, *vs* EOX alone. Of the 553 patients, RAS mutations were found only in 6% (n = 10) of the study population and did appear to benefit from the addition of panitumumab to EOX [186]. A Phase III ENRICH study currently in enrolling in Japan and Korea is studying the addition of nimotuzumab, an EGFR antibody, to irinotecan as second line therapy in patients with EGFR overexpressed gastric or GEJ carcinoma [187]. Apatinib, a VEGFR2 tyrosine kinase inhibitor (TKI), has demonstrated modest activity in a Phase 3 trial conducted in China of a heavily-treated population (received 2 or more lines of prior therapy) with median OS of 6.5 *vs*. 4.8 months in the placebo arm [54].

The Phase II international INTEGRATE trial involving four countries (South Korea, New Zealand, Australia, and Canada) investigated the use of regorafenib (an oral multi-kinase inhibitor of VEGF receptors 1-3, KIT, PDGFR alpha and beta, FGFR 1 and 2) compared to placebo in patients with gastroesophageal cancer that had failed first and second line chemotherapy [188]. A modest survival benefit of 5.8 months in the regorafenib arm compared to 4.5 months in the placebo arm was noted. There were also regional differences with greater PFS in South Koreans. The authors plan to investigate regorafenib in a phase III trial. Another trial is comparing the use of Regorafenib to placebo in patients with locally advanced EC who have undergone surgery and CRT [189].

Currently, trials looking at different molecular-targeted therapy are ongoing and the standard treatment regimen for EC has evolved to include immunotherapy. Many early phase trials targeting anti-PD-1, anti-PDL1, and CTLA-4 are underway in various populations of EC. A Phase 1b trial KEYNOTE-012 included 39 advanced gastric cancers with PD-L1 expression who received pembrolizumab, anti-PD-1 monoclonal antibody, and ORR was 22% with median response duration was 24 weeks. PD-L1 expression was associated with improved PFS [56]. KEYNOTE-028 is an open label Phase IB trial evaluated the role of immunotherapy with pembrolizumab as third line therapy in PD-L1 positive metastatic EC (17 ESCC, 5 EAC). Objective responses were demonstrated in 29% and 40% in ESCC and EAC, respectively [54, 190]. This highlights the need for predictive biomarkers for these agents. As discussed earlier, PD-L1 expression has been found to around 40% in EC. A Phase III study is currently evaluating the role of nivolumab, a PD-1 antibody, in patients with resected EC who underwent preoperative chemoradiation and were diagnosed with residual pathologic disease after surgical excision with negative margins [191]. Another early phase study is investigating the combination of brachytherapy and pembrolizumab in patients with untreated metastatic EC [192]. Further investigations adding checkpoint inhibitors to cytotoxic and/or targeted therapy are in the horizon with hopes of potentiating the effects of immune blockade.

THE PALLIATIVE APPROACH TO PATIENT

Supportive Care

There is increasing evidence that early integration of palliative care in oncology patients leads to improved quality of life and may even increase survival in some patient populations [193]. Therefore, it is paramount that symptoms like pain and nausea in addition to the primary problem of dysphagia be addressed early in the treatment course of these patients. As with all cancers, therapy should be individualized to each patient and should include a multi-modality approach to achieve the best outcome.

Dysphagia

EC can often present with progressive dysphagia, often termed an alarm symptom in older patients. However, once dysphagia is present, it indicates that the mass is either partially or completely occluding the esophageal lumen. This can lead to poor quality of life from pain, nausea, emesis, and weight loss. Moreover, such patients are at high risk for aspiration. Management of dysphagia is largely supportive and based on the severity of symptoms. There are several strategies to treat malignant dysphagia that can be offered to patients with resectable disease as well as metastatic non-resectable disease.

- ***Chemoradiation***
  This is usually preferred for patients who can tolerate chemoradiotherapy and the regimens are described in detail in the previous sections. Several studies have shown that CRT can significantly restore swallowing function with improvement noted as early as 2 weeks after starting therapy [194, 195]. A retrospective case control study in 2008 compared CRT to endoscopic stenting in patients with inoperable ESCC and concluded that both methods effectively relieved dysphagia but that the former group had an increased median survival time of 6 months [196].

- ***Endoscopic Palliation***
  For patients that cannot tolerate surgery or chemoradiation, endoscopic procedures offer immediate relief of malignant dysphagia. This option can also be offered to patients with a high degree of obstruction prior to starting curative therapy as well as to patients with tracheoesophageal fistulas who are at risk for perforation from radiation. Endoscopic palliation includes placement of self-expandable stents, balloon dilatation and local ablative therapy for tumor debulking. According to the 2013 Gastrointestinal Endoscopy guidelines, stenting is the preferred method for palliation of dysphagia and for patients with tracheoesophageal fistulas [197]. A 2009 meta-analysis compared different methods of endoscopic palliation and concluded the same, taking into consideration cost effectiveness, need for re-intervention and length of survival [198]. The role of the stent is to bypass the obstruction or to seal the fistula, leading to immediate relief of symptoms. Metal stents are favored over plastic stents due to lower rate of migration [197, 198]. Covered or partially covered metal stents are preferred to uncovered metal stents due to lower rates of in-stent tumor growth and need for re-intervention [199].

- ***Brachytherapy***
  Brachytherapy refers to the endoscopic placement of small catheters in the esophageal lumen that deliver high doses of radiation to the tumor while relatively sparing the surrounding tissues. A 2004 randomized control trial compared brachytherapy to endoscopic stent placement in patients with inoperable EC and concluded that while stent placement delivered immediate short term relief, brachytherapy provided a more long-lasting improvement in dysphagia with fewer complications [200]. This was also noted in the 2009

meta-analysis mentioned earlier [198]. However, brachytherapy is not widely available and is not an option for patients with fistulas (due to perforation risk). Some studies have combined brachytherapy with EBRT with better quality of life and without significant toxicity [201].

- ***Radiation Therapy***
  While historically popular, radiation therapy alone has fallen out of favor due to high risk of complications (see Radiation Esophagitis below) such as tracheoesophageal fistulas and strictures, which could lead to secondary dysphagia. Moreover, symptomatic relief with radiation therapy can vary and may not provide immediate relief offered by endoscopic palliative methods described previously. However, this modality can be considered in palliative setting in symptomatic patients who are at high risk for procedures due to co-morbidities.

Nausea and Vomiting

Patients with EC may experience nausea and vomiting, both as a result of emetogenic chemotherapy and from mechanical tumor obstruction. Patients can be prescribed a combination of 5-HT3 antagonists, NK-1 antagonists, and corticosteroids for prevention of nausea and vomiting. These are usually administered the day of chemotherapy and continued for the following few days. For palliative treatment of non-specific nausea/vomiting, dopamine antagonists can be used as well. When the symptoms of nausea and vomiting are secondary to mechanical tumor obstruction, patients can be treated as in the case of dysphagia with endoscopic stenting, debulking, palliative radiation, and brachytherapy as described previously.

Bleeding

Gastrointestinal bleeding in patients with EC can be from the tumor itself, mucosal damage from CRT, or more seriously, from an aorto-esophageal fistula. As with any brisk or hemodynamically significant gastrointestinal bleeding, endoscopy may be required to treat the source of bleeding.

Mucositis

Mucositis can develop both from anti-neoplastic agents as well as from radiation. It can affect the entire gastrointestinal tract and lead to severe pain on eating, swallowing and even speaking. Loss of the mucosal barrier causes an increased rate of infection especially by opportunistic species. Treatment and prophylaxis of mucositis include oral cryotherapy, topical anesthetics, mucosal coating agents and oral hygiene.

Radiation Esophagitis

Since a majority of patients with EC undergo radiation as part of their treatment regimen, radiation esophagitis is a common complication. There are two broad categories: acute and chronic esophagitis. Acute radiation esophagitis affects between 30-50% of patients and is often a limiting factor in dose escalation [202 - 205]. Acute esophagitis can occur after 2 weeks of radiation and presents with dysphagia, odynophagia, and chest pain. Symptoms are mostly self-limited but some patients can develop strictures, fistulas, and perforation requiring endoscopic management [204]. Treatment is otherwise supportive and involves topical anesthetics, PPI, and dietary modification. Chronic esophagitis can present months or even years after radiation in about 8-11% of patients [202, 205]. Chronic fibrosis can lead to strictures, fistulas and altered esophageal motility, which can be treated by balloon dilatation, stents, and diet modification, respectively [204].

Pain

Pain is a common complaint among cancer patients and can precipitate from tumor burden or from treatment complications. As with all aspects of supportive care, pain management should be individualized and followed closely to optimize quality of life. Pharmacologic options include NSAIDs as well as short and long acting opioids. Due to the multidimensional aspect of pain, recent data suggest earlier involvement of non-pharmacologic therapy, cognitive-behavioral therapy and spiritual support when applicable [206].

Cachexia

Patients with advanced cancers, often enter a state of hypercatabolism also known as cachexia. This chronic inflammatory environment causes skeletal muscle break down. Patients often experience anorexia and a profound weight loss. Cachexia has been associated with failure of treatment regimens and is accompanied by a poor prognosis. Treatment of cachexia includes appetite stimulants: megestrol, glucocorticoids and anabolic steroids [207]. Artificial nutritional support to bypass an obstructive tumor can be considered, provided that life expectancy is months to years. Consultation with a nutritionist may be helpful in preventing nutritional deficiencies and ensuring adequate calorie intake.

Promising new agents currently undergoing Phase III studies include enobosarm and anamorelin. It is well known that hypogonadism can result in increased fatigue and anorexia, which led to the development of androgen therapy for fatigue and cachexia. A Phase II trial of enobosarm, a selective androgen receptor modulator, demonstrated improvement in lean body mass and physical function in patients with advanced cancer [208]. A Phase III trial investigated enobosarm in patients with advanced non-small cell lung cancer and randomized patients to chemotherapy with and without enobosarm. Preliminary results indicated increase in lean body mass and stair climbing power in the enobosarm arm [209].

Other agents that have been studies include ghrelin and ghrelin analogs. Anamorelin, an oral ghrelin mimetic was recently tested in the RAMONA 1 and 2 trials. The authors randomized patients with non-small cell lung cancer in a 2:1 ratio to Anamorelin *vs* placebo and noted increased lean body mass with no increased adverse effects in the Anamorelin arm [210].

CONCLUSION

In summary, EC is a common worldwide cancer with regional differences in histology and pathogenesis. The key signaling pathways are being further elucidated and explored beyond what is known currently. The approach to EC should involve a multidisciplinary approach. Novel therapies are being developed to help change natural history of EC.

ABBREVIATIONS

5-FU	5-fluorouracil
AC	adjuvant chemotherapy
ADH1B	alcohol dehydrogenase 1B
AGA	American Gastroenterological Association
ALDH2	aldehyde dehydrogenase 2 family
AJCC	American Joint Committee on Cancer
APC	argon plasma coagulation
ASCC1	activating signal co-integrator 1 complex subunit 1
ASGE	American Society for Gastrointestinal Endoscopy
AST	acid suppressive therapy
BE	Barrett's Esophagus
BM	Barrett's Metaplasia
BMI	body mass index
BMT	bimodality therapy
BP	base pair
CAP	College of American Pathologists
cm	centimeters
CCND1	Cyclin D1
CF	cisplatin and fluorouracil
CRC	colon cancer
CRT	chemoradiation
CTHRC1	collagen triple helix repeat containing 1
CTLA-4	cytotoxic T-lymphocyte antigen 4
DCF	Docetaxel, Cisplatin and a fluoropyrimidine
DFS	disease free survival
DPYD	dihydropyrimidine dehydrogenase
EAC	esophageal adenocarcinoma
EBRT	external beam radiation therapy
EC	esophageal cancer
ECF	Epirubicin, Cisplatin, and 5-FU

ECX	Epirubicin, Cisplatin and Capecitabine
EGF	epidermal growth factor
EGFR	epidermal growth factor receptor
EGJ	Esophagogastric junction
EMR	endoscopic mucosal resection
EMT	epithelial to mesenchymal transition
EOF	Epirubicin, Oxaliplatin and 5-FU
EOX	Epirubicin, Oxaliplatin and Capecitabine
ESD	endoscopic submucosal dissection
ESCC	squamous cell carcinoma
EUS	endoscopic ultrasound
FA	Fanconi anemia
FBE	Familial Barrett's Esophagus
FDG	2-[fluorine 18] fluoro-2-deo-y-D-glucose
FISH	fluorescence *in situ* hybridization
FNA	fine-needle aspiration
FOLFIRI	5-FU, Irinotecan, and Leucovorin
FOLFOX	5-FU, Oxaliplatin, and Leucovorin
FOLFIRINOX	5-FU, Oxaliplatin, Irinotecan, and Leuovorin
GEJ	gastroesophageal junction
GERD	gastroesophageal reflux disease
GWAS	genome-wide association studies
H2B	histamine- 2 blockers
HDGC	Hereditary Diffuse Gastric Cancer
HGD	high grade dysplasia
HPV	human papilloma virus
HR	hazard ratio
IF	irinotecan, 5-FU
IGRT	Image Guided Radiotherapy
IHC	Immunohistochemical
IND	indefinite for dysplasia
IMRT	Intensity Modulated Radiotherapy
LES	lower esophageal sphincter
LGD	low grade dysplasia
LVI	lymphovascular invasion
MSR1	macrophage scavenger receptor 1
NBI	narrow-band imaging
nm	nanometers
NSAIDs	nonsteroidal anti-inflammatory drugs
OS	overall survival
PBT	Proton beam therapy
PCR	
PD-L1	Programmed death ligand 1
PD-L2	Programmed death ligand 2
PD-1	Programmed death 1
PDT	photodynamic therapy
PET	positron emission tomography
PET-CR	positron emission tomograph-complete response
PFS	progression-free survival
PMME	primary malignant melanoma of the esophagus
PPI	Proton pump inhibitors
RFA	radiofrequency ablation
RFS	relapse-free survival
RR	response rate
SEER	Surveillance, Epidemiology, and End Results
SM	submucosal
SUV	standard uptake value
T-DM1	ado-trastuzumab emtansine

TGFα	transforming growth factor-α
TGFβ	transforming growth factor β
THE	transhiatal esophagogastrectomy
TIME	Traditional Invasive *vs.* Minimally invasive Esophagectomy
TKI	tyrosine kinase inhibitor
TMT	trimodality therapy
TNF	tumor necrosis factor receptor
TNM	Tumor-Node-Metastasis
TTE	transthoracic esophagogastrectomy
TTP	time to progression
UES	upper esophageal sphincter
UFT	Tegafur
US	United States
VEGF	vascular endothelial growth factors
vs	*vs*
WES	whole exome sequencing
WHO	World Health Organization

CONFLICT OF INTEREST

The authors confirm that they have no conflict of interest to declare for this publication.

ACKNOWLEDGEMENTS

We would like to acknowledge the contributions of Dr. Mamoun Younes for his slides and Dr. Nirav Thosani for his endoscopic pictures.

REFERENCES

[1] Herszényi L, Tulassay Z. Epidemiology of gastrointestinal and liver tumors. Eur Rev Med Pharmacol Sci 2010; 14(4): 249-58.
[PMID: 20496531]

[2] Lambert R, Hainaut P. The multidisciplinary management of gastrointestinal cancer. Epidemiology of oesophagogastric cancer. Best Pract Res Clin Gastroenterol 2007; 21(6): 921-45.
[http://dx.doi.org/10.1016/j.bpg.2007.10.001] [PMID: 18070696]

[3] Napier KJ, Scheerer M, Misra S. Esophageal cancer: A Review of epidemiology, pathogenesis, staging workup and treatment modalities. World J Gastrointest Oncol 2014; 6(5): 112-20.
[http://dx.doi.org/10.4251/wjgo.v6.i5.112] [PMID: 24834141]

[4] Wheeler JB, Reed CE. Epidemiology of esophageal cancer. Surg Clin North Am 2012; 92(5): 1077-87.
[http://dx.doi.org/10.1016/j.suc.2012.07.008] [PMID: 23026270]

[5] Zhang Y. Epidemiology of esophageal cancer. World J Gastroenterol 2013; 19(34): 5598-606.
[http://dx.doi.org/10.3748/wjg.v19.i34.5598] [PMID: 24039351]

[6] Holmes RS, Vaughan TL. Epidemiology and pathogenesis of esophageal cancer. Seminars in radiation oncology. USA: WB Saunders 2007; 17: pp. (1)2-9.
[http://dx.doi.org/10.1016/j.semradonc.2006.09.003]

[7] Younes M, Henson DE, Ertan A, Miller CC. Incidence and survival trends of esophageal carcinoma in the United States: racial and gender differences by histological type. Scand J Gastroenterol 2002; 37(12): 1359-65.
[http://dx.doi.org/10.1080/003655202762671215] [PMID: 12523583]

[8] Zhang HZ, Jin GF, Shen HB. Epidemiologic differences in esophageal cancer between Asian and Western populations. Chinese journal of cancer 2012; 31(6): 281. [http://dx.doi.org/10.5732/cjc.011.10390]

[9] Islami F, Boffetta P, Ren JS, Pedoeim L, Khatib D, Kamangar F. High-temperature beverages and foods and esophageal cancer riska systematic review. Int J Cancer 2009; 125(3): 491-524. [http://dx.doi.org/10.1002/ijc.24445] [PMID: 19415743]

[10] Archer MC. Mechanisms of action of N-nitroso compounds. Cancer Surv 1989; 8(2): 241-50. [PMID: 2696579]

[11] Lukanich JM. Section I: epidemiological review. Semin Thorac Cardiovasc Surg 2003; 15(2): 158-66. [http://dx.doi.org/10.1016/S1043-0679(03)70024-0] [PMID: 12838486]

[12] Liu J, Wang J, Leng Y, Lv C. Intake of fruit and vegetables and risk of esophageal squamous cell carcinoma: a meta-analysis of observational studies. Int J Cancer 2013; 133(2): 473-85. [http://dx.doi.org/10.1002/ijc.28024] [PMID: 23319052]

[13] Shimizu M, Ban S, Odze RD. Squamous dysplasia and other precursor lesions related to esophageal squamous cell carcinoma. Gastroenterol Clin North Am 2007; 36(4): 797-811, v-vi. [http://dx.doi.org/10.1016/j.gtc.2007.08.005] [PMID: 17996791]

[14] Hvid-Jensen F, Pedersen L, Drewes AM, Sørensen HT, Funch-Jensen P. Incidence of adenocarcinoma among patients with Barretts esophagus. N Engl J Med 2011; 365(15): 1375-83. [http://dx.doi.org/10.1056/NEJMoa1103042] [PMID: 21995385]

[15] van Nistelrooij AM, Dinjens WN, Wagner A, Spaander MC, van Lanschot JJ, Wijnhoven BP. Hereditary Factors in Esophageal Adenocarcinoma. Gastrointest Tumors 2014; 1(2): 93-8. [http://dx.doi.org/10.1159/000362575] [PMID: 26675496]

[16] Ohashi S, Miyamoto S, Kikuchi O, Goto T, Amanuma Y, Muto M. Recent advances from basic and clinical studies of esophageal squamous cell carcinoma. Gastroenterology 2015; 149(7): 1700-15. [http://dx.doi.org/10.1053/j.gastro.2015.08.054] [PMID: 26376349]

[17] Wu C, Kraft P, Zhai K, *et al.* Genome-wide association analyses of esophageal squamous cell carcinoma in Chinese identify multiple susceptibility loci and gene-environment interactions. Nat Genet 2012; 44(10): 1090-7. [http://dx.doi.org/10.1038/ng.2411] [PMID: 22960999]

[18] Wu M, Chang SC, Kampman E, *et al.* Single nucleotide polymorphisms of ADH1B, ADH1C and ALDH2 genes and esophageal cancer: a population-based case-control study in China. Int J Cancer 2013; 132(8): 1868-77. [http://dx.doi.org/10.1002/ijc.27803] [PMID: 22930414]

[19] Casson AG, Zheng Z, Evans SC, *et al.* Cyclin D1 polymorphism (G870A) and risk for esophageal adenocarcinoma. Cancer 2005; 104(4): 730-9. [http://dx.doi.org/10.1002/cncr.21229] [PMID: 15971196]

[20] Liu G, Cescon DW, Zhai R, *et al.* p53 Arg72Pro, MDM2 T309G and CCND1 G870A polymorphisms are not associated with susceptibility to esophageal adenocarcinoma. Dis Esophagus 2010; 23(1): 36-9. [http://dx.doi.org/10.1111/j.1442-2050.2009.00960.x] [PMID: 19302219]

[21] Zhuo W, Zhang L, Wang Y, Zhu B, Chen Z. Cyclin D1 G870A polymorphism is a risk factor for esophageal cancer among Asians. Cancer Invest 2012; 30(9): 630-6. [http://dx.doi.org/10.3109/07357907.2012.726385] [PMID: 23020291]

[22] Ellis NA, German J. Molecular genetics of Blooms syndrome. Hum Mol Genet 1996; 5(Spec No) (Suppl. 1): 1457-63. [PMID: 8875252]

[23] Lindor NM, McMaster ML, Lindor CJ, Greene MH. National Cancer Institute, Division of Cancer Prevention, Community Oncology and Prevention Trials Research Group. Concise handbook of familial cancer susceptibility syndromes - second edition. J Natl Cancer Inst Monogr 2008; 38(38): 1-93.
[PMID: 18559331]

[24] Sun X, Elston R, Barnholtz-Sloan J, *et al.* A segregation analysis of Barretts esophagus and associated adenocarcinomas. Cancer Epidemiol Biomarkers Prev 2010; 19(3): 666-74.
[http://dx.doi.org/10.1158/1055-9965.EPI-09-1136] [PMID: 20200424]

[25] Jacquemont C, Taniguchi T. The Fanconi anemia pathway and ubiquitin. BMC Biochem 2007; 8(1) (Suppl. 1): S10.
[http://dx.doi.org/10.1186/1471-2091-8-S1-S10] [PMID: 18047734]

[26] Blaydon DC, Etheridge SL, Risk JM, *et al.* RHBDF2 mutations are associated with tylosis, a familial esophageal cancer syndrome. Am J Hum Genet 2012; 90(2): 340-6.
[http://dx.doi.org/10.1016/j.ajhg.2011.12.008] [PMID: 22265016]

[27] Kuo B, Urma D. Esophagus-anatomy and development. GI Motility online 2006.

[28] Rice TW, Blackstone EH, Rusch VW. 7th edition of the AJCC Cancer Staging Manual: esophagus and esophagogastric junction. Ann Surg Oncol 2010; 17(7): 1721-4.
[http://dx.doi.org/10.1245/s10434-010-1024-1] [PMID: 20369299]

[29] Kim TJ, Kim HY, Lee KW, Kim MS. Multimodality assessment of esophageal cancer: preoperative staging and monitoring of response to therapy. Radiographics 2009; 29(2): 403-21.
[http://dx.doi.org/10.1148/rg.292085106] [PMID: 19325056]

[30] Spechler SJ. Barrett esophagus and risk of esophageal cancer: a clinical review. JAMA 2013; 310(6): 627-36.
[http://dx.doi.org/10.1001/jama.2013.226450] [PMID: 23942681]

[31] Pasricha S, Li N, Bulsiewicz WJ, *et al.* Sex and race and/or ethnicity differences in patients undergoing radiofrequency ablation for Barretts esophagus: results from the U.S. RFA Registry. Gastrointest Endosc 2015; 82(2): 276-84.
[http://dx.doi.org/10.1016/j.gie.2015.01.015] [PMID: 25841575]

[32] Younes M, Lechago J, Chakraborty S, *et al.* Relationship between dysplasia, p53 protein accumulation, DNA ploidy, and Glut1 overexpression in Barrett metaplasia. Scand J Gastroenterol 2000; 35(2): 131-7.
[http://dx.doi.org/10.1080/003655200750024281] [PMID: 10720109]

[33] Younes M, Ertan A, Lechago LV, Somoano JR, Lechago J. p53 Protein accumulation is a specific marker of malignant potential in Barretts metaplasia. Dig Dis Sci 1997; 42(4): 697-701.
[http://dx.doi.org/10.1023/A:1018828207371] [PMID: 9125634]

[34] Kaye PV, Ilyas M, Soomro I, *et al.* Dysplasia in Barretts oesophagus: p53 immunostaining is more reproducible than haematoxylin and eosin diagnosis and improves overall reliability, while grading is poorly reproducible. Histopathology 2016; 69(3): 431-40.
[http://dx.doi.org/10.1111/his.12956] [PMID: 26918780]

[35] Younes M, Lauwers GY, Ertan A, *et al.* The significance of indefinite for dysplasia grading in Barrett metaplasia. Arch Pathol Lab Med 2011; 135(4): 430-2.
[PMID: 21466357]

[36] Sinh P, Anaparthy R, Young PE, *et al.* Clinical outcomes in patients with a diagnosis of indefinite for dysplasia in Barretts esophagus: a multicenter cohort study. Endoscopy 2015; 47(8): 669-74.
[http://dx.doi.org/10.1055/s-0034-1391966] [PMID: 25910065]

[37] Reid BJ, Haggitt RC, Rubin CE, *et al.* Observer variation in the diagnosis of dysplasia in Barretts esophagus. Hum Pathol 1988; 19(2): 166-78.
[http://dx.doi.org/10.1016/S0046-8177(88)80344-7] [PMID: 3343032]

[38] Odze RD. Update on the diagnosis and treatment of Barrett esophagus and related neoplastic precursor lesions. Arch Pathol Lab Med 2008; 132(10): 1577-85.
[PMID: 18834215]

[39] Pophali P, Halland M. Barretts oesophagus: diagnosis and management. BMJ 2016; 353: i2373.
[http://dx.doi.org/10.1136/bmj.i2373] [PMID: 27169585]

[40] Tomizawa Y, Wang KK. Screening, surveillance, and prevention for esophageal cancer. Gastroenterol Clin North Am 2009; 38(1): 59-73, viii.
[http://dx.doi.org/10.1016/j.gtc.2009.01.014] [PMID: 19327567]

[41] Katz PO, Gerson LB, Vela MF. Guidelines for the diagnosis and management of gastroesophageal reflux disease. Am J Gastroenterol 2013; 108(3): 308-28.
[http://dx.doi.org/10.1038/ajg.2012.444] [PMID: 23419381]

[42] Moore M, Afaneh C, Benhuri D, Antonacci C, Abelson J, Zarnegar R. Gastroesophageal reflux disease: A review of surgical decision making. World J Gastrointest Surg 2016; 8(1): 77-83.
[http://dx.doi.org/10.4240/wjgs.v8.i1.77] [PMID: 26843915]

[43] Hopkins J, Switzer NJ, Karmali S. Update on novel endoscopic therapies to treat gastroesophageal reflux disease: A review. World J Gastrointest Endosc 2015; 7(11): 1039-44.
[PMID: 26322157]

[44] Lazarus B, Chen Y, Wilson FP, *et al.* Proton pump inhibitor use and the risk of chronic kidney disease. JAMA Intern Med 2016; 176(2): 238-46.
[http://dx.doi.org/10.1001/jamainternmed.2015.7193] [PMID: 26752337]

[45] Gomm W, von Holt K, Thomé F, *et al.* Association of proton pump inhibitors with risk of dementia: a pharmacoepidemiological claims data analysis. JAMA Neurol 2016; 73(4): 410-6.
[http://dx.doi.org/10.1001/jamaneurol.2015.4791] [PMID: 26882076]

[46] Carlson N, Lechago J, Richter J, *et al.* Acid suppression therapy may not alter malignant progression in Barretts metaplasia showing p53 protein accumulation. Am J Gastroenterol 2002; 97(6): 1340-5.
[http://dx.doi.org/10.1111/j.1572-0241.2002.05770.x] [PMID: 12094847]

[47] Ertan A, Zaheer I, Correa AM, Thosani N, Blackmon SH. Photodynamic therapy *vs* radiofrequency ablation for Barretts dysplasia: efficacy, safety and cost-comparison. World J Gastroenterol 2013; 19(41): 7106-13.
[http://dx.doi.org/10.3748/wjg.v19.i41.7106] [PMID: 24222954]

[48] Wolf WA, Pasricha S, Cotton C, *et al.* Incidence of esophageal adenocarcinoma and causes of mortality after radiofrequency ablation of Barretts esophagus. Gastroenterology 2015; 149(7): 1752-1761.e1.
[http://dx.doi.org/10.1053/j.gastro.2015.08.048] [PMID: 26327132]

[49] Pasricha S, Bulsiewicz WJ, Hathorn KE, *et al.* Durability and predictors of successful radiofrequency ablation for Barretts esophagus. Clin Gastroenterol Hepatol 2014; 12(11): 1840-7.e1.
[http://dx.doi.org/10.1016/j.cgh.2014.04.034] [PMID: 24815329]

[50] Navarro-Ballester A, De Lázaro-De Molina S, Gaona-Morales J. Primary Malignant Melanoma of the Esophagus: A Case Report and Review of the Literature. Am J Case Rep 2015; 16: 491-5.
[http://dx.doi.org/10.12659/AJCR.894041] [PMID: 26212619]

[51] Ye ZY, Cao QH, Liu F, *et al.* Primary Esophageal Extranasal NK/T Cell Lymphoma With Biphasic Morphology: A Case Report and Literature Review. Medicine (Baltimore) 2015; 94(28): e1151.
[http://dx.doi.org/10.1097/MD.0000000000001151] [PMID: 26181557]

[52] Saito T, Mitomi H, Yao T. Molecular pathology and potential therapeutic targets in esophageal basaloid squamous cell carcinoma. Int J Clin Exp Pathol 2015; 8(3): 2267-73.
[PMID: 26045734]

[53] Clemons NJ, Phillips WA, Lord RV. Signaling pathways in the molecular pathogenesis of adenocarcinomas of the esophagus and gastroesophageal junction. Cancer Biol Ther 2013; 14(9): 782-95.
[http://dx.doi.org/10.4161/cbt.25362] [PMID: 23792587]

[54] Wang VE, Grandis JR, Ko AH. New Strategies in Esophageal Carcinoma: Translational Insights from Signaling Pathways and Immune Checkpoints. American Association for Cancer Research 2016. clincanres-0292.

[55] Wei Q, Chen L, Sheng L, Nordgren H, Wester K, Carlsson J. EGFR, HER2 and HER3 expression in esophageal primary tumours and corresponding metastases. Int J Oncol 2007; 31(3): 493-9.
[PMID: 17671674]

[56] Raufi AG, Klempner SJ. Immunotherapy for advanced gastric and esophageal cancer: preclinical rationale and ongoing clinical investigations. J Gastrointest Oncol 2015; 6(5): 561-9.
[PMID: 26487950]

[57] Domper Arnal MJ, Ferrández Arenas Á, Lanas Arbeloa Á. Esophageal cancer: Risk factors, screening and endoscopic treatment in Western and Eastern countries. World J Gastroenterol 2015; 21(26): 7933-43.
[PMID: 26185366]

[58] Varghese TK Jr, Hofstetter WL, Rizk NP, *et al.* The society of thoracic surgeons guidelines on the diagnosis and staging of patients with esophageal cancer. Ann Thorac Surg 2013; 96(1): 346-56.
[http://dx.doi.org/10.1016/j.athoracsur.2013.02.069] [PMID: 23752201]

[59] Washington K, Berlin J, Branton P. Protocol for the Examination of Specimens from Patients with Carcinoma of the Esophagus. College of American Pathologists (CAP). Available from: http://www.cap.org/ShowProperty?nodePath=/UCMCon/Contribution%20Folders/WebContent/pdf/esophagus-13protocol-3112.pdf. , 2016 [June 6, 2016.];

[60] Wei Q, Chen L, Sheng L, Nordgren H, Wester K, Carlsson J. EGFR, HER2 and HER3 expression in esophageal primary tumours and corresponding metastases. Int J Oncol 2007; 31(3): 493-9.
[PMID: 17671674]

[61] Moelans CB, van Diest PJ, Milne AN. Her-2/neu testing and therapy in gastroesophageal adenocarcinoma. Pathology research international 2010.

[62] Chirieac LR, Swisher SG, Ajani JA, *et al.* Posttherapy pathologic stage predicts survival in patients with esophageal carcinoma receiving preoperative chemoradiation. Cancer 2005; 103(7): 1347-55.
[http://dx.doi.org/10.1002/cncr.20916] [PMID: 15719440]

[63] Wu TT, Chirieac LR, Abraham SC, *et al.* Excellent interobserver agreement on grading the extent of residual carcinoma after preoperative chemoradiation in esophageal and esophagogastric junction carcinoma: a reliable predictor for patient outcome. Am J Surg Pathol 2007; 31(1): 58-64.
[http://dx.doi.org/10.1097/01.pas.0000213312.36306.cc] [PMID: 17197919]

[64] Monjazeb AM, Riedlinger G, Aklilu M, *et al.* Outcomes of patients with esophageal cancer staged with [^{1}□F]fluorodeoxyglucose positron emission tomography (FDG-PET): can postchemoradiotherapy FDG-PET predict the utility of resection? J Clin Oncol 2010; 28(31): 4714-21.
[http://dx.doi.org/10.1200/JCO.2010.30.7702] [PMID: 20876421]

[65] Wang Z, Li Y, Ahmad A, *et al.* Targeting miRNAs involved in cancer stem cell and EMT regulation: An emerging concept in overcoming drug resistance. Drug Resist Updat 2010; 13(4-5): 109-18.
[http://dx.doi.org/10.1016/j.drup.2010.07.001] [PMID: 20692200]

[66] Valeri N, Gasparini P, Braconi C, *et al.* MicroRNA-21 induces resistance to 5-fluorouracil by down-regulating human DNA MutS homolog 2 (hMSH2). Proc Natl Acad Sci USA 2010; 107(49): 21098-103.
[http://dx.doi.org/10.1073/pnas.1015541107] [PMID: 21078976]

[67] Wang P, Zhuang L, Zhang J, *et al.* The serum miR-21 level serves as a predictor for the chemosensitivity of advanced pancreatic cancer, and miR-21 expression confers chemoresistance by targeting FasL. Mol Oncol 2013; 7(3): 334-45. [http://dx.doi.org/10.1016/j.molonc.2012.10.011] [PMID: 23177026]

[68] Komatsu S, Ichikawa D, Kawaguchi T, *et al.* Circulating miR-21 as an independent predictive biomarker for chemoresistance in esophageal squamous cell carcinoma. Am J Cancer Res 2016; 6(7): 1511-23. [PMID: 27508093]

[69] Wang Y, Zhao Y, Herbst A, *et al.* miR-221 Mediates Chemoresistance of Esophageal Adenocarcinoma by Direct Targeting of DKK2 Expression. Ann Surg 2016; 264(5): 804-14. [http://dx.doi.org/10.1097/SLA.0000000000001928] [PMID: 27501171]

[70] Sun J, Song K, Feng X, Gao S. MicroRNA-367 is a potential diagnostic biomarker for patients with esophageal squamous cell carcinoma. Biochem Biophys Res Commun 2016; 473(2): 363-9. [http://dx.doi.org/10.1016/j.bbrc.2016.01.042] [PMID: 26777997]

[71] Sun J, Song K, Feng X, Gao S. MicroRNA-367 is a potential diagnostic biomarker for patients with esophageal squamous cell carcinoma. Biochem Biophys Res Commun 2016; 473(2): 363-9. [http://dx.doi.org/10.1016/j.bbrc.2016.01.042] [PMID: 26777997]

[72] Zhou S, Yang B, Zhao Y, Xu S, Zhang H, Li Z. Prognostic value of microRNA-100 in esophageal squamous cell carcinoma. J Surg Res 2014; 192(2): 515-20.

[73] Takahashi H, Arimura Y, Masao H. Endoscopic submucosal dissection is superior to conventional endoscopic resection as a curative treatment for early SCC of the esophagus. Gastrointest Endosc 2010; 72: 255-64.

[74] Alvarez Herrero L, van Vilsteren FG, Pouw RE, *et al.* Endoscopic radiofrequency ablation combined with endoscopic resection for early neoplasia in Barretts esophagus longer than 10 cm. Gastrointest Endosc 2011; 73(4): 682-90. [http://dx.doi.org/10.1016/j.gie.2010.11.016] [PMID: 21292262]

[75] Pech O, May A, Manner H, *et al.* Long-term efficacy and safety of endoscopic resection for patients with mucosal adenocarcinoma of the esophagus. Gastroenterology 2014; 146(3): 652-660.e1. [http://dx.doi.org/10.1053/j.gastro.2013.11.006] [PMID: 24269290]

[76] Zehetner J, DeMeester SR, Hagen JA, *et al.* Endoscopic resection and ablation *versus* esophagectomy for high-grade dysplasia and intramucosal adenocarcinoma. J Thorac Cardiovasc Surg 2011; 141(1): 39-47. [http://dx.doi.org/10.1016/j.jtcvs.2010.08.058] [PMID: 21055772]

[77] Worrell S, DeMeester SR. Endoscopic Resection and Ablation for Early-Stage Esophageal Cancer. Thorac Surg Clin 2016; 26(2): 173-6. [http://dx.doi.org/10.1016/j.thorsurg.2015.12.005] [PMID: 27112256]

[78] Berry MF, Zeyer-Brunner J, Castleberry AW, *et al.* Treatment modalities for T1N0 esophageal cancers: a comparative analysis of local therapy *versus* surgical resection. J Thorac Oncol 2013; 8(6): 796-802. [http://dx.doi.org/10.1097/JTO.0b013e3182897bf1] [PMID: 24614244]

[79] Schölvinck D, Künzli H, Meijer S, *et al.* Management of patients with T1b esophageal adenocarcinoma: a retrospective cohort study on patient management and risk of metastatic disease. Surg Endosc 2016; 1-2.

[80] Altorki N, Skinner D. Should en bloc esophagectomy be the standard of care for esophageal carcinoma? Ann Surg 2001; 234(5): 581-7. [http://dx.doi.org/10.1097/00000658-200111000-00001] [PMID: 11685019]

[81] Omloo JM, Lagarde SM, Hulscher JB, *et al.* Extended transthoracic resection compared with limited transhiatal resection for adenocarcinoma of the mid/distal esophagus: five-year survival of a randomized clinical trial. Ann Surg 2007; 246(6): 992-1000. [http://dx.doi.org/10.1097/SLA.0b013e31815c4037] [PMID: 18043101]

[82] Song L, Liu Y, Wang Z, Ren WG, Liu XY. Curative effect comparison between Ivor-Lewis esophagectomy and left transthoracic esophagectomy in treatment of middle thoracic esophagus carcinoma. Hepatogastroenterology 2012; 59(115): 738-41. [PMID: 22024231]

[83] Chang AC, Ji H, Birkmeyer NJ, Orringer MB, Birkmeyer JD. Outcomes after transhiatal and transthoracic esophagectomy for cancer. Ann Thorac Surg 2008; 85(2): 424-9. [http://dx.doi.org/10.1016/j.athoracsur.2007.10.007] [PMID: 18222237]

[84] Zingg U, McQuinn A, DiValentino D, *et al.* Minimally invasive *versus* open esophagectomy for patients with esophageal cancer. Ann Thorac Surg 2009; 87(3): 911-9. [http://dx.doi.org/10.1016/j.athoracsur.2008.11.060] [PMID: 19231418]

[85] Markar SR, Karthikesalingam A, Thrumurthy S, Low DE. Volume-outcome relationship in surgery for esophageal malignancy: systematic review and meta-analysis 20002011. J Gastrointest Surg 2012; 16(5): 1055-63. [http://dx.doi.org/10.1007/s11605-011-1731-3] [PMID: 22089950]

[86] Rodgers M, Jobe BA, ORourke RW, Sheppard B, Diggs B, Hunter JG. Case volume as a predictor of inpatient mortality after esophagectomy. Arch Surg 2007; 142(9): 829-39. [http://dx.doi.org/10.1001/archsurg.142.9.829] [PMID: 17875837]

[87] Kuo EY, Chang Y, Wright CD. Impact of hospital volume on clinical and economic outcomes for esophagectomy. Ann Thorac Surg 2001; 72(4): 1118-24. [http://dx.doi.org/10.1016/S0003-4975(01)02962-9] [PMID: 11603422]

[88] Luketich JD, Pennathur A, Franchetti Y, *et al.* Minimally invasive esophagectomy: results of a prospective phase II multicenter trial-the eastern cooperative oncology group (E2202) study. Ann Surg 2015; 261(4): 702-7. [http://dx.doi.org/10.1097/SLA.0000000000000993] [PMID: 25575253]

[89] Cuesta MA, Biere SS, van Berge Henegouwen MI, van der Peet DL. Randomised trial, Minimally Invasive Oesophagectomy *versus* open oesophagectomy for patients with resectable oesophageal cancer. J Thorac Dis 2012; 4(5): 462-4. [PMID: 23050108]

[90] Peyre CG, Hagen JA, DeMeester SR, *et al.* Predicting systemic disease in patients with esophageal cancer after esophagectomy: a multinational study on the significance of the number of involved lymph nodes. Ann Surg 2008; 248(6): 979-85. [http://dx.doi.org/10.1097/SLA.0b013e3181904f3c] [PMID: 19092342]

[91] Groth SS, Virnig BA, Whitson BA, *et al.* Determination of the minimum number of lymph nodes to examine to maximize survival in patients with esophageal carcinoma: data from the Surveillance Epidemiology and End Results database. J Thorac Cardiovasc Surg 2010; 139(3): 612-20. [http://dx.doi.org/10.1016/j.jtcvs.2009.07.017] [PMID: 19709685]

[92] Yuan F, Qingfeng Z, Jia W, *et al.* Influence of Metastatic Status and Number of Removed Lymph Nodes on Survival of Patients With Squamous Esophageal Carcinoma. Medicine (Baltimore) 2015; 94(48): e1973. [http://dx.doi.org/10.1097/MD.0000000000001973] [PMID: 26632887]

[93] Zheng YZ, Zhao W, Hu Y, *et al.* Aggressive surgical resection does not improve survival in operable esophageal squamous cell carcinoma with N23 status. World journal of gastroenterology. WJG 2015; 21(28): 8644. [http://dx.doi.org/10.3748/wjg.v21.i28.8644] [PMID: 26229406]

[94] National Comprehensive Cancer Network (NCCN). *NCCN Clinical Practice Guidelines in Oncology. Esophageal and Esophagogastric Junctions Cancers Version 2.2016.* July 2016; National Comprehensive Cancer Network. [Abstract available at https://www.nccn.org/professionals/physician_gls/pdf/esophageal.pdf].

[95] Tessier W, Gronnier C, Messager M, *et al.* Does timing of surgical procedure after neoadjuvant chemoradiation affect outcomes in esophageal cancer? Ann Thorac Surg 2014; 97(4): 1181-9. [http://dx.doi.org/10.1016/j.athoracsur.2013.12.026] [PMID: 24529482]

[96] Kim JY, Correa AM, Vaporciyan AA, *et al.* Does the timing of esophagectomy after chemoradiation affect outcome? Ann Thorac Surg 2012; 93(1): 207-12. [http://dx.doi.org/10.1016/j.athoracsur.2011.05.021] [PMID: 21962263]

[97] Chiu CH, Chao YK, Chang HK, *et al.* Interval between neoadjuvant chemoradiotherapy and surgery for esophageal squamous cell carcinoma: does delayed surgery impact outcome? Ann Surg Oncol 2013; 20(13): 4245-51. [http://dx.doi.org/10.1245/s10434-013-3139-7] [PMID: 23959050]

[98] Parekh K, Fairchild T, Van Natta T. Timing of esophagectomy after completion of neoadjuvant therapy affects anastomotic leak rates. Interact Cardiovasc Thorac Surg 2008; 7 (Suppl. 2): S185-6.

[99] Franko J, Voynov G, Goldman CD. Esophagectomy Timing After Neoadjuvant Therapy for Distal Esophageal Adenocarcinoma. Ann Thorac Surg 2016; 101(3): 1123-30. [http://dx.doi.org/10.1016/j.athoracsur.2015.09.044] [PMID: 26652139]

[100] Markar SR, Karthikesalingam A, Thrumurthy S, Low DE. Volume-outcome relationship in surgery for esophageal malignancy: systematic review and meta-analysis 20002011. J Gastrointest Surg 2012; 16(5): 1055-63. [http://dx.doi.org/10.1007/s11605-011-1731-3] [PMID: 22089950]

[101] Rodgers M, Jobe BA, ORourke RW, Sheppard B, Diggs B, Hunter JG. Case volume as a predictor of inpatient mortality after esophagectomy. Arch Surg 2007; 142(9): 829-39. [http://dx.doi.org/10.1001/archsurg.142.9.829] [PMID: 17875837]

[102] Kuo EY, Chang Y, Wright CD. Impact of hospital volume on clinical and economic outcomes for esophagectomy. Ann Thorac Surg 2001; 72(4): 1118-24. [http://dx.doi.org/10.1016/S0003-4975(01)02962-9] [PMID: 11603422]

[103] Bailey SH, Bull DA, Harpole DH, *et al.* Outcomes after esophagectomy: a ten-year prospective cohort. Ann Thorac Surg 2003; 75(1): 217-22. [http://dx.doi.org/10.1016/S0003-4975(02)04368-0] [PMID: 12537219]

[104] Biere SS, Maas KW, Cuesta MA, van der Peet DL. Cervical or thoracic anastomosis after esophagectomy for cancer: a systematic review and meta-analysis. Dig Surg 2011; 28(1): 29-35. [http://dx.doi.org/10.1159/000322014] [PMID: 21293129]

[105] Kassis ES, Kosinski AS, Ross P Jr, Koppes KE, Donahue JM, Daniel VC. Predictors of anastomotic leak after esophagectomy: an analysis of the society of thoracic surgeons general thoracic database. Ann Thorac Surg 2013; 96(6): 1919-26. [http://dx.doi.org/10.1016/j.athoracsur.2013.07.119] [PMID: 24075499]

[106] Petrovich Z, Langholz B, Formenti S, Luxton G, Astrahan M. Management of carcinoma of the esophagus: the role of radiotherapy. Am J Clin Oncol 1991; 14(1): 80-6. [http://dx.doi.org/10.1097/00000421-199102000-00018] [PMID: 1702923]

[107] Wobbes T, Baron B, Paillot B, *et al.* Prospective randomised study of split-course radiotherapy *versus* cisplatin plus split-course radiotherapy in inoperable squamous cell carcinoma of the oesophagus. Eur J Cancer 2001; 37(4): 470-7. [http://dx.doi.org/10.1016/S0959-8049(00)00399-3] [PMID: 11267856]

[108] al-Sarraf M, Martz K, Herskovic A, *et al.* Progress report of combined chemoradiotherapy *versus* radiotherapy alone in patients with esophageal cancer: an intergroup study. J Clin Oncol 1997; 15(1): 277-84.
[PMID: 8996153]

[109] Minsky BD, Pajak TF, Ginsberg RJ, *et al.* INT 0123 (Radiation Therapy Oncology Group 9405) phase III trial of combined-modality therapy for esophageal cancer: high-dose *versus* standard-dose radiation therapy. J Clin Oncol 2002; 20(5): 1167-74.
[http://dx.doi.org/10.1200/JCO.20.5.1167] [PMID: 11870157]

[110] Noronha V, Prabhash K, Joshi A, *et al.* Clinical Outcome in Definitive Concurrent Chemoradiation With Weekly Paclitaxel and Carboplatin for Locally Advanced Esophageal and Junctional Cancer. Oncol Res 2016; 23(4): 183-95.
[http://dx.doi.org/10.3727/096504016X14537290676865] [PMID: 27053347]

[111] Ling TC, Slater JM, Nookala P, *et al.* Analysis of intensity-modulated radiation therapy (IMRT), proton and 3D conformal radiotherapy (3D-CRT) for reducing perioperative cardiopulmonary complications in esophageal cancer patients. Cancers (Basel) 2014; 6(4): 2356-68.
[http://dx.doi.org/10.3390/cancers6042356] [PMID: 25489937]

[112] Chuong MD, Hallemeier CL, Jabbour SK, *et al.* Improving outcomes for esophageal cancer using proton beam therapy. Int J Radiat Oncol Biol Phys 2016; 95(1): 488-97.
[http://dx.doi.org/10.1016/j.ijrobp.2015.11.043]

[113] M.D. Anderson Cancer Center. Proton Beam Therapy (PBT) *Vs* Intensity-Modulated Radiation Therapy (IMRT) Trial. In: ClinicalTrials.gov [Internet]. Bethesda (MD): National Library of Medicine (US). 2000- [Cited 2016 August 21]. Available from: https://clinicaltrials.gov/ct2/show/NCT01512589 NLM Identifier: NCT01512589.

[114] Diasio RB, Johnson MR. Dihydropyrimidine dehydrogenase: its role in 5-fluorouracil clinical toxicity and tumor resistance. Clin Cancer Res 1999; 5(10): 2672-3.
[PMID: 10537327]

[115] Grem JL, Shoemaker DD, Petrelli NJ, Douglass HO Jr. Severe life-threatening toxicities observed in study using leucovorin with 5-fluorouracil. J Clin Oncol 1987; 5(10): 1704.
[PMID: 3309201]

[116] Shan K, Lincoff AM, Young JB. Anthracycline-induced cardiotoxicity. Ann Intern Med 1996; 125(1): 47-58.
[http://dx.doi.org/10.7326/0003-4819-125-1-199607010-00008] [PMID: 8644988]

[117] Cunningham D, Starling N, Rao S, *et al.* Upper Gastrointestinal Clinical Studies Group of the National Cancer Research Institute of the United Kingdom. Capecitabine and oxaliplatin for advanced esophagogastric cancer. N Engl J Med 2008; 358(1): 36-46.
[http://dx.doi.org/10.1056/NEJMoa073149] [PMID: 18172173]

[118] van Hagen P, Hulshof MC, van Lanschot JJ, *et al.* CROSS Group. Preoperative chemoradiotherapy for esophageal or junctional cancer. N Engl J Med 2012; 366(22): 2074-84.
[http://dx.doi.org/10.1056/NEJMoa1112088] [PMID: 22646630]

[119] Mariette C, Dahan L, Mornex F, *et al.* Surgery alone *versus* chemoradiotherapy followed by surgery for stage I and II esophageal cancer: final analysis of randomized controlled phase III trial FFCD 9901. J Clin Oncol 2014; 32(23): 2416-22.
[http://dx.doi.org/10.1200/JCO.2013.53.6532] [PMID: 24982463]

[120] Adelstein DJ, Rice TW, Rybicki LA, *et al.* Does paclitaxel improve the chemoradiotherapy of locoregionally advanced esophageal cancer? A nonrandomized comparison with fluorouracil-based therapy. J Clin Oncol 2000; 18(10): 2032-9.
[PMID: 10811667]

[121] Kim DW, Blanke CD, Wu H, *et al.* Phase II study of preoperative paclitaxel/cisplatin with radiotherapy in locally advanced esophageal cancer. Int J Radiat Oncol Biol Phys 2007; 67(2): 397-404. [ic].
[http://dx.doi.org/10.1016/j.ijrobp.2006.08.062] [PMID: 17097833]

[122] Sjoquist KM, Burmeister BH, Smithers BM, *et al.* Australasian Gastro-Intestinal Trials Group. Survival after neoadjuvant chemotherapy or chemoradiotherapy for resectable oesophageal carcinoma: an updated meta-analysis. Lancet Oncol 2011; 12(7): 681-92. [alTrials.gov].
[http://dx.doi.org/10.1016/S1470-2045(11)70142-5] [PMID: 21684205]

[123] Kidane B, Coughlin S, Vogt K, Malthaner R. Preoperative chemotherapy for resectable thoracic esophageal cancer. Cochrane Database Syst Rev 2015; (5): CD001556.
[PMID: 25988291]

[124] Stahl M, Stuschke M, Lehmann N, *et al.* Chemoradiation with and without surgery in patients with locally advanced squamous cell carcinoma of the esophagus. J Clin Oncol 2005; 23(10): 2310-7.
[http://dx.doi.org/10.1200/JCO.2005.00.034] [PMID: 15800321]

[125] Bedenne L, Michel P, Bouché O, *et al.* Chemoradiation followed by surgery compared with chemoradiation alone in squamous cancer of the esophagus: FFCD 9102. J Clin Oncol 2007; 25(10): 1160-8.

[126] Sudo K, Xiao L, Wadhwa R, *et al.* Importance of surveillance and success of salvage strategies after definitive chemoradiation in patients with esophageal cancer. J Clin Oncol 2014; 32(30): 3400-5.
[http://dx.doi.org/10.1200/JCO.2014.56.7156]

[127] Shridhar R, Freilich J, Hoffe SE, *et al.* Single-institution retrospective comparison of preoperative *versus* definitive chemoradiotherapy for adenocarcinoma of the esophagus. Ann Surg Oncol 2014; 21(12): 3744-50.
[http://dx.doi.org/10.1245/s10434-014-3795-2] [PMID: 24854492]

[128] Macdonald JS, Smalley SR, Benedetti J, *et al.* Chemoradiotherapy after surgery compared with surgery alone for adenocarcinoma of the stomach or gastroesophageal junction. N Engl J Med 2001; 345(10): 725-30.
[http://dx.doi.org/10.1056/NEJMoa010187]

[129] Smalley SR, Benedetti JK, Haller DG, *et al.* Updated analysis of SWOG-directed intergroup study 0116: a phase III trial of adjuvant radiochemotherapy *versus* observation after curative gastric cancer resection. J Clin Oncol 2012; 30(19): 2327-33.
[http://dx.doi.org/10.1200/JCO.2011.36.7136] [PMID: 22585691]

[130] Adelstein DJ, Rice TW, Rybicki LA, *et al.* Mature results from a phase II trial of postoperative concurrent chemoradiotherapy for poor prognosis cancer of the esophagus and gastroesophageal junction. J Thorac Oncol 2009; 4(10): 1264-9.
[http://dx.doi.org/10.1097/JTO.0b013e3181b26f8e] [PMID: 19668013]

[131] Kim GJ, Koshy M, Hanlon AL, *et al.* The benefit of chemotherapy in esophageal cancer patients with residual disease after trimodality therapy. Am J Clin Oncol 2016; 39(2): 136-41.
[http://dx.doi.org/10.1097/COC.0000000000000036] [PMID: 24487417]

[132] Burt BM, Groth SS, Sada YH, *et al.* Utility of Adjuvant Chemotherapy After Neoadjuvant Chemoradiation and Esophagectomy for Esophageal Cancer. Ann Surg 2016.
[http://dx.doi.org/10.1097/SLA.0000000000001954] [PMID: 27501170]

[133] Blackham AU, Yue B, Almhanna K, *et al.* The prognostic value of residual nodal disease following neoadjuvant chemoradiation for esophageal cancer in patients with complete primary tumor response. J Surg Oncol 2015; 112(6): 597-602.
[http://dx.doi.org/10.1002/jso.24050] [PMID: 26394724]

[134] Cunningham D, Allum WH, Stenning SP, *et al.* MAGIC Trial Participants. Perioperative chemotherapy *versus* surgery alone for resectable gastroesophageal cancer. N Engl J Med 2006; 355(1): 11-20.
[http://dx.doi.org/10.1056/NEJMoa055531] [PMID: 16822992]

[135] Ychou M, Boige V, Pignon JP, *et al.* Perioperative chemotherapy compared with surgery alone for resectable gastroesophageal adenocarcinoma: an FNCLCC and FFCD multicenter phase III trial. J Clin Oncol 2011; 29(13): 1715-21.
[http://dx.doi.org/10.1200/JCO.2010.33.0597] [PMID: 21444866]

[136] University Hospital Freiburg. Perioperative Chemotherapy Compared To Neoadjuvant Chemoradiation in Patients With Adenocarcinoma of the Esophagus (ESOPEC) In: ClinicalTrials.gov [Internet]. Bethesda (MD): National Library of Medicine (US). 2000- [Cited 2016 August 21]. Available from: https://clinicaltrials.gov/ct2/show/NCT02509286 NLM: NCT02509286.

[137] Gwynne S, Hurt C, Evans M, Holden C, Vout L, Crosby T. Definitive chemoradiation for oesophageal cancera standard of care in patients with non-metastatic oesophageal cancer. Clin Oncol (R Coll Radiol) 2011; 23(3): 182-8.
[http://dx.doi.org/10.1016/j.clon.2010.12.001] [PMID: 21232928]

[138] Versteijne E, van Laarhoven HW, van Hooft JE, *et al.* Definitive chemoradiation for patients with inoperable and/or unresectable esophageal cancer: locoregional recurrence pattern. Dis Esophagus 2015; 28(5): 453-9.
[http://dx.doi.org/10.1111/dote.12215] [PMID: 24725186]

[139] Petrovich Z, Langholz B, Formenti S, Luxton G, Astrahan M. Management of carcinoma of the esophagus: the role of radiotherapy. Am J Clin Oncol 1991; 14(1): 80-6.
[http://dx.doi.org/10.1097/00000421-199102000-00018] [PMID: 1702923]

[140] Wobbes T, Baron B, Paillot B, *et al.* Prospective randomised study of split-course radiotherapy *versus* cisplatin plus split-course radiotherapy in inoperable squamous cell carcinoma of the oesophagus. Eur J Cancer 2001; 37(4): 470-7.
[http://dx.doi.org/10.1016/S0959-8049(00)00399-3] [PMID: 11267856]

[141] Caspers RJ, Welvaart K, Verkes RJ, Hermans J, Leer JW. The effect of radiotherapy on dysphagia and survival in patients with esophageal cancer. Radiother Oncol 1988; 12(1): 15-23.
[http://dx.doi.org/10.1016/0167-8140(88)90188-0] [PMID: 2457230]

[142] Wang H, Ryu J, Gandara D, *et al.* A phase II study of paclitaxel, carboplatin, and radiation with or without surgery for esophageal cancer. J Thorac Oncol 2007; 2(2): 153-7.
[http://dx.doi.org/10.1097/JTO.0b013e31802bff75] [PMID: 17410032]

[143] Ruppert BN, Watkins JM, Shirai K, *et al.* Cisplatin/Irinotecan *versus* carboplatin/paclitaxel as definitive chemoradiotherapy for locoregionally advanced esophageal cancer. Am J Clin Oncol 2010; 33(4): 346-52.
[http://dx.doi.org/10.1097/COC.0b013e3181aaca26] [PMID: 19841574]

[144] Sharma R, Yang GY, Nava HR, *et al.* A single institution experience with neoadjuvant chemoradiation (CRT) with irinotecan (I) and cisplatin (C) in locally advanced esophageal carcinoma (LAEC). ASCO Annual Meeting Proceedings. 27(15S): e15619.

[145] Ajani JA, Winter K, Okawara GS, *et al.* Phase II trial of preoperative chemoradiation in patients with localized gastric adenocarcinoma (RTOG 9904): quality of combined modality therapy and pathologic response. J Clin Oncol 2006; 24(24): 3953-8.
[http://dx.doi.org/10.1200/JCO.2006.06.4840] [PMID: 16921048]

[146] Conroy T, Galais MP, Raoul JL, *et al.* Fédération Francophone de Cancérologie Digestive and UNICANCER-GI Group. Definitive chemoradiotherapy with FOLFOX *versus* fluorouracil and cisplatin in patients with oesophageal cancer (PRODIGE5/ACCORD17): final results of a randomised, phase 2/3 trial. Lancet Oncol 2014; 15(3): 305-14.
[http://dx.doi.org/10.1016/S1470-2045(14)70028-2] [PMID: 24556041]

[147] Siegel R, Ward E, Brawley O, Jemal A. Cancer statistics, 2011: the impact of eliminating socioeconomic and racial disparities on premature cancer deaths. CA Cancer J Clin 2011; 61(4): 212-36.
[http://dx.doi.org/10.3322/caac.20121] [PMID: 21685461]

[148] Sudo K, Xiao L, Wadhwa R, *et al.* Importance of surveillance and success of salvage strategies after definitive chemoradiation in patients with esophageal cancer. J Clin Oncol 2014; 32(30): 3400-5.
[http://dx.doi.org/10.1200/JCO.2014.56.7156] [PMID: 25225435]

[149] Sudo K, Taketa T, Correa AM, *et al.* Locoregional failure rate after preoperative chemoradiation of esophageal adenocarcinoma and the outcomes of salvage strategies. J Clin Oncol 2013; 31(34): 4306-10.
[http://dx.doi.org/10.1200/JCO.2013.51.7250] [PMID: 24145339]

[150] Lou F, Sima CS, Adusumilli PS, *et al.* Esophageal cancer recurrence patterns and implications for surveillance. J Thorac Oncol 2013; 8(12): 1558-62.
[http://dx.doi.org/10.1097/01.JTO.0000437420.38972.fb] [PMID: 24389438]

[151] Abate E, DeMeester SR, Zehetner J, *et al.* Recurrence after esophagectomy for adenocarcinoma: defining optimal follow-up intervals and testing. J Am Coll Surg 2010; 210(4): 428-35.
[http://dx.doi.org/10.1016/j.jamcollsurg.2010.01.006] [PMID: 20347734]

[152] Enzinger PC, Mayer RJ. Esophageal cancer. N Engl J Med 2003; 349(23): 2241-52.
[http://dx.doi.org/10.1056/NEJMra035010] [PMID: 14657432]

[153] Wagner AD, Grothe W, Haerting J, Kleber G, Grothey A, Fleig WE. Chemotherapy in advanced gastric cancer: a systematic review and meta-analysis based on aggregate data. J Clin Oncol 2006; 24(18): 2903-9.
[http://dx.doi.org/10.1200/JCO.2005.05.0245] [PMID: 16782930]

[154] Ajani JA, Ilson DH, Daugherty K, Pazdur R, Lynch PM, Kelsen DP. Activity of taxol in patients with squamous cell carcinoma and adenocarcinoma of the esophagus. J Natl Cancer Inst 1994; 86(14): 1086-91.
[http://dx.doi.org/10.1093/jnci/86.14.1086] [PMID: 7912736]

[155] Ajani JA. Contributions of chemotherapy in the treatment of carcinoma of the esophagus: results and commentary. InSeminars in oncology 1994; 21(4): 474.

[156] Bleiberg H, Conroy T, Paillot B, *et al.* Randomised phase II study of cisplatin and 5-fluorouracil (5-FU) *versus* cisplatin alone in advanced squamous cell oesophageal cancer. Eur J Cancer 1997; 33(8): 1216-20.
[http://dx.doi.org/10.1016/S0959-8049(97)00088-9] [PMID: 9301445]

[157] Koizumi W, Narahara H, Hara T, *et al.* S-1 plus cisplatin *versus* S-1 alone for first-line treatment of advanced gastric cancer (SPIRITS trial): a phase III trial. Lancet Oncol 2008; 9(3): 215-21.
[http://dx.doi.org/10.1016/S1470-2045(08)70035-4] [PMID: 18282805]

[158] Ohtsu A, Shimada Y, Shirao K, *et al.* Japan Clinical Oncology Group Study (JCOG9205). Randomized phase III trial of fluorouracil alone *versus* fluorouracil plus cisplatin *versus* uracil and tegafur plus mitomycin in patients with unresectable, advanced gastric cancer: The Japan Clinical Oncology Group Study (JCOG9205). J Clin Oncol 2003; 21(1): 54-9.
[http://dx.doi.org/10.1200/JCO.2003.04.130] [PMID: 12506170]

[159] Cunningham D, Starling N, Rao S, *et al.* Upper Gastrointestinal Clinical Studies Group of the National Cancer Research Institute of the United Kingdom. Capecitabine and oxaliplatin for advanced esophagogastric cancer. N Engl J Med 2008; 358(1): 36-46.
[http://dx.doi.org/10.1056/NEJMoa073149] [PMID: 18172173]

[160] Takahashi H, Arimura Y, Yamashita K, *et al.* Phase I/II study of docetaxel/cisplatin/fluorouracil combination chemotherapy against metastatic esophageal squamous cell carcinoma. J Thorac Oncol 2010; 5(1): 122-8.

[http://dx.doi.org/10.1097/JTO.0b013e3181c1ffd5] [PMID: 19898259]

[161] Van Cutsem E, Moiseyenko VM, Tjulandin S, *et al.* V325 Study Group. Phase III study of docetaxel and cisplatin plus fluorouracil compared with cisplatin and fluorouracil as first-line therapy for advanced gastric cancer: a report of the V325 Study Group. J Clin Oncol 2006; 24(31): 4991-7. [http://dx.doi.org/10.1200/JCO.2006.06.8429] [PMID: 17075117]

[162] Shah MA, Janjigian YY, Stoller R, *et al.* Randomized multicenter phase II study of modified docetaxel, cisplatin, and fluorouracil (DCF) *vs* DCF plus growth factor support in patients with metastatic gastric adenocarcinoma: A study of the US Gastric Cancer Consortium. J Clin Oncol 2015; JCO-2015.

[163] Kim M, Keam B, Kim TM, *et al.* Phase II Study of Irinotecan and Cisplatin Combination Chemotherapy in Metastatic, Unresectable Esophageal Cancer. Cancer research and treatment 2016.

[164] Dank M, Zaluski J, Barone C, *et al.* Randomized phase III study comparing irinotecan combined with 5-fluorouracil and folinic acid to cisplatin combined with 5-fluorouracil in chemotherapy naive patients with advanced adenocarcinoma of the stomach or esophagogastric junction. Ann Oncol 2008; 19(8): 1450-7. [http://dx.doi.org/10.1093/annonc/mdn166] [PMID: 18558665]

[165] Guimbaud R, Louvet C, Ries P, *et al.* Prospective, randomized, multicenter, phase III study of fluorouracil, leucovorin, and irinotecan *versus* epirubicin, cisplatin, and capecitabine in advanced gastric adenocarcinoma: a French intergroup (Fédération Francophone de Cancérologie Digestive, Fédération Nationale des Centres de Lutte Contre le Cancer, and Groupe Coopérateur Multidisciplinaire en Oncologie) study. J Clin Oncol 2014; 32(31): 3520-6. [http://dx.doi.org/10.1200/JCO.2013.54.1011] [PMID: 25287828]

[166] Washington University School of Medicine. Combination Chemotherapy in Treating Patients With Advanced Stomach, Gastroesophageal, or Esophageal Cancer (FOLFIRINOX). In: ClinicalTrials.gov [Internet]. Bethesda (MD): National Library of Medicine (US). 2000- [Cited 2016 August 21]. Available from: https://clinicaltrials.gov/ct2/show/NCT01928290 NLM: NCT01928290.

[167] Kato K, Tahara M, Hironaka S, *et al.* A phase II study of paclitaxel by weekly 1-h infusion for advanced or recurrent esophageal cancer in patients who had previously received platinum-based chemotherapy. Cancer Chemother Pharmacol 2011; 67(6): 1265-72. [http://dx.doi.org/10.1007/s00280-010-1422-x] [PMID: 20703479]

[168] Muro K, Hamaguchi T, Ohtsu A, *et al.* A phase II study of single-agent docetaxel in patients with metastatic esophageal cancer. Ann Oncol 2004; 15(6): 955-9. [http://dx.doi.org/10.1093/annonc/mdh231] [PMID: 15151954]

[169] Hong YS, Song SY, Lee SI, *et al.* A phase II trial of capecitabine in previously untreated patients with advanced and/or metastatic gastric cancer. Ann Oncol 2004; 15(9): 1344-7. [http://dx.doi.org/10.1093/annonc/mdh343] [PMID: 15319239]

[170] Janowitz T, Thuss-Patience P, Marshall A, *et al.* Chemotherapy *vs* supportive care alone for relapsed gastric, gastroesophageal junction, and oesophageal adenocarcinoma: a meta-analysis of patient-level data. Br J Cancer 2016; 114(4): 381-7. [http://dx.doi.org/10.1038/bjc.2015.452] [PMID: 26882063]

[171] Wong SK, Chiu PW, Leung SF, *et al.* Concurrent chemoradiotherapy or endoscopic stenting for advanced squamous cell carcinoma of esophagus: a case-control study. Ann Surg Oncol 2008; 15(2): 576-82. [http://dx.doi.org/10.1245/s10434-007-9679-y] [PMID: 18057993]

[172] Ikeda E, Kojima T, Kaneko K, *et al.* Efficacy of concurrent chemoradiotherapy as a palliative treatment in stage IVB esophageal cancer patients with dysphagia. Jpn J Clin Oncol 2011; 41(8): 964-72. [http://dx.doi.org/10.1093/jjco/hyr088] [PMID: 21742654]

[173] Hudis CA. Trastuzumab mechanism of action and use in clinical practice. N Engl J Med 2007; 357(1): 39-51.
[http://dx.doi.org/10.1056/NEJMra043186] [PMID: 17611206]

[174] Ross JS, McKenna BJ. The HER-2/neu oncogene in tumors of the gastrointestinal tract. Cancer Invest 2001; 19(5): 554-68.
[http://dx.doi.org/10.1081/CNV-100103852] [PMID: 11458821]

[175] Rossi E, Grisanti S, Villanacci V, *et al.* HER-2 overexpression/amplification in Barretts oesophagus predicts early transition from dysplasia to adenocarcinoma: a clinico-pathologic study. J Cell Mol Med 2009; 13(9B): 3826-33.
[http://dx.doi.org/10.1111/j.1582-4934.2008.00517.x] [PMID: 19292734]

[176] Bang YJ, Van Cutsem E, Feyereislova A, *et al.* ToGA Trial Investigators. Trastuzumab in combination with chemotherapy *versus* chemotherapy alone for treatment of HER2-positive advanced gastric or gastro-oesophageal junction cancer (ToGA): a phase 3, open-label, randomised controlled trial. Lancet 2010; 376(9742): 687-97.
[http://dx.doi.org/10.1016/S0140-6736(10)61121-X] [PMID: 20728210]

[177] National Cancer Institute. Radiation Therapy, Paclitaxel, and Carboplatin with or without Trastuzumab in treating patients with Esophageal Cancer. In: ClinicalTrials.gov [Internet]. Bethesda (MD): National Library of Medicine (US). 2000- [Cited 2016 August 21]. Available from: https://clinicaltrials.gov/ct2/show/NCT01196390?term=NCT01196390&rank=1 NLM: NCT0119-6390.

[178] Ferrara N, Davis-Smyth T. The biology of vascular endothelial growth factor. Endocr Rev 1997; 18(1): 4-25.
[http://dx.doi.org/10.1210/edrv.18.1.0287] [PMID: 9034784]

[179] Yoon HH, Bendell JC, Braiteh FS, *et al.* Ramucirumab (RAM) plus FOLFOX as front-line therapy (Rx) for advanced gastric or esophageal adenocarcinoma (GE-AC): randomized, double-blind, multicenter phase 2 trial. InASCO Annual Meeting Proceedings. 32(15): 4004.

[180] Fuchs CS, Tomasek J, Yong CJ, *et al.* REGARD Trial Investigators. Ramucirumab monotherapy for previously treated advanced gastric or gastro-oesophageal junction adenocarcinoma (REGARD): an international, randomised, multicentre, placebo-controlled, phase 3 trial. Lancet 2014; 383(9911): 31-9.
[http://dx.doi.org/10.1016/S0140-6736(13)61719-5] [PMID: 24094768]

[181] Wilke H, Muro K, Van Cutsem E, *et al.* RAINBOW Study Group. Ramucirumab plus paclitaxel *versus* placebo plus paclitaxel in patients with previously treated advanced gastric or gastro-oesophageal junction adenocarcinoma (RAINBOW): a double-blind, randomised phase 3 trial. Lancet Oncol 2014; 15(11): 1224-35.
[http://dx.doi.org/10.1016/S1470-2045(14)70420-6] [PMID: 25240821]

[182] Hecht JR, Bang YJ, Qin SK, *et al.* Lapatinib in Combination With Capecitabine Plus Oxaliplatin in Human Epidermal Growth Factor Receptor 2–Positive Advanced or Metastatic Gastric, Esophageal, or Gastroesophageal Adenocarcinoma: TRIO-013/LOGiC—A Randomized Phase III Trial. J Clin Oncol 2015; JCO-2015.
[PMID: 26628478]

[183] Ohtsu A, Shah MA, Van Cutsem E, *et al.* Bevacizumab in combination with chemotherapy as first-line therapy in advanced gastric cancer: a randomized, double-blind, placebo-controlled phase III study. J Clin Oncol 2011; 29(30): 3968-76.
[http://dx.doi.org/10.1200/JCO.2011.36.2236] [PMID: 21844504]

[184] Enzinger PC, Burtness BA, Niedzwiecki D, *et al.* CALGB 80403 (Alliance)/E1206: A Randomized Phase II Study of Three Chemotherapy Regimens Plus Cetuximab in Metastatic Esophageal and Gastroesophageal Junction Cancers. J Clin Oncol 2016; 34(23): 2736-42.
[http://dx.doi.org/10.1200/JCO.2015.65.5092] [PMID: 27382098]

[185] Al-Shamsi HO, Alhazzani W, Wolff RA. Extended RAS testing in metastatic colorectal cancer-Refining the predictive molecular biomarkers. J Gastrointest Oncol 2015; 6(3): 314-21. [PMID: 26029459]

[186] Waddell T, Chau I, Cunningham D, *et al.* Epirubicin, oxaliplatin, and capecitabine with or without panitumumab for patients with previously untreated advanced oesophagogastric cancer (REAL3): a randomised, open-label phase 3 trial. Lancet Oncol 2013; 14(6): 481-9. [http://dx.doi.org/10.1016/S1470-2045(13)70096-2] [PMID: 23594787]

[187] Kuhnil Pharmaceutical Co., Ltd. Phase 3 Study of Nimotuzumab and Irinotecan as Second Line With Advanced or Recurrect Gastric and Gastroesophageal Junction Cancer. In: ClinicalTrials.gov [Internet]. Bethesda (MD): National Library of Medicine (US). 2000- [Cited 2016 August 21]. Available from: https://clinicaltrials.gov/ct2/show/NCT01813253 NLM: NCT01813253.

[188] Pavlakis N, Sjoquist KM, Martin AJ, *et al.* Regorafenib for the Treatment of Advanced Gastric Cancer (INTEGRATE): A Multinational Placebo-Controlled Phase II Trial. J Clin Oncol 2016; 34(23): 2728-35. [http://dx.doi.org/10.1200/JCO.2015.65.1901] [PMID: 27325864]

[189] Academic and Community Cancer Research United. Study of Adjuvant Regorafenib *vs.* Placebo in Patients with Node Positive Esophageal Cancer that completed Pre-operative Therapy. In: ClinicalTrials.gov [Internet]. Bethesda (MD): National Library of Medicine (US). 2000- [Cited 2016 August 21]. Available from: https://clinicaltrials.gov/ct2/show/NCT02234180?term=NCT022-34180&rank=1 NLM: NCT02234180.

[190] Bennouna J, Shen L, Enzinger PC, *et al.* KEYNOTE-181: Phase 3, open-label study of second-line pembrolizumab *vs* single-agent chemotherapy in patients with advanced/metastatic esophageal adenocarcinoma. ASCO Annual Meeting Proceedings. 34(15): TPS4140.

[191] Bristol-Myers Squibb. Study of Adjuvant Nivolumab or placebo in subjects with Resected Esophageal or Gastroesophageal Junction Cancer (CheckMate 577). In: ClinicalTrials.gov [Internet]. Bethesda (MD): National Library of Medicine (US). 2000- [Cited 2016 August 21]. Available from https://clinicaltrials.gov/ct2/show/NCT02743494?term=CA209-577&rank=1 NLM: NCT02743494.

[192] Washington University School of Medicine. Pembrolizumab with Locally Delivered Radiation Therapy for the Initial Treatment of Metastatic Esophageal Cancers. In: ClinicalTrials.gov [Internet]. Bethesda (MD): National Library of Medicine (US). 2000- [Cited 2016 August 21]. Available from https://clinicaltrials.gov/ct2/show/NCT02642809?term=NCT02642809&rank=1 NLM: NCT02642-809.

[193] Temel JS, Greer JA, Muzikansky A, *et al.* Early palliative care for patients with metastatic non-smal--cell lung cancer. N Engl J Med 2010; 363(8): 733-42. [http://dx.doi.org/10.1056/NEJMoa1000678] [PMID: 20818875]

[194] Ikeda E, Kojima T, Kaneko K, *et al.* Efficacy of concurrent chemoradiotherapy as a palliative treatment in stage IVB esophageal cancer patients with dysphagia. Jpn J Clin Oncol 2011; 41(8): 964-72. [http://dx.doi.org/10.1093/jjco/hyr088] [PMID: 21742654]

[195] Coia LR, Soffen EM, Schultheiss TE, Martin EE, Hanks GE. Swallowing function in patients with esophageal cancer treated with concurrent radiation and chemotherapy. Cancer 1993; 71(2): 281-6. [http://dx.doi.org/10.1002/1097-0142(19930115)71:2<281::AID-CNCR2820710202>3.0.CO;2-0] [PMID: 8422619]

[196] Wong SK, Chiu PW, Leung SF, *et al.* Concurrent chemoradiotherapy or endoscopic stenting for advanced squamous cell carcinoma of esophagus: a case-control study. Ann Surg Oncol 2008; 15(2): 576-82. [http://dx.doi.org/10.1245/s10434-007-9679-y] [PMID: 18057993]

[197] Evans JA, Early DS, Chandraskhara V, *et al.* ASGE Standards of Practice Committee, American Society for Gastrointestinal Endoscopy. The role of endoscopy in the assessment and treatment of

esophageal cancer. Gastrointest Endosc 2013; 77(3): 328-34.
[http://dx.doi.org/10.1016/j.gie.2012.10.001] [PMID: 23410694]

[198] Sreedharan A, Harris K, Crellin A, Forman D, Everett SM. WITHDRAWN: Interventions for dysphagia in oesophageal cancer. Cochrane Database Syst Rev 2011; (2): CD005048.
[PMID: 21328271]

[199] Saranovic Dj, Djuric-Stefanovic A, Ivanovic A, Masulovic D, Pesko P. Fluoroscopically guided insertion of self-expandable metal esophageal stents for palliative treatment of patients with malignant stenosis of esophagus and cardia: comparison of uncovered and covered stent types. Dis Esophagus 2005; 18(4): 230-8.
[http://dx.doi.org/10.1111/j.1442-2050.2005.00484.x] [PMID: 16128779]

[200] Homs MY, Steyerberg EW, Eijkenboom WM, *et al.* Single-dose brachytherapy *versus* metal stent placement for the palliation of dysphagia from oesophageal cancer: multicentre randomised trial. Lancet 2004; 364(9444): 1497-504.
[http://dx.doi.org/10.1016/S0140-6736(04)17272-3] [PMID: 15500894]

[201] Homs MY, Steyerberg EW, Eijkenboom WM, *et al.* Single-dose brachytherapy *versus* metal stent placement for the palliation of dysphagia from oesophageal cancer: multicentre randomised trial. Lancet 2004; 364(9444): 1497-504.
[http://dx.doi.org/10.1016/S0140-6736(04)17272-3] [PMID: 15500894]

[202] Curran WJ Jr, Paulus R, Langer CJ, *et al.* Sequential *vs.* concurrent chemoradiation for stage III non-small cell lung cancer: randomized phase III trial RTOG 9410. J Natl Cancer Inst 2011; 103(19): 1452-60.
[http://dx.doi.org/10.1093/jnci/djr325] [PMID: 21903745]

[203] Byhardt RW, Scott C, Sause WT, *et al.* Response, toxicity, failure patterns, and survival in five Radiation Therapy Oncology Group (RTOG) trials of sequential and/or concurrent chemotherapy and radiotherapy for locally advanced non–small-cell carcinoma of the lung. Int J Radiat Oncol Biol Phys 1998; 42(3): 469-78.

[204] Coia LR, Myerson RJ, Tepper JE. Late effects of radiation therapy on the gastrointestinal tract. Int J Radiat Oncol Biol Phys 1995; 31(5): 1213-36.
[http://dx.doi.org/10.1016/0360-3016(94)00419-L]

[205] Maguire PD, Sibley GS, Zhou SM, *et al.* Clinical and dosimetric predictors of radiation-induced esophageal toxicity. Int J Radiat Oncol Biol Phys 1999; 45(1): 97-103.
[http://dx.doi.org/10.1016/S0360-3016(99)00163-7]

[206] Luckett T, Davidson PM, Green A, Boyle F, Stubbs J, Lovell M. Assessment and management of adult cancer pain: a systematic review and synthesis of recent qualitative studies aimed at developing insights for managing barriers and optimizing facilitators within a comprehensive framework of patient care. J Pain Symptom Manage 2013; 46(2): 229-53.
[http://dx.doi.org/10.1016/j.jpainsymman.2012.07.021] [PMID: 23159681]

[207] Miller S, McNutt L, McCann MA, McCorry N, Bort□Marti S. Use of corticosteroids for anorexia in palliative medicine: a systematic review. J Palliat Med 2014; 17(4): 482-5.
[http://dx.doi.org/10.1089/jpm.2013.0324] [PMID: 24702642]

[208] Dobs AS, Boccia RV, Croot CC, *et al.* Effects of enobosarm on muscle wasting and physical function in patients with cancer: a double-blind, randomised controlled phase 2 trial. Lancet Oncol 2013; 14(4): 335-45.
[http://dx.doi.org/10.1016/S1470-2045(13)70055-X] [PMID: 23499390]

[209] GTx. Phase III Study of the Effect of GTx-024 on Muscle Wasting in Patients With Non-Small Cell Lung Cancer (NSCLC).In: ClinicalTrials.gov [Internet]. Bethesda (MD): National Library of Medicine (US). 2000- [Cited 2016 August 21]. Available from: https://clinicaltrials.gov/show/NCT01355484. NLM: NCT01355484.

[210] Temel JS, Abernethy AP, Currow DC, *et al.* Anamorelin in patients with non-small-cell lung cancer and cachexia (ROMANA 1 and ROMANA 2): results from two randomised, double-blind, phase 3 trials. Lancet Oncol 2016; 17(4): 519-31.
[http://dx.doi.org/10.1016/S1470-2045(15)00558-6] [PMID: 26906526]

CHAPTER 3

Androgen Deprivation Therapy for Prostate Cancer

Patricia Tai[1,*], **Evgeny Sadikov**[1], **Asim Amjad**[1], **Nelson Leong**[1], **Arbind Dubey**[3], **Wojciech Dolata**[2], **Miroslav Jancewicz**[2] and **Rashmi Koul**[3]

Departments of [1]Radiation Oncology, and [2]Medical Oncology, Allan Blair Cancer Centre, Regina, Canada; [3]Department of Radiation Oncology, CancerCare Manitoba, Winnipeg, Canada

Abstract: In the past, androgen deprivation therapy (ADT) was used for the conservative treatment of prostatic cancer, but now also used in the setting of neoadjuvant and adjuvant treatment in combination with radiotherapy. Another use is for loco-regional or distant recurrence after primary treatment of surgery or radiotherapy. ADT is an alternative for local failure after radical treatment and it compares favorably with cryotherapy or high-intensity focused ultrasound therapy. Traditionally gonadotropin releasing hormone (GnRH) agonists are used. A new class of agent in clinical use is the gonadotrophin antagonist degarelix. Newer choices for castrate resistant prostate cancer include abiraterone and enzalutamide. The emphasis of this review is on drug discovery, design and clinical trials. The indication and rationale for choosing the appropriate first and second line drugs will be discussed for easy access at point of care. This chapter summarizes the recent developments and the controversies to be explored in the future which will be of interest to all health care professionals, colleagues in the pharmaceutical industry, family physicians, urologists, radiation and medical oncologists. We also add our clinical experience of use of different ADT throughout this review to make it practical for bedside management. Common questions from physicians and patients are answered in this review.

Keywords: Androgen deprivation therapy, Anti-androgens, Agonist, Antagonist, Adjuvant, Biochemical failure, Clinical trials, Degarelix, Gonadotropin-releasing hormone, Metastasis, Prostate cancer, Prostate-specific antigen, Primary treatment.

INTRODUCTION

Adenocarcinoma of the prostate is a hormone-sensitive tumor. In 1941, Higgins published the first observational study of effectiveness of orchiectomy (removal

* **Corresponding author Professor Patricia Tai:** Department of Radiation Oncology, University of Saskatchewan, Allan Blair Cancer Centre, Regina, Canada; Tel: (306) 766 -2296; E-mail: patricia.tai@saskcancer.ca

Atta-ur-Rahman and M. Iqbal Choudhary (Eds.)

of testes) or estrogen on patients with metastatic prostate cancer [1]. Recent research found the biological basis that explains the phenomenon. There are androgen receptors on the tumors cells and the genes involved are also elucidated [2]. Almost all prostate cancer cells express receptors for male hormones (androgen) and androgen stimulates the growth of prostate cancer cells.

The emphasis of this review is on drug discovery, research findings and design of clinical trials. The rationale for choosing the appropriate drugs will be discussed in this chapter for easy access at point of care. This chapter summarizes the recent developments and the issues to be explored in the future which will be of interest to family physicians, urologists, radiation and medical oncologists.

WHAT ARE THE INDICATIONS OF ADT?

Chemoprevention

5-alpha-reductase inhibitors such as finasteride have been shown to decrease androgenic stimulation of the prostate, often used in benign prostatic hyperplasia. In clinical studies, 5-alpha-reductase inhibitors suppress serum and intra-prostatic levels of dihydrotestosterone, an important promoter of prostate cancer, leading to reduction in prostate size and suppression of glandular cell activity as measured by prostate specific antigen (PSA) secretion [3]. In addition, 5-alpha-reductase inhibitors have demonstrated an excellent safety profile and tolerance in controlled clinical trials. No significant metabolic effects have been observed in gonadotropin secretion, spermatogenesis, serum lipids or glucose tolerance. The efficacy and safety of 5-alpha-reductase inhibitors in published studies strongly supports investigating their use for chemoprevention of prostate cancer.

The Southwest Oncology Group (SWOG) S9207 study assessed the hypothesis that finasteride can reduce the prevalence of prostate cancer. It randomized over 18,000 healthy men, aged 55 and older, to either finasteride (5 mg/day) or placebo to be taken for seven years [4]. Low and intermediate-risk prostate cancers were less frequent among those who took finasteride than the placebo group [5, 6], with no difference in overall survival after 18 years of follow-up [7].

Similarly, the Reduction by Dutasteride of Prostate Cancer Events (REDUCE) trial also demonstrated overall decrease in prostate cancer incidence [8, 9]. For those with low-risk prostate cancers, the Reduction by Dutasteride of clinical progression Events in Expectant Management (REDEEM) trial showed that rates for either pathological progression or treatment intervention were lowered to 38% for dutasteride as compared to 48% for placebo [10].

These drugs can affect the quality of life with effects of sexual activity. Post-finasteride syndrome has been noted recently with effect on cognitive function [11].

Treatment of Prostate Cancer (Fig. 1)

Hormonal therapy nowadays is based on ADT and no longer on estrogen. The clinical scenario for its use was in the conservative treatment of prostatic cancer as primary treatment when patients are unwilling or unfit to undergo radical, definitive treatments of either surgery or radiotherapy due to co-morbidities or life-expectancy of less than 10 years. Radiotherapy (RT) is only available in specialized tertiary centers which are concentrated in large cities. Patients in rural areas may be unwilling or unable to afford to travel for radiotherapy.

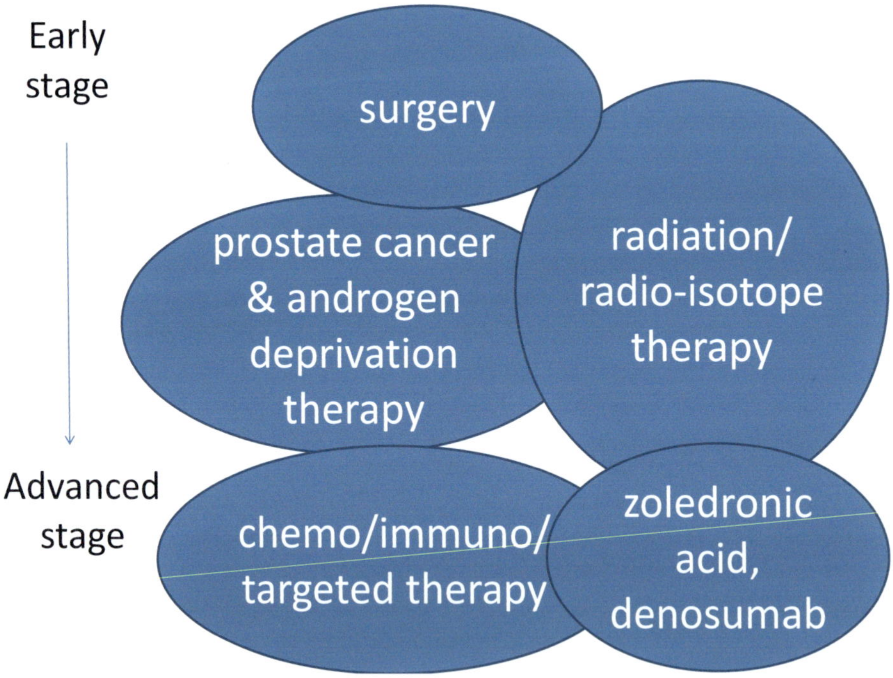

Fig. (1). Indications of androgen deprivation therapy in combination with other modalities.

In the past few decades, ADT is also given in the setting of neoadjuvant and adjuvant treatment in combination with radiotherapy. Patients with advanced prostate cancers are treated with ADT with or without radiotherapy. Bolla *et al.* of the European Organization for Research and Treatment of Cancer (EORTC) published the first study to show a survival benefit of 3 years from goserelin combined with radiotherapy [12].

Another use of ADT is in loco-regional or distant relapse after primary treatment of surgery or radiotherapy. Local failure can be treated with cryotherapy or high-intensity focused ultrasound therapy. However due to potential complications, many patients and physicians use ADT instead.

ADT as Primary Treatment

Although primary ADT is not commonly used in the United States, some patients in other countries may prefer it due to convenience. The disadvantage is difficulty to justify the non-curative treatment when hormone resistance develops later.

Is primary ADT alone enough for prostate cancer treatment within the life-time of patients? The National Cancer Institute of Canada (NCIC PR.3) has joined the Medical Research Council (MRC PR07) of United Kingdom in the INT T94-0110 trial [13]. The trial demonstrates a significant survival benefit from the addition of radiation therapy to the treatment of patients with cancer of the prostate who are receiving total androgen blockade in terms of overall survival, time to progression, symptomatic local control and quality of life. Similarly, the STAMPEDE trial showed failure-free survival benefit of local radiotherapy for both node negative and node positive patients without distant metastasis [14]. The STAMPEDE trial compared the addition of docetaxel, zoledronic acid, or both to first-line long-term ADT in prostate cancer and radiotherapy was given to some patients.

ADT Combined with Surgery

This treatment combination is controversial. The Mayo Clinic studied 22 patients with clinical stage B2 (T2c) or C (T3) prostate cancer who underwent down-staging ADT before radical prostatectomy [15]. For each patient with ADT, another matched patient who had not received preoperative ADT was chosen. Results show ADT has little or no benefit for decreasing the extent of tumor or pathological stage. Another study reported more difficulties and blood loss after pre-operative ADT [16].

These findings are contrary to the experience from Quebec [17]: the volume of the prostate gland decreased by approximately 48% as assessed by the transrectal ultrasound (TRUS) and digital rectal examination after three months of flutamide and a GnRH agonist. The down-staging with an atrophic prostate gland made dissection of the prostate much easier from the prostatic apex and the posterolateral neurovascular bundle. In fact, tumor was not detected in 12 of the 50 prostatectomy. After neoadjuvant ADT and surgery, patients require a median time of 7.5 months for recovery of sexual function.

ADT Combined with Radiotherapy

ADT is often used as an adjunctive treatment in combination with RT (before, during, and after) for a total duration of 6 months to life-long in studies for intermediate and high risk (high Gleason grade and/or high PSA) prostate cancer. ADT enhances the effectiveness of RT by reducing the number of cancer cells that have to be killed by radiotherapy, making the cancer cells more sensitive to radiation, decrease the prostate volume, improving tumor oxygenation and spatial cooperation to kill micro-metastases. ADT shrinks down the prostate volume before external beam radiotherapy or brachytherapy and hence a better radiation dose distribution is possible.

RTOG 8307 was one of the first trials, which indicated that combined ADT and RT is beneficial [18]. It compared megestrol acetate with diethylostilbestrol with an improved outcome compared to historical study control group.

The benefit of the combined treatment modalities was confirmed by the Radiation Therapy Oncology Group (RTOG) 8531 and 8610 studies [19]. Both also answered the questions of how long should hormonal therapy be given and who will benefit from it. Patients were randomised to receive long-term hormones (LTH) on RTOG 8531 and received goserelin starting the last week of external beam radiotherapy to life-long treatment versus no ADT. Patients treated with short-term hormones (STH) on RTOG 8610 received goserelin and flutamide two months prior to and during radiotherapy. Statistically significant improvements in biochemical no evidence of disease control, distant metastases failure and cause-specific failure were demonstrated for LTH *versus* STH. In those patients receiving LTH, the benefit was only observed in centrally reviewed Gleason scores of 7 with scores 8-10 cancers [19].

There is evidence for benefit of ADT when combined with brachytherapy, in a study with similar subset of patients [20]. Low risk patients defined by PSA $\leq$ 10 ng/ml, stage $\leq$ T2a, and Gleason score $\leq$ 6 did not benefit from neoadjuvant ADT. All other patients as a group have a significantly lower positive biopsy rate of 3.4% *versus* 21.1% with and without prior ADT ($P = 0.003$).

Gaudet M *et al.* in Quebec, Canada conducted a randomized study of 60 prostate cancer patients with low and intermediate-risk prostate cancer and prostate volume > 50 cc. He found 3 months of bicalutamide 50 mg and dutasteride 0.5 mg daily to be non-inferior to 3 months of LHRH agonist with one month of bicalutamide for prostate volume reduction prior to I-125 permanent implant brachytherapy [21], although about 1/6 of the bicalutamide+dutasteride group needed longer than 3 months. However the combination has less sexual toxicity than the LHRH agonist group, and now used in many Canadian centers.

Nowadays at the British Columbia Cancer Agency of Canada, high-tier intermediate risk prostate cancer is treated with six months of ADT and seed brachytherapy [22]. High risk patients have ADT, pelvic radiotherapy and seed brachytherapy.

Combined radiotherapy and ADT have more toxicity than radiotherapy alone. Dose-escalated radiotherapy (66, 70, 74 Gy) and ADT independently increase urethral stricture in the Trans-Tasman Radiation Oncology Group (TROG) 03.04 Randomised Androgen Deprivation and Radiotherapy (RADAR) trial [23, 24]. This study randomized 1071 patients with locally advanced prostate cancer to 6 *versus* 18 months of androgen suppression plus radiotherapy, with or without 18 months of zoledronic acid. It shows no difference between the 6 and 18 months of ADT.

Hormonal Therapy Combined with Chemotherapy

The STAMPEDE trial involved 2962 patients *with high-risk, locally advanced, metastatic or recurrent* prostate cancer who are starting first-line long-term hormone therapy [25]. They were randomized to standard of care (SOC) only, SOC plus zoledronic acid (SOC + ZA), SOC plus docetaxel (SOC + Doc), or SOC with both zoledronic acid and docetaxel (SOC + ZA + Doc). The addition of docetaxel to first line long-term ADT (SOC + Doc) has a median survival of 81 months, which is indeed excellent news for prostate cancer patients. However due to 52% grade 3-5 toxicity, it should be considered for fit patients only. Zoledronic acid confers no overall survival benefit for hormone-sensitive cancer and is not funded for this indication. It is however funded for castrate-resistant cancer.

The ChemoHormonal therapy *versus* Androgen Ablation Randomized Trial for Extensive Disease in prostate cancer (CHAARTED) study shows that addition of docetaxel at the start of ADT in *metastatic* patients resulted in significantly superior survival than ADT alone: 57.6 *versus* 44 months [26].

Other Adjunctive Treatments

Patients should be advised to take vitamin D 1000 I.U. and calcium 1200 mg per day. The best source is through the diet and to meet the requirements, an oral supplement can be taken. When calcium supplements are taken, it should be spaced apart from other drugs by 2 hours and not more than 500 mg each time for better absorption.

Cancer and Acute Leukemia Group B (CALGB) 90202 demonstrated that zoledronic acid for hormone-sensitive metastatic prostate cancer does not decrease skeletal-related events or survival [27, 28]. Similarly, for high-risk localized prostate cancer, Zometa European Study (ZEUS) showed that it does not prevent bony metastases [29]. Calcium and renal function should be monitored during zoledronic acid use since at least 480 cases of acute renal failure had been reported in the literature [30].

The other drug, denosumab has several advantages over zoledronic acid. It only requires monitoring of calcium [31]. Denosumab is a fully human monoclonal antibody that inhibits RANK Ligand (RANKL) [32]. It is more effective than zoledronic acid to prevent skeletal-related events [33, 34]. However, there is more osteonecrosis of the jaw.

For bulky primary prostate cancer, transurethral resection can decrease the risk of hormone refractory prostate cancer among patients with metastatic hormone sensitive disease [35]. Similarly patients given any form of treatment for local control will have less obstructive symptoms later on. Even for hormone-naïve patients with pelvic node disease, Messing's study of prostatectomy and immediate ADT/orchiectomy has better survival results than other studies which left the prostate cancer primary without resection [36].

WHICH ADT TO USE?

Experience of ADT for adjuvant or salvage treatment is based on its effect on metastatic disease. Prostate cancer responds to androgen hormonal ablation with bilateral orchiectomy. The following summarizes development of different choices of ADT.

Bilateral Orchiectomy

This simple surgery removes 80% of circulating testosterone (but in prostate gland only 60% of testosterone is from circulation). The advantage is fast onset. For many years, orchiectomy was the standard of care, an approach that is not preferred by patients, due to psychological impact of disfigurement, irreversibility, perception of invasiveness, risk of infection and bleeding in elderly with multiple co-morbidities. It produces menopausal symptoms including increased risk of cardiovascular complications, peripheral arterial disease (hazard ratio, HR 1.13) and venous thromboembolism (HR 1.27) according to the American Surveillance Epidemiology End Result (SEER) database [37].

Estrogen and Progesterone

Estrogen therapy was used as ADT but is associated with side effects, such as hot flushes and gynecomastia, which frequently leads to treatment cessation. It is seldom used nowadays due to high risk of thrombosis, cardiovascular complications and the availability of better ADT options.

Diethylstilboestrol (DES) is an androgen receptor competitor. It decreases luteinizing hormone (LH) secretion by an effect on the testosterone synthesis pathway. Early study showed that 1 mg per day was not enough to achieve castration level, and about 3 mg per day is effective to control prostate cancer.

In hormone relapsed prostate cancer, a small randomized study of 28 patients showed that DES compared to flutamide (antiandrogen to be discussed in later section) significantly decreased prostatic-specific antigen (PSA) although the overall survival benefit does not reach statistical significance [38].

Progesterone is also used nowadays, in the form of megestrol (megace) to treat hot flashes (40 mg once to twice daily) and as a secondary ADT (160 mg per day) when total androgen blockade fails.

Steroidal Anti-androgen: Cyproterone Acetate (Androcur)

It suppresses the hypothalamus-pituitary axis by a negative feedback mechanism to inhibit the secretion of LH resulting in decreased production of testicular testosterone. It also has a peripheral action of blocking the binding of dihydrotesterone to specific receptors on prostate cancer cells.

The typical dose is 50 mg twice a day (BID) or thrice a day (TID). The metabolism is primarily hepatic. Cyproterone acetate is metabolized by the CYP3A4 enzyme, forming the active metabolite 15beta-hydroxycyproterone acetate, which retains its antiandrogen activity, but has reduced progesterone activity. It may cause elevation of bilirubin, transaminases, calcium, and lipid profile.

The disadvantages are a small risk of gynecomastia, thrombosis, cardiovascular complications due to fluid retention. Tachyphylaxis is another issue, with rapid appearance of progressive diminished response. Caution should be exercise for use in patients with pre-existing liver disease, diabetes, cardiac problems. Monitoring of blood sugar, liver function test and lipid profile is recommended.

Non-steroidal Anti-androgens

After orchiectomy and estrogens were developed, oral antiandrogens then became available. It is not as effective as luteinizing hormone-releasing hormone (LHRH) agonists which appeared on the market later on. They act by two mechanisms: inhibition of androgen binding to the androgen receptor, and inhibition of androgen-independent activation of the receptor [39]. The latter happens in different pathways, including inhibiting nuclear co-activators, activating cosuppressors, and inhibiting transcription of a variety of androgen-regulated genes. Therefore it is more accurate to call anti-androgen as androgen-receptor antagonists.

Since these anti-androgens block receptor binding and androgen uptake, dihydrotestosterone level in prostate cancer cells are decreased. The latter causes a compensatory increase in luteinizing hormone (LH) release and hence testosterone level. They can cause gynecomastia, which is prevented by LHRH.

Flutamide (Brand name: euflex) appeared to be the first in the market. It may cause hepatotoxicity but the incidence is as low as two patients with clinical liver disease (0.18%) and four patients with elevation of transaminase to four times of normal (0.36%) among 1,091 patients [40]. The author recommends liver function test at 2 and 4 weeks after flutamide is started. In fact it is prudent to monitor liver function test for all anti-androgens.

Bicalutamide (Brand name: casodex) is available later. It is the most commonly used anti-androgen nowadays due to its effectiveness and better tolerance by patients. It is less likely to cause hormone-resistance than flutamide. The pill contains lactose. The most common complication is diarrhea, which unfortunately resulted in early acute renal failure in one of our patients.

Typical dose is 50 mg/day and mostly used to prevent flare or combined with gonadotropin agonist or antagonist for maximal androgen blockade. Adjuvant bicalutamide studies after prostatectomy demonstrated its effectiveness in European and American guidelines.

Bicalutamide being a competitive inhibitor of androgen at the androgen receptor, a higher dose can give better higher response rate. Studies have shown that higher doses of bicalutamide 150 mg once daily are nearly as effective as castration, leuprolide or goserelin [41]. But another interesting publication on bicalutamide 150 mg daily monotherapy showed that it is less effective than castration in patients with metastatic disease with a difference in median survival of six weeks [42]. However it has shown a benefit in terms of quality of life and subjective response when compared to castration and that it has an acceptable tolerance [43, 44].

The combination of bicalutamide (150 mg/day) with finasteride (5 mg/day) is used to preserve sexual function in about half of the treated patients [45]. Finasteride also confers additional androgen blockade.

High-dose bicalutamide might reduce the risk of osteoporosis, but may be associated with an increased risk for fluid retention, heart failure, and blood clots.

Bicalutamide is used by some physicians to delay the risk for cancer progression in an adjuvant setting in high-risk patients but may not benefit low-risk patients and may also expose them to a greater risk for fluid retention and blood clots.

For patients who had PSA rising above nadir of previous antiandrogen, bicalutamide 150 mg induced a PSA decline in 17 of 38 patients (44.7%): 7/17 (18.4%) dropped to ≥ 85% of initial PSA and 10 (26.3%) ≥ 50% but <85% . The response last for a median duration of 18.5 months for partial and 37.4 months for complete responders. The median time to metastasis was 52.5 months for responders and 15.7 months for non-responders (Log-Rank test 9.3, P =0.002) [46]. When patients fail on combined flutamide and gonadotrophin agonist, change to bicalutamide 150 mg/day brought on response in 22.5% of patients. It was well tolerated, except with more hot flashes [47].

Nilutamide (nilandron in the United States and anandron in Canada) is another anti-androgen option. It is generally used as second line therapy. If patients have anti-androgen withdrawal response before, there will be a 100% chance of response compared to 18% chance for those without response to anti-androgen withdrawal [48]. It is not available in the formulary at least in some provinces of Canada. Nilutamide can cause mild and reversible visual side effects (31–58%) including delayed ocular adaptation to darkness and impaired color vision and interstitial pneumonitis (0.77–2.4%) [49].

PSA decline by anti-androgen withdrawal had been described by many studies, typically the drug was given after orchiectomy or with LHRH analog. In the SWOG 9426 study, Sartor *et al.* reported on 210 patients, of which 1/5 responded with PSA drop to half or more [50].

LHRH Agonist

LH release depends on pulsatile release of LHRH. LHRH analog produces a continuous level of LHRH which causes an initial increase in LH release (flare can be prevented, although not totally by anti-androgen) followed by down regulation of LHRH receptors in pituitary & then decrease in LH release and hence testosterone (3 - 4 weeks) [51]. Various groups have studied the effects of androgen blockade administered as monotherapy and as combination therapy: LHRH analogue plus antiandrogen. Clinicians should cover the flare period by an anti-androgen for 2-4 weeks when starting any patient on GnRH agonist. The anti-androgen should be given 1 week prior or the same day as the start of GnRH agonist. Our group had seen spinal cord compression, deep vein thrombosis and acute urinary retentions due to flare among patients treated by community urologists.

The first LHRH analog developed was goserelin (zoladex) given as 3.6 mg monthly subcutaneous deport or 10.8 mg every (q) 3 months (m). Later leuprolide (lupron) 7.5 mg intramuscular (IM) monthly, 22.5 mg every (q) 3 months (m), 30 mg q4m became available. The other leuprolide (eligard) in addition has a 45 mg q6m depot available and is chosen by patients who need to travel for long vacations. It is noted that granuloma can develop around Lupron depot, with or without signs of inflammation, so clinicians should try to change to goserelin.

LHRH analogs have been used due to its reversibility and patient preference. However, recently orchiectomy is being advocated again due to lower cost, risks of fractures, peripheral arterial disease, and cardiac-related complications than GnRH agonists [52]. But the irreversibility, surgical risks and psychological impact are not preferred by patients.

GnRH Antagonist

Traditionally LHRH analogs have been used for more than 3 decades. A new class of agent in clinical use is the gonadotrophin antagonist. A GnRH antagonist such as degarelix (firmagon) has the advantage of rapid reduction of testosterone and is preferred to GnRH agonists in situations when early response is important. The lack of flare reaction, as compared to GnRH agonists, is particularly desirable as it would not aggravate the problem (spinal cord compression, bone pain or urinary obstruction).

The first trial CS21 was led by Klotz *et al.* (2008), a 12-month open-label randomized study on the use of degarelix 240 mg for 1 month then maintenance 80 or 160 mg *versus* 7.5 mg leuprolide monthly in different stages of prostate cancer [53]. At 3 days after starting treatment, the median testosterone levels were =<0.5 ng/mL in 96.1% and 95.5% of patients in the degarelix 240/80 mg and 240/160 mg groups, respectively. Some patients in the leuprolide group had testosterone surge (defined as a testosterone increase of >= 15% from baseline, on any 2 days during the first 2 weeks): the median testosterone levels increased by 65% from baseline by day 3 (6.30 ng/mL). Of the 201 patients in the leuprolide group, 23 (11%) received concomitant bicalutamide for flare protection at the start of treatment, of which 17/23 (74%) still had a testosterone surge. For the remaining 178 patients in the leuprolide group who did not receive bicalutamide, 144 (81%) had a surge in testosterone.

The study CS21A, a 5-year extension trial suggested that patients could be safely switched from GnRH agonist to degarelix treatment with sustained efficacy, as measured by biochemical markers [54]. There is a significant reduction of PSA progression hazard rate. The follicle-stimulating hormone (FSH) was suppressed more by degarelix than GnRH agonists. The above published report had a median

27.5 month follow-up only, however a later paper reported long-term safety and efficacy of degarelix up to 5 years [55].

Two recent pooled data analyses from 5 and 6 randomized studies on degarelix suggested improved disease control, quality of life, less urinary tract symptoms, decreased risk of cardiovascular diseases and overall survival when compared with leuprolide, a GnRH agonist [56, 57].

In the literature, most degarelix studies are from America, Canada and Europe. Our experience in Regina, Canada noted [58]:

- Communication with patients, local nurses and family doctors regarding benefits and risks is important. Verbal instructions and written material should be provided to patients so they are not frightened by the red swelling after degarelix, nor family doctor prescribes antibiotics or order expensive scans.
- The antidepressant, citalopram, quetiapine and amiodarone are found in Lexi-Comp to have interaction with GnRH antagonist and agonist due to prolongation of QT interval in electrocardiogram (ECG) [59]. Patients who cannot change to sertraline, another antidepressant without drug interaction, can be monitored with ECG, although there is no formal recommendation of frequency of ECG.
- Even when the testosterone is at castrate level (testosterone <0.69 ng/L) with degarelix monotherapy at the time of PSA relapse, adding antiandrogen to degarelix can still lower the PSA.
- When patients have mild urinary obstruction, degarelix can help to avoid procedure of stent or nephrostomy [60]. But if the hydronephrosis is severe, degarelix will not help and the procedure should be performed soon without waiting for degarelix response.
- When switching from a combination of LHRH analog and anti-androgen, PSA was less likely to respond with degarelix alone and hence it will be more efficient, without any time delay to switch to combined degarelix and anti-androgen.

Degarelix has less risk of thrombosis, skeletal-related events, better FSH, PSA, and cancer control than GnRH analogs. There are many potential advantages of degarelix over GnRH analog:

- Compared to leuprolide, it provides a better control of the bone formation marker serum alkaline phosphatase (ALP) in patients with metastatic disease [61].
- Pickles *et al.* (2012) described the problem of incomplete testosterone suppression with GnRH agonists: the risk of a breakthrough > 32 ng/dL (1.1 nmol/L) was 6.6%, and > 50 ng/dL (1.7 nmol/L) was 3.4% [62]. Repeated breakthroughs occurred in 16% of patients. The 5-year biochemical no evidence

of disease (bNED) duration was inferior in those with breakthroughs of 1.1 – 1.7 nmol/L *versus* those without (58% *vs* 73%, respectively; $P = 0.048$).

- Tombal *et al.* (2005) also reported that about 5% to 17% patients on GnRH agonists fail to achieve a castrate testosterone level of 50 ng/dL (1.7 nmol/L) or less [63]. These are clinically relevant as there is a relationship between testosterone suppression and androgen-independent progression: breakthrough testosterone increases predict decreased progression-free survival (PFS) [64].

WHAT ARE THE SECOND LINE ADT?

Most prostate cancer cells either die or go into a dormant phase when the blood level of the male hormone, called testosterone, and its far more potent derivative, called dihydrotestostrone, are dramatically lowered. This phase of so-called "androgen-dependent" prostate cancer can be quite variable, lasting from only a few months to as long as 20 years.

In the second phase of hormonal treatment, the tumor can grow even though the male hormone level is low. During this phase, the tumor cells still can be controlled by discontinuing some drugs that were being taken previously or by switching to a different drug. This administration and withdrawal of hormones is called secondary hormonal therapy.

The principle behind secondary hormonal therapy is that while the patient is taking a hormone (such as bicalutamide) that blocks the growth of the cancer, the cancer cells can mutate or change in a way that actually make the bicalutamide stimulate their growth rather than suppress it. In this situation, simply stopping the bicalutamide can have a beneficial withdrawal effect and may lower the PSA for a period of 3 to 9 months in 20% to 50% of cases.

After a while, the PSA will again begin to rise. When this rise occurs, other similar drugs of the antiandrogen family, such as flutamide, nilutamide, or megestrol, may be started, and the PSA may again decrease for a period of time. If the cancer cells again mutate and become stimulated to grow by the new drug, the new drug may be stopped and again, in some cases, the PSA will again decrease.

In the old days, we could sometimes use a variety of drugs, switching from one to another, to achieve possibly an additional response. When antiandrogen drugs no longer work, it is possible in some cases, to achieve additional responses with other hormonal agents, such as stilphostrol (diethylstilbesterol diphosphate), or estrogens. However, nowadays with more potent second line ADT, we do not need to do these switches if the health care system can afford the more expensive new drugs.

Ketoconazole is an inhibitor of androgen synthesis and require the additional use of cortisone-like medications, because they suppress the production of cortisol by the adrenal glands. The typical dose of ketoconazole is 200mg increasing to 400mg three time per day alone or combine with prednisone.

Megestrol acetate 160 mg per day is another choice. It should be avoided in patients with heart disease, high blood pressure, or diabetes. Another second line ADT is glucocorticoids: prednisone 5 mg twice daily. Prednisone can be combined with abiraterone, mitoxantrone, docetaxel and sunitinib [65] as in Cancer Care Ontario guidelines [66].

Castrate-Resistant Prostate Cancer (CRPC)

Many men on ADT eventually will have biochemical, radiographic, and/or symptomatic progression despite conventionally defined castrate levels of testosterone (<50 ng/ml or <1.7 nmol/L) [67]. This state is now referred to as castration-resistant prostate cancer (CRPC) [68]. Some of them only have biochemical recurrence. Other patients have metastases and are further divided into asymptomatic or symptomatic.

The great majority of patients do not develop symptoms of metastatic prostate cancer (such as pain or weight loss) until the PSA has reached a level of 100 to 300. Some patients with very advanced disease have PSA levels in the thousands and yet have little symptoms from our experience. Each tumor is somewhat unique in its behavior, as is each patient. Measurement of PSA levels is the best way of determining the response of therapy. In general, if the PSA level can be decreased by 50%, survival is usually prolonged. A few agents are effective for CRPC patients [69, 70].

Even after prostate cancer cells reach the stage at which they are no longer responsive to hormone therapy, they still may be sensitive to treatment with radiation (including radium-223 [71, 72] and strontium-89), chemotherapy (docetaxel, cabazitaxel), enzalutamide, abiraterone or experimental drugs [73].

TRAPEZE is a British randomised study of 757 patients on effectiveness and cost of chemotherapy with zoledronic acid, strontium-89, or both, on bony mCRPC [74]. None of the arms improved overall survival. Strontium-89 costs more than zoledronic acid. The generic form of zoledronic acid costs only 1/5 of the Zometa (brand name) in Britain, and is favored in Canada as well for the similar reason. Zoledronic acid, but not strontium-89 significantly decreased skeletal-related events to only two-third compared with those not given zoledronic acid [75].

A few of our patients developed pancytopenia after four milli-curies, the standard dose of strontium-89 and became transfusion dependent. Zoledronic acid is easily monitored with calcium and renal function.

For CRPC, biopsy is indicated to detect any neuroendocrine or dedifferentiation that supports the use of cisplatin and etoposide. The specimen can be subjected to next-generation and whole exome sequencing, by which breast cancer gene 2 (BRCA2) and other DNA damage repair gene alterations are detected more frequently [76].

Ketoconazole (Nizoral) Plus Steroid

It is an antifungal agent which inhibits adrenal androgen production and hence it is active as salvage treatment for prostate cancer. Later more effective drugs were found, see below. The typical dose is 200 to 400 mg three times per day. Patients may have nausea and vomiting within a few hours of administration. Rash, fatigue and generalized weakness are the other side effects. Nowadays it is used only if the newer drugs below are not available for symptomatic mCRPC with good performance status and previous docetaxel chemotherapy.

Enzalutamide (Xtandi)

This second-generation androgen receptor (AR) antagonist was called MDV3100 before. It directly binds to the AR thus blocking the androgen. It also blocks translocation of the AR complex in the nucleus and the binding of the complex to the deoxyribonucleic acid (DNA), resulting in apoptosis and slowing down cancer growth. In contrast to other anti-androgens (*e.g.* bicalutamide), enzalutamide does not act as a partial AR agonist [77]. The other advantage is not requiring the co-administration of steroid.

The AFFIRM study showed that 1199 patients with mCRPC after first line docetaxel and given enzalutamide had a median survival of 18.4 months compared to 13.6 months in the placebo group, *i.e.* overall survival gain of 4.8 months [78]. The androgen receptor inhibitor is approved for use in the salvage setting for castrate resistant prostate cancer who failed docetaxel.

This is followed by the PREVAIL study on 1717 chemotherapy-naïve patients with mCRPC had a median overall survival of 35.3 months with enzalutamide, compared to 31.3 months with placebo, *i.e.* overall survival gain of 4 months [79, 80]. Enzalutamide significantly improves radiographic progression-free survival of patients with or without nodal or visceral disease, low or high volume bone metastases. It is also well tolerated by patients [81]. It is effective in elderly aged 75 years or older [82] although patients should be warned about a higher risk of falls. It also delays the commencement of chemotherapy which is more toxic and inconvenient than the oral enzalutamide.

Currently PR17 (ENZAMET) trial tests its use in initial ADT combined with total androgen blockade in metastatic prostate cancer [83]. Chemotherapy use is up to the investigators. International sites open so far include America, Canada, United Kingdom, Ireland, Australia, New Zealand. Accrual is completed in spring 2017. The typical dose is 160 mg to be taken orally once daily. Its main side effects are seizures (0.9%), fatigue (39.7%), and diarrhea (26.6%) [84, 85]. Therefore it should not be used in patients with a high risk or a history of seizure.

Abiraterone (Zytiga, Abiratas, Abretone, Abirapro)

It is a CYP17A1 inhibitor that decreases androgen production. The typical dose of abiraterone is 1000 mg plus prednisone 5 mg twice daily by mouth [86, 87]. The first study is COU-AA-301 on its beneficial use of 1195 mCRPC patients with prior docetaxel [86]. The TTP, PFS and OS are all increased. The second study of COU-AA-301 involved 1088 mCRPC patients without prior chemotherapy [88]. The updated analysis of COU-AA-302 confirms the safety of abiraterone [89].

At PSA progression on abiraterone and prednisone, up to 40% patients have a durable PSA response when switched to oral dexamethasone 0.5 mg daily [90]. Table **1** helps clinicians to select patients for enzalutamide or abiraterone as recently discussed in the Annual Canadian Urological Association of June 2016 [91].

TAK-700 (Orteronel)

2353 patients on the ELM-PC 4 study were randomized to TAK-700 with prednisone *versus* placebo with prednisone [92]. Only the radiographic progression-free interval was significantly increased but not overall survival. It is associated with 17% risk of increase in lipase, 10% risk of increased amylase and pancreatitis. It is no longer being developed as treatment for CRPC. The RTOG 1115 study of ADT and dose-escalated radiotherapy with or without TAK-700 as neoadjuvant treatment had been closed also [93].

WHAT ARE THE CONTROVERSIES OF ADT?

Hormonal therapy has a few controversies. First is whether a combined blockade of male hormones from the testicles and those from the adrenal glands is better than just blocking the hormones from the testicles only. Hormones from the testicles are responsible for more than 90% of male hormones in the body. We shall examine the evidence that combined blockade is slightly more effective and in which subgroups of cancer patients.

Another area of controversy is related to the timing of treatment, *i.e.*, whether hormonal therapy should be given early *versus* later when there are documented metastases or related symptoms. In the past several studies with limitations in design have shown no advantage for early hormonal therapy; however, recently a survival advantage was found for early treatment in selected men with prostate cancer.

Next is the controversy of intermittent *versus* continuous hormonal therapy. The advantage of intermittent hormonal therapy is that it gives the patient "holidays" to recover from the adverse side effects of continuous hormonal therapy. However it is argued that testosterone recovery in the non-treatment interval is less than expected and so does the improvement in quality of life. The great majority of patients respond to intermittent hormonal therapy. Recent randomized trials show that a selected group of patients benefit the most (please see section on intermittent ADT for details).

The last controversy is the cardiovascular side effects of ADT. Does it matter? Do patients die from it instead of prostate cancer? In other words is the treatment worse than the disease. The reader can go to the respective sections of the controversies.

Maximum Androgen Blockade (MAB)

This is achieved by a combination of orchiectomy or LHRH agonist/antagonist with anti-androgen, so called total/maximum androgen blockade (TAB/MAB). The National Cancer Institute Intergroup protocol 0036, which is the largest cooperative study to date of patients with advanced prostatic cancer, showed that combination therapy with leuprolide and flutamide *versus* leuprolide alone offered greater benefit in both time to disease progression and median survival while circumventing tumor flare and its associated symptoms [94]. The subgroup of good performance status, minimal disease subset particularly benefit from the total androgen blockade *versus* leuprolide alone. Thus, combination therapy for total androgen ablation becomes an important treatment option for adjuvant and salvage treatment. However, some may choose to use monotherapy due to expense, side effects and some published studies of flutamide showing no extra benefit to total androgen blockade [95, 96].

There are two European Organization for Research and Treatment of Cancer (EORTC) studies which tested maximal androgen blockade (MAB) *versus* orchiectomy: 30843 and 30853. EORTC 30843 randomized patients with advanced, metastatic prostate cancer to a combination of the LHRH agonist buserelin (nasal spray) and cyproterone acetate, either continuously or only during the first 2 weeks, compared with orchiectomy. Cyproterone was used to prevent flare response from buserelin and hot flashes. The three arms showed no difference in response rate, time to progression (subjective and objective) and survival [97, 98]. On the other hand, EORTC 30853 showed that patients with advanced, metastatic prostate cancer on goserelin plus flutamide lived significantly longer than those given orchiectomy alone [99, 100]. It was deduced that the survival advantage of MAB in EORTC 30853 was limited to patients with a good prognosis - 164/302 (54%) of the patients) [101]. While in EORTC 30843, only 93/337 patients (28%) had a good prognosis so there were insufficient number statistically to show and difference, *i.e.* patients in EORTC 30843 tend to have a worse prognosis than patients in EORTC 30853.

Individual data from 22 randomized studies of 5710 patients was analyzed by the Prostate Cancer Trialists' Collaborative Group was published in 2010 [102].The results for cyproterone acetate, used in 1/5 of all patients, was somewhat discouraging when used for maximum androgen blockade (MAB). The 5-year survival MAB was 15.4% *vs* 18.1% for androgen suppression (logrank 2p=0.04). In the literature, MAB is associated with a better medium overall survival & disease-free survival in the subgroup without symptoms and with minimal bone metastases (<5 total number of metastases, PSA <100 ng/L, testosterone <300 ng/mL or 3.4 nmol/L) and good performance status, compared with orchiectomy or LHRH alone [103].

Within the class of non-steroidal anti-androgens, the ligand-independent activation is inhibited to different extent. Over the last three decades, more than 27 clinical trials have addressed the benefit of MAB *versus* monotherapy. Most of these trials have evaluated flutamide or nilutamide. The Prostate Cancer Trialists' Collaborative Group meta-analysis suggested a modest survival benefit of MAB with a 3%-5% mortality reduction at 5 years [104]. The Cochrane Collaborative Review Group on Prostate Diseases demonstrated a 3.7 to 7 months absolute increase in survival duration by MAB [105]. MAB with bicalutamide results in 20% less risk of death than monotherapy so it is more effective. In prostate cancer patients at high risk for mortality (based on extent of disease or prostate-specific antigen kinetics), combination therapy with bicalutamide should be considered in preference to monotherapy. The Prostate Cancer Trialists' Collaborative Group meta-analysis also showed that MAB with steroidal anti-androgen (cyproterone acetate) decreases survival than monotherapy.

Adverse side effects are more common with combined blockade, and any advantage must be balanced against the potential for increased costs and side effects, like hot flashes, thromboembolism, and diarrhea.

Timing of ADT

Neoadjuvant ADT and Radiotherapy

The issue of timing of ADT with respect to radiotherapy was tested in the previously described RTOG trial 9413, in which 1323 men with clinically localized disease and an estimated risk of nodal metastases of at least 15 percent were randomly assigned to whole pelvic (WPRT) or prostate alone RT [106 - 108]. All men were then further randomized to neoadjuvant plus concurrent ADT (goserelin or leuprolide plus flutamide) administered for two months before and during RT (four months total), or adjuvant ADT with the same drugs given for the same length of time, but only after the completion of RT. The majority of enrolled men had T2c or higher stage disease, a serum PSA <30 ng/mL, and a Gleason score of 7 or higher (thus, they would fall into the intermediate-risk and high-risk categories). With a median follow-up of 59 months from treatment completion, when all four treatment arms were compared, men undergoing WPRT plus neoadjuvant and concurrent RT had a significant progression-free survival advantage. In the subset of men with intermediate risk disease (PSA <30 ng/mL and Gleason score 7 to 10 or PSA >=30, Gleason score 2 to 6) undergoing WPRT, those receiving neoadjuvant and concurrent RT had a significantly higher four-year progression-free survival rate (64 *versus* 49 percent, p = 0.014) compared to men receiving adjuvant ADT. There was no advantage to short-term neoadjuvant as compared to adjuvant ADT in those undergoing prostate only RT. These data suggest a favorable biologic interaction between WPRT and short-term neoadjuvant ADT.

Another RTOG study 9910 showed that 8 and 28 weeks of ADT prior to radiotherapy have no difference in cause-specific or overall survival rates [109]. Therefore 8 weeks of neoadjuvant ADT is still the standard of care in North America.

Total Duration of ADT with Radiotherapy

The EORTC 22863 used three years of ADT after completion of radiotherapy with a 5-year overall survival of 79%, compared to only 63% in the radiotherapy alone arm.

Another EORTC study compared 6 months *versus* 3 years showed that the shorter treatment duration has inferior survival outcome [110]. ADT was started on the same day of radiotherapy in EORTC study. The timing of ADT is different in America where it is given as a neoadjuvant treatment of two months then extended after radiotherapy as an adjuvant treatment. Another difference is the total duration of ADT.

RTOG study 9202 used ADT for two years after external beam radiotherapy and 5-year overall survival was 80% compared to 69% for radiotherapy alone arm. A practical point is that in Europe, the lack of prostate cancer screening resulted in a higher disease burden than the Americans who have opportunistic PSA screening by family doctors. In the clinic, we tend to use a longer duration, i.e. 3years for those patients with palpable bulky disease.

Our interpretation is that previous studies did not use dose-escalated radiotherapy with intensity-modulated technique, *e.g.* RTOG 8531 [111]. The conclusion of the optimal duration of ADT is still unanswered in the setting of dose-escalated radiotherapy.

Early Versus Late ADT for Metastatic Prostate Cancer

The National Cancer Institute (NCI) study [112] suggested that early total androgen blockade may be advantageous to delayed treatment for patients with metastatic prostate cancer. An analogy can be drawn between patients who have rising PSA after failure of the primary treatment and it is possible that early treatment may improve survival but we need randomized trials to confirm this suggestion.

Prostate cancer is an androgen-dependent tumor and deprivation of androgen hormone has been the mainstay in the management of patients with distant metastases. Despite an initial response rate of about 80%, predictable and irreversible resistance to androgen deprivation will occur in the vast majority of patients. This progression from initial response is attributed to the fact that surviving tumor cells become androgen-independent [113].

Most of the older studies favor earlier start of ADT but the delayed or observation arm were given ADT until really late. The British Medical Research Council randomized 938 patients with locally advanced or asymptomatic metastatic disease, found that the deferred group had more complications like urinary obstruction, pathological fractures [114]. Similarly, Messing *et al.* in the updated report of 98 patients with median follow-up of 11.9 years found benefit of immediate ADT by orchiectomy or LHRH analog in node-positive prostate cancer patients after prostatectomy and node dissection compared to deferred group till distant metastases or symptomatic recurrence [115]. In addition, EORTC 30891 showed a modest benefit from immediate ADT for patients with T0-4 N0-2 M0 prostate cancer [116]. At a longer median follow-up of 12.8 years, deferred ADT has a significantly worse overall survival, hazard ratio of 1.21 than deferred ADT. However the time to hormone-resistance between the two groups are the same [117].

In contrast to the above, the Population data of Cancer of the Prostate Strategic Urologic Research Endeavour (CaPSURE) study did not demonstrate any survival difference between those who commence ADT within 3 months of PSA relapse *versus* deferred until metastases, symptoms or shortening of PSA doubling time (PSAD) [118]. For elderly patients who do not have curative local treatment, early ADT has a better TTP, CSS but similar OS than delayed ADT [119]. The author concluded that deferred ADT can avoid side effects. The urologist Walsh, *et al.* favors delayed ADT due to cost and complications [120].

In an opinion statement from Hussain *et al.*, early ADT upon the diagnosis of metastatic prostate cancer is recommended as the standard practice. This can decrease complications like spinal cord compression [121]. For non-metastatic patients, it is better to start ADT early for aggressive disease in terms of fast doubling time, or bulky disease.

Intermittent ADT (IHT)

Intermittent androgen deprivation therapy has been studied in animal models. In the androgen-dependent tumour models, investigators found that apoptosis could be re-induced and that this approach prolonged, indeed almost tripled, the mean time to androgen-independent status [122, 123].

Currently there is increasing evidence suggesting that progression to androgen-independence is an adaptive process secondary to androgen withdrawal. In studying mechanisms of progression, Bruchovsky found that, in the androgen-dependent *shionogi* carcinoma model, androgen withdrawal alters the ratio of stem cells in the tumor cell population [124]. Initially there is an elimination of differentiated cells and a decrease in the proportion of tumourigenic stem cell. At the time of progression and recurrence a marked 20-fold increase in the proportion of total stem cells and 500-fold increase in the proportion of androgen-independent stem cells was noted. These data suggest that progression begins early in the disease course secondary to lack of androgen-induced differentiation of the parent stem cells with resultant loss of apoptotic potential [124]. If androgens are replaced before progression begins, the surviving stem cells should give rise to an androgen-dependent tumor susceptible to further hormonal manipulation [124].

Clinical data indicates that a satisfactory palliative response can be achieved in patients who have restarted androgen deprivation therapy following a period without any therapy. Prolonged therapy-free intervals of several months could be achieved without apparent adverse effect on survival [125]. This experience in metastatic disease is utilized in the salvage treatment of rising PSA after failure of the primary treatment. It is understood that this salvage treatment is not curative but its use is justified because many of these patients are elderly, and salvage prostatectomy or brachytherapy or cryotherapy has severe treatment morbidity.

In addition, despite the most advanced imaging techniques, it is possible these patients may have micro-metastases in the lymph nodes or distant organs. The intermittent androgen deprivation approach is meant to provide treatment to control the tumor, with a potential for prolonged therapy-free intervals resulting in improved quality of life, delay in progression to androgen independence, and reduced cost of therapy. Additionally, the men may gain relief from distressing side effects, especially hot flashes, and to regain potency.

The duration of induction therapy is crucial for the success of this approach. The induction duration should be the time required for maximal tumor suppression as represented by PSA nadirs. Current data indicates that 50-80% of metastatic patients will achieve a nadir PSA by 3-8 months following hormonal therapy [126 - 128].

For non-metastatic disease, a phase III study of the National Cancer Institute of Canada (PR.7) IHT was non-inferior to continuous therapy with respect to overall survival [129]. IHT is not advisable for highly aggressive cancer (Gleason 8-10, PDA doubling time <6 months). Induction ADT can be given as 3-9 months of gonadotrophin-releasing antagonist alone or LHRH analog plus bicalutamide 50 mg daily for 10 days (1 day before and 9 days after). By the end of the induction period, the PSA level usually falls to <4 ng/mL, then the ADT can be held. The cycle is repeated when PSA rises back to 10 ng/mL. One will observe that the cycle lengths get shorter and shorter. By the time patient can be off treatment for < 6 months, he should be put on continuous ADT. We recommend measuring the PSA every 2-3 months.

For metastatic prostate cancer, continuous ADT remains the standard of care. The South-West Oncology Group study (INT-0162/SWOG-9346/NCIC PR.8) survival of patients on IHT is not comparable to continuous therapy as the confidence interval of survival cross the upper boundary of non-inferiority [130]. In metastatic hormone-sensitive prostate cancer, Hussain *et al.* found that after 6-7 months of induction ADT, the median survivals were 75, 44 and 13 months if PSA fell to <=0.2, >0.2-4 and > 4 ng/mL, respectively [131]. In the study the trigger to start another cycle of ADT was PSA rising back to 20m ng/mL or more.

Recovery of Testosterone in Intermittent ADT

After 6 months of luteinizing hormone-releasing hormone (LHRH) analogue treatment, 90% of patients had a normalization of testosterone level within 18 weeks [132]. A median 12.9 weeks was needed for recovery of testosterone above castrate level, and older patients needed more time for recovery. Therefore the quality of life improvement for intermittent ADT is less than expected.

More Cardiovascular Complications with IHT- A Surprise

Bone, endocrine and cognitive complications are not significantly reduced by IHT in the S9346 study [133]. There is significantly more 10-year cumulative incidence of ischemic and thrombotic events: 24% for continuous and 33% for IHT (P = 0.02). Each time the LHRH agonist is started, T-cells are activated and promote destabilization of vascular plaque.

SIDE EFFECTS OF ADT

Possible side effects of hormonal therapy [134] include hot flashes (that can be treated with megestrol acetate, cyproterone acetate, gabapentin, and venlafaxine), osteoporosis and fractures, sexual dysfunction, increased body fat (11%), decreased muscle mass (4%), adverse changes in cholesterol and triglycerides, increased fasting blood glucose and hemoglobin A1c with an increased risk for diabetes, changes in arterial compliance with an increased risk of heart attack, breast enlargement with some medications that have estrogen or progesterone-like properties (this side-effect can be minimized by pre-treatment irradiation of the breasts, tamoxifen, or surgery), dry skin, dry eyes, hair loss, anemia, loss of energy, cognitive dysfunction, depression, and vertigo.

Individual drugs have their specific side effects. For instance, flutamide can cause diarrhea and liver dysfunction while nilutamide can cause visual problems and interstitial pneumonia. Casodex hepatotoxicity has been reported [135]. Therefore routine monitoring of liver function test is necessary. When the transaminases are two times of normal, they should be stopped.

Cardiovascular Toxicity

ADT increases the risk of cardiovascular disease and thromboembolism [136], especially for those with baseline problem already [137]. Significantly more cardiovascular events are seen in retrospective studies but not randomized studies. A speculation is that randomized studies select patients with lesser co-morbidities, including cardiovascular risks. The question is whether there is excessive death from cardiovascular toxicity than cancer death. So far the benefit of the combined ADT and radiotherapy for high-risk patients outweighs the risk. To prevent cardiovascular events, oral daily aspirin 81 mg is recommended by cardiologists. We also encourage communication between oncologists and cardiologists to facilitate multidisciplinary care.

Gynecomastia

Men starting long-term ADT can receive prophylactic RT to both breast buds within first month, 8Gy in 1 treatment using orthovoltage or electron. Another alternative is prophylactic tamoxifen 20 mg/d which does not appear to affect disease control based on PSA suppression [138].

Osteoporosis and Fractures

Osteoporosis is common in prostate cancer patients receiving long-term continuous hormonal therapy, especially slender white men, men with positive family history of osteoporosis, and men taking steroids. There is a 5- to 10- fold increased loss of bone during first year of treatment. Dual energy x-ray absorptiometry of the hip is the gold-standard diagnostic test for measuring bone loss.

Smoking and alcohol cessation, weight bearing exercise, vitamin D3 and calcium supplements are also helpful in preventing osteoporosis. Monitoring of bone densitometry is advisable with baseline which determines subsequent frequency according to national guidelines [139]. If the patient is at moderate risk of bone fracture in 10 years, the on-going ADT should be taken into account.

Patients with moderate to high risk of fracture in 10 years should be put on oral bisphosphonates (*e.g.* clodronate [140, 141], etidronate, alendronate). After dental consultation to avoid future risk of osteonecrosis of the jaw, intravenous zoledronic acid can prevent osteoporosis even when given yearly [142] but is not funded for such indication in Canada. It improves the bone mineral study results [143]. Typical dose is 4 mg intravenously every 3-4 weeks with dose reduction according to creatinine clearance. Unfortunately so far no survival benefit of zoledronic acid has been found in studies. Bisphosponates are funded in Canada for mCRPC to decrease skeletal events including need for radiotherapy, and spinal cord compression. It must be used with caution in patients who had extensive dental work, as it can cause deterioration of the jawbone, called osteonecrosis of the mandible.

WHAT WOULD PATIENTS ASK THEIR DOCTOR?

“How long can I live?” is the most common question we heard in the clinic. Within 5 years of initial diagnosis, about 1/10 to 1/5 of men will progress to metastatic castration-resistant prostate cancer [144]. Patients with node-positive disease treated with ADT and radiotherapy has a 10-year overall survival of about 50% [108]. For hormone-naïve patients with bone metastases in the past, the median time to progression with bilateral orchiectomy or medical castration is 12-

18 months, and the median time to survival is 24-36 months. Nowadays results from randomized studies achieved an overall survival of 57.6 to 65 months with ADT+6 cycles of docetaxel. For non-metastatic castrate resistant prostate cancer (CRPC) patients treated with palliative radiotherapy >40 Gy, the median survival is 48 months [145]. For metastatic CRPC patients, the median survival is 15 months with cabazitaxel or abiraterone, *i.e.* a gain of around 4 months compared to those without the drug [86, 146].

"How expensive are those drugs?" is also a very first common question. The answer will depend on the country, health coverage and negotiated price. In Canada, it is covered in the universal Medicare system.

"Will I become a woman?" is perhaps the next most common question. The patient may have less male baldness, gynecomastia, less body hair, smaller testes but the voice will remain the same.

FUTURE RESEARCH

Areas of future study include androgen receptor signaling pathway, tumor biomarkers, genetic mutation, follicular stimulating hormone, early use of second or third line drugs, proper sequencing of ADT and chemotherapy, etc.

Androgen Receptor Signaling Pathway

Molecular profiling may help to select the best therapy for a particular patient. One example is the androgen-receptor splice variant 7 (AR-V7), a truncated receptor with missing the C-terminus, which carries the ligand binding domain. AR-V7 can either hetero- or homo-dimerize with other androgen-receptor splice variants, and has activity even in the absence of androgens to produce messenger ribonucleic acid (mRNA). Circulating tumor cells expressing AR-V7 have no response to abiraterone or enzalutamide [147].

Third-generation AR-targeting agents at early stage of development are galeterone, ODM-204, and EPI-506. Galeterone and ODM-204 both target the androgen receptor and also prevent the biosynthesis of androgens, *i.e.* combined inhibitive effects of enzalutamide plus abiraterone. In addition galeterone can also degrade the androgen receptor. Therefore they could be more effective than monotherapy abiraterone or enzalutamide.

Open-label phase I and II studies: Androgen Receptor Modulation Optimized for Response-1 (ARMOR1) and ARMOR2 were performed in treatment-naive nonmetastatic or metastatic CRPC [148]. Galeterone was then hypothesized to be more effective against prostate cancer cells with AR-V7. The phase 3 trial,

ARMOR-3 randomized treatment-naïve mCPRC patients with AR-V7 to either galeterone or enzalutamide [149]. Unfortunately the trial was discontinued due to lack of radiographic progression-free survival improvement with galeterone, compared to enzalutamide.

ODM-204 inhibits both CYP17A1 and AR. It has demonstrated efficacy in animal models and the first clinical trial is currently underway in England [150].

Genetic Mutation

A landmark paper in 2015 demonstrated an 88% response rate to olaparib in patients with DNA-repair defects, including BRCA2 [151]. Poly adenosine diphosphate ribose polymerase (PARP) inhibitors are very effective in prostate cancer with BRCA1 and 2 mutations [152]. More studies are needed in future for poly-ADP ribose polymerase (PARP) inhibitors, platinum agents, and other double strand break-inducing DNA damaging agents in patients with DNA-repair alterations.

Prostate cancers can also adapt the PI3K/AKT pathway and become resistant to ADT. Researches on targeting both AR and PI3K/AKT signaling may lead to a breakthrough. There is a published study to elucidate the effect of PI3K/AKT inhibitors on the expressions of full length AR (AR-FL) and its splice variant (AR-V7) [153]. It alters AR gene transcription initiation and RNA splicing.

CONCLUSIONS

Neoadjuvant hormonal therapy can improve disease-free survival and local control when given before RT; it has only decreased positive surgical margins when given prior to radical prostatectomy. Although hormonal therapy given immediately after either radical prostatectomy or radiation therapy is highly effective, the side effects of persistent long-term use must be weighed for each patient.

Hormonal therapy has been considered to be the standard treatment at the time of cancer progression after definitive therapy, and many of the randomised trials have essentially compared adjuvant therapy to delayed therapy. Historical trials using adjuvant hormonal therapy have been limited due to difficulties in clinical staging, as well as toxicities attributed to the formulations used. More recently, hormonal therapy has been found to delay disease progression, increase disease-free survival, and decrease morbidity and mortality when given immediately after prostatectomy or radiation therapy in selected patients.

Practice changing discussion in this reviews include: (1) gonadotrophin-releasing hormone antagonist has better survival and our experience is shared, (2) increased thromboembolism with intermittent hormonal therapy, and (3) no survival benefit of zoledronic acid has been found in studies. The recommendation is for use in mCRPC only to prevent skeletal events like pathological fracture, and spinal cord compression.

CONFLICT OF INTEREST

The authors confirm that they have no conflict of interest to declare for this publication.

ACKNOWLEDGEMENTS

Declared none.

REFERENCES

[1] Huggins C, Stevens RE Jr, Hodges CV. The effect of castration on advanced carcinoma of the prostate gland. Arch Surg 1941; 43: 209. [http://dx.doi.org/10.1001/archsurg.1941.01210140043004]

[2] Fialova B, Luzna P, Gursky J, Langova K, Kolar Z, Trtkova KS. Epigenetic modulation of AR gene expression in prostate cancer DU145 cells with the combination of sodium butyrate and 5-Aza-2-deoxycytidine. Oncol Rep 2016; 36(4): 2365-74. [PMID: 27499010]

[3] Gormley GJ. Chemoprevention strategies for prostate cancer: the role of 5 alpha-reductase inhibitors. J Cell Biochem Suppl 1992; 16H: 113-7. [http://dx.doi.org/10.1002/jcb.240501226] [PMID: 1283894]

[4] Feigl P, Blumenstein B, Thompson I, *et al.* Design of the Prostate Cancer Prevention Trial (PCPT). Control Clin Trials 1995; 16(3): 150-63. [http://dx.doi.org/10.1016/0197-2456(94)00XXX-M] [PMID: 7540965]

[5] Kaplan SA, Roehrborn CG, Meehan AG, *et al.* PCPT: Evidence that finasteride reduces risk of most frequently detected intermediate- and high-grade (Gleason score 6 and 7) cancer. Urology 2009; 73(5): 935-9. [http://dx.doi.org/10.1016/j.urology.2008.09.079] [PMID: 19328538]

[6] Unger JM, Till C, Thompson IM Jr, *et al.* Long-term Consequences of Finasteride *vs* Placebo in the Prostate Cancer Prevention Trial. J Natl Cancer Inst 2016; 108(12): djw168. [http://dx.doi.org/10.1093/jnci/djw168] [PMID: 27565902]

[7] Thompson IM Jr, Goodman PJ, Tangen CM, *et al.* Long-term survival of participants in the prostate cancer prevention trial. N Engl J Med 2013; 369(7): 603-10. [http://dx.doi.org/10.1056/NEJMoa1215932] [PMID: 23944298]

[8] Andriole GL, Bostwick DG, Brawley OW, *et al.* REDUCE Study Group. Effect of dutasteride on the risk of prostate cancer. N Engl J Med 2010; 362(13): 1192-202. [http://dx.doi.org/10.1056/NEJMoa0908127] [PMID: 20357281]

[9] Grubb RL, Andriole GL, Somerville MC, Mahoney C, Manyak MJ, Castro R. The REDUCE Follow-Up Study: low rate of new prostate cancer diagnoses observed during a 2-year, observational, followup study of men who participated in the REDUCE trial. J Urol 2013; 189(3): 871-7. [http://dx.doi.org/10.1016/j.juro.2012.09.099] [PMID: 23021996]

[10] Fleshner NE, Lucia MS, Egerdie B, *et al.* Dutasteride in localised prostate cancer management: the REDEEM randomised, double-blind, placebo-controlled trial. Lancet 2012; 379(9821): 1103-11. [http://dx.doi.org/10.1016/S0140-6736(11)61619-X] [PMID: 22277570]

[11] Ganzer CA, Jacobs AR, Iqbal F. Persistent sexual, emotional, and cognitive impairment post-finasteride: a survey of men reporting symptoms. Am J Men Health 2015; 9(3): 222-8. [http://dx.doi.org/10.1177/1557988314538445] [PMID: 24928450]

[12] Bolla M, Gonzalez D, Warde P, *et al.* Improved survival in patients with locally advanced prostate cancer treated with radiotherapy and goserelin. N Engl J Med 1997; 337(5): 295-300. [http://dx.doi.org/10.1056/NEJM199707313370502] [PMID: 9233866]

[13] Brundage M, Sydes MR, Parulekar WR, *et al.* Impact of radiotherapy when added to androgen-deprivation therapy for locally advanced prostate cancer: long-term quality-of-life outcomes from the NCIC CTG PR3/MRC PR07 randomized trial. J Clin Oncol 2015; 33(19): 2151-7. [http://dx.doi.org/10.1200/JCO.2014.57.8724] [PMID: 26014295]

[14] James ND, Spears MR, Clarke NW, *et al.* STAMPEDE Investigators. STAMPEDE Investigators. Failure-free survival and radiotherapy in patients with newly diagnosed nonmetastatic prostate cancer: data from patients in the control arm of the STAMPEDE trial. JAMA Oncol 2016; 2(3): 348-57. [http://dx.doi.org/10.1001/jamaoncol.2015.4350] [PMID: 26606329]

[15] Oesterling JE, Andrews PE, Suman VJ, Zincke H, Myers RP. Preoperative androgen deprivation therapy: artificial lowering of serum prostate specific antigen without downstaging the tumor. J Urol 1993; 149(4): 779-82. [PMID: 7681117]

[16] Van Poppel H, Ameye F, Oyen R, Van De Voorde W, Baert L. Neo-adjuvant hormonotherapy does not facilitate radical prostatectomy. Acta Urol Belg 1992; 60(3): 73-82. [PMID: 1492636]

[17] Monfette G, Dupont A, Labrie F, *et al.* Multiple advantages before and after radical prostatectomy with combined endocrine therapy. In: Altwein JE, Faul P, Schneider W, Eds. Incidental carcinoma of the prostate. Berlin: Springer 1991; pp. 246-53. [http://dx.doi.org/10.1007/978-3-642-76129-4_37]

[18] [1 December 2016]; Available at: https://www.rtog.org/ClinicalTrials/ProtocolTable

[19] Horwitz EM, Winter K, Hanks GE, Lawton CA, Russell AH, Machtay M. Subset analysis of RTOG 8531 and 8610 indicates an advantage for long-term *vs.* short-term adjuvant hormones for patients with locally advanced nonmetastatic prostate cancer treated with radiation therapy. Int J Radiat Oncol Biol Phys 2001; 49(4): 947-56. [http://dx.doi.org/10.1016/S0360-3016(00)01443-7] [PMID: 11240235]

[20] Stone NN, Stock RG, Unger P. Effects of neoadjuvant hormonal therapy on prostate biopsy results after (125)I and (103)Pd seed implantation. Mol Urol 2000; 4(3): 163-8.

[21] Gaudet M, Vigneault É, Foster W, Meyer F, Martin AG. Randomized non-inferiority trial of Bicalutamide and Dutasteride *versus* LHRH agonists for prostate volume reduction prior to I-125 permanent implant brachytherapy for prostate cancer. Radiother Oncol 2016; 118(1): 141-7.

[22] Herbert C, Morris WJ, Keyes M, *et al.* Outcomes following iodine-125 brachytherapy in patients with Gleason 7, intermediate risk prostate cancer: a population-based cohort study. Radiother Oncol 2012; 103(2): 228-32. [http://dx.doi.org/10.1016/j.radonc.2012.01.006] [PMID: 22326573]

[23] Denham JW, Joseph D, Lamb DS, *et al.* Short-term androgen suppression and radiotherapy *versus* intermediate-term androgen suppression and radiotherapy, with or without zoledronic acid, in men with locally advanced prostate cancer (TROG 03.04 RADAR): an open-label, randomised, phase 3 factorial trial. Lancet Oncol 2014; 15(10): 1076-89. [http://dx.doi.org/10.1016/S1470-2045(14)70328-6] [PMID: 25130995]

[24] Denham JW, Steigler A, Joseph D, *et al.* Radiation dose escalation or longer androgen suppression for locally advanced prostate cancer? Data from the TROG 03.04 RADAR trial. Radiother Oncol 2015; 115(3): 301-7.
[http://dx.doi.org/10.1016/j.radonc.2015.05.016] [PMID: 26072289]

[25] James ND, Sydes MR, Clarke NW, *et al.* STAMPEDE investigators. Addition of docetaxel, zoledronic acid, or both to first-line long-term hormone therapy in prostate cancer (STAMPEDE): survival results from an adaptive, multiarm, multistage, platform randomised controlled trial. Lancet 2016; 387(10024): 1163-77.
[http://dx.doi.org/10.1016/S0140-6736(15)01037-5] [PMID: 26719232]

[26] Sweeney CJ, Chen YH, Carducci M, *et al.* Chemohormonal therapy in metastatic hormone-sensitive prostate cancer. N Engl J Med 2015; 373(8): 737-46.
[http://dx.doi.org/10.1056/NEJMoa1503747] [PMID: 26244877]

[27] Smith MR, Halabi S, Ryan CJ, *et al.* Randomized controlled trial of early zoledronic acid in men with castration-sensitive prostate cancer and bone metastases: results of CALGB 90202 (alliance). J Clin Oncol 2014; 32(11): 1143-50.
[http://dx.doi.org/10.1200/JCO.2013.51.6500] [PMID: 24590644]

[28] Kimura T, Egawa S. Words of Wisdom. Re: Randomized controlled trial of early zoledronic acid in men with castration-sensitive prostate cancer and bone metastases: results of CALGB 90202 (Alliance). Eur Urol 2016; 69(4): 754-5.
[http://dx.doi.org/10.1016/j.eururo.2016.01.019] [PMID: 26972498]

[29] Wirth M, Tammela T, Cicalese V, *et al.* Prevention of bone metastases in patients with high-risk nonmetastatic prostate cancer treated with zoledronic acid: efficacy and safety results of the Zometa European Study (ZEUS). Eur Urol 2015; 67(3): 482-91.
[http://dx.doi.org/10.1016/j.eururo.2014.02.014] [PMID: 24630685]

[30] Edwards BJ, Usmani S, Raisch DW, *et al.* Acute kidney injury and bisphosphonate use in cancer: a report from the research on adverse drug events and reports (RADAR) project. J Oncol Pract 2013; 9(2): 101-6.
[http://dx.doi.org/10.1200/JOP.2011.000486] [PMID: 23814519]

[31] Lipton A, Fizazi K, Stopeck AT, *et al.* Superiority of denosumab to zoledronic acid for prevention of skeletal-related events: a combined analysis of 3 pivotal, randomised, phase 3 trials. Eur J Cancer 2012; 48(16): 3082-92.
[http://dx.doi.org/10.1016/j.ejca.2012.08.002] [PMID: 22975218]

[32] Heidenreich A, Bastian PJ, Bellmunt J, *et al.* European Association of Urology. EAU guidelines on prostate cancer. Part II: Treatment of advanced, relapsing, and castration-resistant prostate cancer. Eur Urol 2014; 65(2): 467-79.
[http://dx.doi.org/10.1016/j.eururo.2013.11.002] [PMID: 24321502]

[33] Smith MR, Saad F, Coleman R, *et al.* Denosumab and bone-metastasis-free survival in men with castration-resistant prostate cancer: results of a phase 3, randomised, placebo-controlled trial. Lancet 2012; 379(9810): 39-46.
[http://dx.doi.org/10.1016/S0140-6736(11)61226-9] [PMID: 22093187]

[34] Fizazi K, Carducci M, Smith M, *et al.* Denosumab *versus* zoledronic acid for treatment of bone metastases in men with castration-resistant prostate cancer: a randomised, double-blind study. Lancet 2011; 377(9768): 813-22.
[http://dx.doi.org/10.1016/S0140-6736(10)62344-6] [PMID: 21353695]

[35] Saad F. CUOG lecture: from diagnosis to death: optimizing outcomes in high-risk prostate cancer. Can Urol Assoc J 2016; 10(5-6): S1-1.

[36] Messing EM, Manola J, Sarosdy M, Wilding G, Crawford ED, Trump D. Immediate hormonal therapy compared with observation after radical prostatectomy and pelvic lymphadenectomy in men with node-positive prostate cancer. N Engl J Med 1999; 341(24): 1781-8.

[http://dx.doi.org/10.1056/NEJM199912093412401] [PMID: 10588962]

[37] Hu JC, Williams SB, OMalley AJ, Smith MR, Nguyen PL, Keating NL. Androgen-deprivation therapy for nonmetastatic prostate cancer is associated with an increased risk of peripheral arterial disease and venous thromboembolism. Eur Urol 2012; 61(6): 1119-28. [http://dx.doi.org/10.1016/j.eururo.2012.01.045] [PMID: 22336376]

[38] Burns-Cox N, Basketter V, Higgins B, Holmes S. Prospective randomised trial comparing diethylstilboestrol and flutamide in the treatment of hormone relapsed prostate cancer. Int J Urol 2002; 9(8): 431-4. [http://dx.doi.org/10.1046/j.1442-2042.2002.00495.x] [PMID: 12225339]

[39] Klotz L. Maximal androgen blockade for advanced prostate cancer. Best Pract Res Clin Endocrinol Metab 2008; 22(2): 331-40. [http://dx.doi.org/10.1016/j.beem.2008.01.004] [PMID: 18471790]

[40] Gomez JL, Dupont A, Cusan L, *et al.* Incidence of liver toxicity associated with the use of flutamide in prostate cancer patients. Am J Med 1992; 92(5): 465-70. [http://dx.doi.org/10.1016/0002-9343(92)90741-S] [PMID: 1349790]

[41] Wirth MP, See WA, McLeod DG, Iversen P, Morris T, Carroll K. Casodex Early Prostate Cancer Trialists Group. Bicalutamide 150 mg in addition to standard care in patients with localized or locally advanced prostate cancer: results from the second analysis of the early prostate cancer program at median followup of 5.4 years. J Urol 2004; 172(5 Pt 1): 1865-70. [http://dx.doi.org/10.1097/01.ju.0000140159.94703.80] [PMID: 15540740]

[42] Tyrrell CJ, Kaisary AV, Iversen P, *et al.* A randomised comparison of Casodex (bicalutamide) 150 mg monotherapy *versus* castration in the treatment of metastatic and locally advanced prostate cancer. Eur Urol 1998; 33(5): 447-56. [http://dx.doi.org/10.1159/000019634] [PMID: 9643663]

[43] [1 December 2016];2016 Available at: https://uroweb.org/guideline/prostate-cancer/

[44] [1 December 2016]; Available at: http://www.auanet.org/education/guidelines/prostate-cancer.cfm

[45] Tay MH, Kaufman DS, Regan MM, *et al.* Finasteride and bicalutamide as primary hormonal therapy in patients with advanced adenocarcinoma of the prostate. Ann Oncol 2004; 15(6): 974-8. [http://dx.doi.org/10.1093/annonc/mdh221] [PMID: 15151957]

[46] Lodde M, Lacombe L, Fradet Y. Salvage therapy with bicalutamide 150 mg in nonmetastatic castration-resistant prostate cancer. Urology 2010; 76(5): 1189-93. [http://dx.doi.org/10.1016/j.urology.2009.12.057] [PMID: 20303155]

[47] Joyce R, Fenton MA, Rode P, *et al.* High dose bicalutamide for androgen independent prostate cancer: effect of prior hormonal therapy. J Urol 1998; 159(1): 149-53. [http://dx.doi.org/10.1016/S0022-5347(01)64039-4] [PMID: 9400459]

[48] Kassouf W, Tanguay S, Aprikian AG. Nilutamide as second line hormone therapy for prostate cancer after androgen ablation fails. J Urol 2003; 169(5): 1742-4. [http://dx.doi.org/10.1097/01.ju.0000057795.97626.66] [PMID: 12686822]

[49] Seigneur J, Trechot PF, Hubert J, Lamy P. Pulmonary complications of hormone treatment in prostate carcinoma. Chest 1988; 93(5): 1106. [http://dx.doi.org/10.1378/chest.93.5.1106] [PMID: 3129240]

[50] Sartor AO, Tangen CM, Hussain MH, *et al.* Southwest Oncology Group. Antiandrogen withdrawal in castrate-refractory prostate cancer: a Southwest Oncology Group trial (SWOG 9426). Cancer 2008; 112(11): 2393-400. [http://dx.doi.org/10.1002/cncr.23473] [PMID: 18383517]

[51] Crawford ED. Challenges in the management of prostate cancer. Br J Urol 1992; 70 (Suppl. 1): 33-8. [http://dx.doi.org/10.1111/j.1464-410X.1992.tb15865.x] [PMID: 1467876]

[52] Sun M, Choueiri TK, Hamnvik OP, *et al.* Comparison of gonadotropin-releasing hormone agonists and orchiectomy of androgen-deprivation therapy. JAMA Oncol 2016; 2(4): 500-7. [http://dx.doi.org/10.1001/jamaoncol.2015.4917] [PMID: 26720632]

[53] Klotz L, Boccon-Gibod L, Shore ND, *et al.* The efficacy and safety of degarelix: a 12-month, comparative, randomized, open-label, parallel-group phase III study in patients with prostate cancer. BJU Int 2008; 102(11): 1531-8. [http://dx.doi.org/10.1111/j.1464-410X.2008.08183.x] [PMID: 19035858]

[54] Crawford ED, Tombal B, Miller K, *et al.* A phase III extension trial with a 1-arm crossover from leuprolide to degarelix: comparison of gonadotropin-releasing hormone agonist and antagonist effect on prostate cancer. J Urol 2011; 186(3): 889-97. [http://dx.doi.org/10.1016/j.juro.2011.04.083] [PMID: 21788033]

[55] Crawford ED, Shore ND, Moul JW, *et al.* Long-term tolerability and efficacy of degarelix: 5-year results from a phase III extension trial with a 1-arm crossover from leuprolide to degarelix. Urology 2014; 83(5): 1122-8. [http://dx.doi.org/10.1016/j.urology.2014.01.013] [PMID: 24661333]

[56] Albertsen PC, Klotz L, Tombal B, Grady J, Olesen TK, Nilsson J. Cardiovascular morbidity associated with gonadotropin releasing hormone agonists and an antagonist. Eur Urol 2014; 65(3): 565-73. [http://dx.doi.org/10.1016/j.eururo.2013.10.032] [PMID: 24210090]

[57] Klotz L, Miller K, Crawford ED, *et al.* Disease control outcomes from analysis of pooled individual patient data from five comparative randomised clinical trials of degarelix *versus* luteinising hormone-releasing hormone agonists. Eur Urol 2014; 66(6): 1101-8. [http://dx.doi.org/10.1016/j.eururo.2013.12.063] [PMID: 24440304]

[58] Sadikov E, Dubey A, Amjad A, *et al.* Real world experience of degarelix: a gonadotropin-releasing hormone antagonist in prostate cancer.

[59] [2 February 2017]; Available at: http://www.uptodate.com/crlsql/interact/frameset.jsp

[60] Tai P, Amjad A, Koul R, Sadikov E, Dubey A. Luteinizing hormone-releasing hormone antagonists for urinary obstruction in prostate cancer. Can Urol Assoc J 2013; 7(9-10): E648-50. [http://dx.doi.org/10.5489/cuaj.412] [PMID: 24409216]

[61] Tombal B, Miller K, Boccon-Gibod L, *et al.* Additional analysis of the secondary end point of biochemical recurrence rate in a phase 3 trial (CS21) comparing degarelix 80 mg *versus* leuprolide in prostate cancer patients segmented by baseline characteristics. Eur Urol 2010; 57(5): 836-42. [http://dx.doi.org/10.1016/j.eururo.2009.11.029] [PMID: 19962227]

[62] Pickles T, Hamm J, Morris WJ, Schreiber WE, Tyldesley S. Incomplete testosterone suppression with luteinizing hormone-releasing hormone agonists: does it happen and does it matter? BJU Int 2012; 110 (11 Pt B): E500-7.

[63] Tombal B, Berges R. How good do current GNRH agonists control testosterone? Can this be improved with Eligard? Eur Urol 2005; 4S: 30. [http://dx.doi.org/10.1016/j.eursup.2005.08.004]

[64] Morote J, Orsola A, Planas J, *et al.* Redefining clinically significant castration levels in patients with prostate cancer receiving continuous androgen deprivation therapy. J Urol 2007; 178(4 Pt 1): 1290-5. [http://dx.doi.org/10.1016/j.juro.2007.05.129] [PMID: 17698136]

[65] Ou Y, Michaelson MD, Sengeløv L, *et al.* Randomized, placebo controlled, phase III trial of sunitinib in combination with prednisone (SU+P) *versus* prednisone (P) alone in men with progressive metastatic castration-resistant prostate cancer (MCRPC). J Clin Oncol 2011; 29(15) (Suppl.): 4515. [abstract]. [http://dx.doi.org/10.1200/jco.2011.29.15_suppl.4515]

[66] [1 December 2016]; Available at: https://www.cancercare.on.ca/common/pages/UserFile.aspx?fileId=318883

[67] Smith MR, Kabbinavar F, Saad F, *et al.* Natural history of rising serum prostate-specific antigen in men with castrate nonmetastatic prostate cancer. J Clin Oncol 2005; 23(13): 2918-25. [http://dx.doi.org/10.1200/JCO.2005.01.529] [PMID: 15860850]

[68] Scher HI, Heller G. Clinical states in prostate cancer: toward a dynamic model of disease progression. Urology 2000; 55(3): 323-7. [http://dx.doi.org/10.1016/S0090-4295(99)00471-9] [PMID: 10699601]

[69] Roviello G, Sigala S, Sandhu S, *et al.* Role of the novel generation of androgen receptor pathway targeted agents in the management of castration-resistant prostate cancer: A literature based meta-analysis of randomized trials. Eur J Cancer 2016; 61: 111-21. [http://dx.doi.org/10.1016/j.ejca.2016.04.002] [PMID: 27162152]

[70] Perletti G, Monti E, Marras E, *et al.* Efficacy and safety of second-line agents for treatment of metastatic castration-resistant prostate cancer progressing after docetaxel. A systematic review and meta-analysis. Arch Ital Urol Androl 2015; 87(2): 121-9. [http://dx.doi.org/10.4081/aiua.2015.2.121] [PMID: 26150028]

[71] Parker C, Nilsson S, Heinrich D, *et al.* ALSYMPCA Investigators. Alpha emitter radium-223 and survival in metastatic prostate cancer. N Engl J Med 2013; 369(3): 213-23. [http://dx.doi.org/10.1056/NEJMoa1213755] [PMID: 23863050]

[72] Saad F, Carles J, Gillessen S, *et al.* Radium-223 International Early Access Program Investigators. Radium-223 and concomitant therapies in patients with metastatic castration-resistant prostate cancer: an international, early access, open-label, single-arm phase 3b trial. Lancet Oncol 2016; 17(9): 1306-16. [http://dx.doi.org/10.1016/S1470-2045(16)30173-5] [PMID: 27473888]

[73] Bahl A, Masson S, Birtle A, Chowdhury S, de Bono J. Second-line treatment options in metastatic castration-resistant prostate cancer: a comparison of key trials with recently approved agents. Cancer Treat Rev 2014; 40(1): 170-7. [http://dx.doi.org/10.1016/j.ctrv.2013.06.008] [PMID: 23958310]

[74] James N, Pirrie S, Pope A, *et al.* TRAPEZE: a randomised controlled trial of the clinical effectiveness and cost-effectiveness of chemotherapy with zoledronic acid, strontium-89, or both, in men with bony metastatic castration-refractory prostate cancer. Health Technol Assess 2016; 20(53): 1-288. [http://dx.doi.org/10.3310/hta20530] [PMID: 27434595]

[75] James ND, Pirrie SJ, Pope AM, *et al.* Clinical Outcomes and Survival Following Treatment of Metastatic Castrate-Refractory Prostate Cancer With Docetaxel Alone or With Strontium-89, Zoledronic Acid, or Both: The TRAPEZE Randomized Clinical Trial. JAMA Oncol 2016; 2(4): 493-9. [http://dx.doi.org/10.1001/jamaoncol.2015.5570] [PMID: 26794729]

[76] Robinson D, Van Allen EM, Wu YM, *et al.* Integrative clinical genomics of advanced prostate cancer. Cell 2015; 161(5): 1215-28. [http://dx.doi.org/10.1016/j.cell.2015.05.001] [PMID: 26000489]

[77] Maeda H, Saito A. [Enzalutamide-a novel androgen receptor inhibitor that provides treatment options for patients with castration-resistant prostate cancer]. Gan To Kagaku Ryoho 2014; 41(7): 805-10. [PMID: 25131864]

[78] Scher HI, Fizazi K, Saad F, *et al.* AFFIRM Investigators. Increased survival with enzalutamide in prostate cancer after chemotherapy. N Engl J Med 2012; 367(13): 1187-97. [http://dx.doi.org/10.1056/NEJMoa1207506] [PMID: 22894553]

[79] Beer TM, Armstrong AJ, Rathkopf DE, *et al.* PREVAIL Investigators. Enzalutamide in metastatic prostate cancer before chemotherapy. N Engl J Med 2014; 371(5): 424-33. [http://dx.doi.org/10.1056/NEJMoa1405095] [PMID: 24881730]

[80] Beer TM, Armstrong AJ, Rathkopf D, *et al.* Enzalutamide in Men with Chemotherapy-naïve Metastatic Castration-resistant Prostate Cancer: Extended Analysis of the Phase 3 PREVAIL Study. Eur Urol 2017; 71(2): 151-4. [http://dx.doi.org/10.1016/j.eururo.2016.07.032] [PMID: 27477525]

[81] Evans CP, Higano CS, Keane T, *et al.* The PREVAIL Study: Primary Outcomes by Site and Extent of Baseline Disease for Enzalutamide-treated Men with Chemotherapy-naïve Metastatic Castration-resistant Prostate Cancer. Eur Urol 2016; 70(4): 675-83. [http://dx.doi.org/10.1016/j.eururo.2016.03.017] [PMID: 27006332]

[82] Graff JN, Baciarello G, Armstrong AJ, *et al.* Efficacy and safety of enzalutamide in patients 75 years or older with chemotherapy-naive metastatic castration-resistant prostate cancer: results from PREVAIL. Ann Oncol 2016; 27(2): 286-94. [http://dx.doi.org/10.1093/annonc/mdv542] [PMID: 26578735]

[83] Available at: https://www.ctg.queensu.ca/news/pr17-enzamet-trial-enzalutamide-prostate-cancer

[84] [1 October 2016]; Available at: http://www.rxlist.com/xtandi-side-effects-drug-center.htm

[85] Sternberg CN, de Bono JS, Chi KN, *et al.* Improved outcomes in elderly patients with metastatic castration-resistant prostate cancer treated with the androgen receptor inhibitor enzalutamide: results from the phase III AFFIRM trial. Ann Oncol 2014; 25(2): 429-34. [http://dx.doi.org/10.1093/annonc/mdt571] [PMID: 24478320]

[86] de Bono JS, Logothetis CJ, Molina A, *et al.* COU-AA-301 Investigators. Abiraterone and increased survival in metastatic prostate cancer. N Engl J Med 2011; 364(21): 1995-2005. [http://dx.doi.org/10.1056/NEJMoa1014618] [PMID: 21612468]

[87] de Bono JS, Oudard S, Ozguroglu M, *et al.* TROPIC Investigators. Prednisone plus cabazitaxel or mitoxantrone for metastatic castration-resistant prostate cancer progressing after docetaxel treatment: a randomised open-label trial. Lancet 2010; 376(9747): 1147-54. [http://dx.doi.org/10.1016/S0140-6736(10)61389-X] [PMID: 20888992]

[88] Morris MJ, Molina A, Small EJ, *et al.* Radiographic progression-free survival as a response biomarker in metastatic castration-resistant prostate cancer: COU-AA-302 results. J Clin Oncol 2015; 33(12): 1356-63. [http://dx.doi.org/10.1200/JCO.2014.55.3875] [PMID: 25624432]

[89] Rathkopf DE, Smith MR, de Bono JS, *et al.* Updated interim efficacy analysis and long-term safety of abiraterone acetate in metastatic castration-resistant prostate cancer patients without prior chemotherapy (COU-AA-302). Eur Urol 2014; 66(5): 815-25. [http://dx.doi.org/10.1016/j.eururo.2014.02.056] [PMID: 24647231]

[90] Lorente D, Omlin A, Ferraldeschi R, *et al.* Tumour responses following a steroid switch from prednisone to dexamethasone in castration-resistant prostate cancer patients progressing on abiraterone. Br J Cancer 2014; 111(12): 2248-53. [http://dx.doi.org/10.1038/bjc.2014.531] [PMID: 25314055]

[91] Gillessen S, Omlin A, Attard G, *et al.* Management of patients with advanced prostate cancer: recommendations of the St Gallen Advanced Prostate Cancer Consensus Conference (APCCC) 2015. Ann Oncol 2015; 26(8): 1589-604. [http://dx.doi.org/10.1093/annonc/mdv257] [PMID: 26041764]

[92] Saad F, Fizazi K, Jinga V, *et al.* ELM-PC 4 investigators. Orteronel plus prednisone in patients with chemotherapy-naive metastatic castration-resistant prostate cancer (ELM-PC 4): a double-blind, multicentre, phase 3, randomised, placebo-controlled trial. Lancet Oncol 2015; 16(3): 338-48. [http://dx.doi.org/10.1016/S1470-2045(15)70027-6] [PMID: 25701170]

[93] [1 December 2016]; Available at: www.rtog.org

[94] Crawford ED, Allen JA. Treatment of newly diagnosed state D2 prostate cancer with leuprolide and flutamide or leuprolide alone, phase III, intergroup study 0036. J Steroid Biochem Mol Biol 1990; 37(6): 961-3.
[http://dx.doi.org/10.1016/0960-0760(90)90450-Y] [PMID: 2126738]

[95] Boccardo F, Pace M, Rubagotti A, *et al.* The Italian Prostatic Cancer Project (PONCAP) Study Group. Goserelin acetate with or without flutamide in the treatment of patients with locally advanced or metastatic prostate cancer. Eur J Cancer 1993; 29A(8): 1088-93.
[http://dx.doi.org/10.1016/S0959-8049(05)80293-X] [PMID: 8518017]

[96] Marshall V, Thompson P, Raghavan D, *et al.* First report of Australian multicenter randomised prostate cancer trial: flutamide does not add to the effect of orchiectomy for metastatic prostate cancer. Proc Annu Meet Am Assoc Cancer Res 1992; 33: A1316.

[97] de Voogt HJ, Studer U, Schröder FH, Klijn JG, de Pauw M, Sylvester R. European Organization for Research and Treatment of Cancer (EROTC) Genito-Urinary Tract Cancer Cooperative Group. Maximum androgen blockade using LHRH agonist buserelin in combination with short-term (two weeks) or long-term (continuous) cyproterone acetate is not superior to standard androgen deprivation in the treatment of advanced prostate cancer. Final analysis of EORTC GU Group Trial 30843. Eur Urol 1998; 33(2): 152-8.
[http://dx.doi.org/10.1159/000019547] [PMID: 9519356]

[98] de Voogt HJ, Klijn JG, Studer U, Schröder F, Sylvester R, De Pauw M. Orchidectomy *versus* Buserelin in combination with cyproterone acetate, for 2 weeks or continuously, in the treatment of metastatic prostatic cancer. Preliminary results of EORTC-trial 30843. J Steroid Biochem Mol Biol 1990; 37(6): 965-9.
[http://dx.doi.org/10.1016/0960-0760(90)90451-P] [PMID: 2149509]

[99] Robinson MR. EORTC protocol 30805: a phase III trial comparing orchidectomy *versus* orchidectomy and cyproterone acetate and low dose stilboestrol in the management of metastatic carcinoma of the prostate. Prog Clin Biol Res 1988; 260: 101-10.
[PMID: 2966402]

[100] Robinson MR, Smith PH, Richards B, Newling DW, de Pauw M, Sylvester R. The final analysis of the EORTC Genito-Urinary Tract Cancer Co-Operative Group phase III clinical trial (protocol 30805) comparing orchidectomy, orchidectomy plus cyproterone acetate and low dose stilboestrol in the management of metastatic carcinoma of the prostate. Eur Urol 1995; 28(4): 273-83.
[PMID: 8575493]

[101] Sylvester RJ, Denis L, de Voogt H. European Organization for Research and Treatment of Cancer (EORTC) Genito-Urinary Tract Cancer Cooperative Group. The importance of prognostic factors in the interpretation of two EORTC metastatic prostate cancer trials. Eur Urol 1998; 33(2): 134-43.
[http://dx.doi.org/10.1159/000019545] [PMID: 9519354]

[102] Prostate Cancer Trialists Collaborative Group. Maximum androgen blockade in advanced prostate cancer: an overview of the randomised trials. Lancet 2000; 355(9214): 1491-8.
[http://dx.doi.org/10.1016/S0140-6736(00)02163-2] [PMID: 10801170]

[103] Crawford ED, Eisenberger MA, McLeod DG, *et al.* A controlled trial of leuprolide with and without flutamide in prostatic carcinoma. N Engl J Med 1989; 321(7): 419-24.
[http://dx.doi.org/10.1056/NEJM198908173210702] [PMID: 2503724]

[104] Chodak G, Gomella L, Phung H. Combined androgen blockade in advanced prostate cancer: looking back to move forward. Clin Genitourin Cancer 2007; 5(6): 371-8.
[http://dx.doi.org/10.3816/CGC.2007.n.019] [PMID: 17956709]

[105] Schmitt B, Wilt TJ, Schellhammer PF, *et al.* Combined androgen blockade with nonsteroidal antiandrogens for advanced prostate cancer: a systematic review. Urology 2001; 57(4): 727-32.
[http://dx.doi.org/10.1016/S0090-4295(00)01086-4] [PMID: 11306391]

[106] Roach M III, DeSilvio M, Lawton C, *et al.* Radiation Therapy Oncology Group 9413. Phase III trial

comparing whole-pelvic versus prostate-only radiotherapy and neoadjuvant versus adjuvant combined androgen suppression: Radiation Therapy Oncology Group 9413. J Clin Oncol 2003; 21(10): 1904-11. [http://dx.doi.org/10.1200/JCO.2003.05.004] [PMID: 12743142]

[107] Roach M III, DeSilvio M, Valicenti R, *et al.* Whole-pelvis, mini-pelvis, or prostate-only external beam radiotherapy after neoadjuvant and concurrent hormonal therapy in patients treated in the Radiation Therapy Oncology Group 9413 trial. Int J Radiat Oncol Biol Phys 2006; 66(3): 647-53. [http://dx.doi.org/10.1016/j.ijrobp.2006.05.074] [PMID: 17011443]

[108] Lawton CA, DeSilvio M, Roach M III, *et al.* An update of the phase III trial comparing whole pelvic to prostate only radiotherapy and neoadjuvant to adjuvant total androgen suppression: updated analysis of RTOG 9413, with emphasis on unexpected hormone/radiation interactions. Int J Radiat Oncol Biol Phys 2007; 69(3): 646-55. [http://dx.doi.org/10.1016/j.ijrobp.2007.04.003] [PMID: 17531401]

[109] Pisansky TM, Hunt D, Gomella LG, *et al.* Duration of androgen suppression before radiotherapy for localized prostate cancer: radiation therapy oncology group randomized clinical trial 9910. J Clin Oncol 2015; 33(4): 332-9. [http://dx.doi.org/10.1200/JCO.2014.58.0662] [PMID: 25534388]

[110] Bolla M, de Reijke TM, Van Tienhoven G, *et al.* EORTC Radiation Oncology Group and Genito-Urinary Tract Cancer Group. Duration of androgen suppression in the treatment of prostate cancer. N Engl J Med 2009; 360(24): 2516-27.

[111] Souhami L, Bae K, Pilepich M, Sandler H. Impact of the duration of adjuvant hormonal therapy in patients with locally advanced prostate cancer treated with radiotherapy: a secondary analysis of RTOG 8531. J Clin Oncol 2009; 27(13): 2137-43. [http://dx.doi.org/10.1200/JCO.2008.17.4052] [PMID: 19307511]

[112] Eisenberqer M, Crawford ED, McCleod D, *et al.* A comparison of leuprolide and flutamide *vs* leuprolide alone in newly diagnosed stage D2 prostate cancer: prognostic and therapeutic importance of the minimal disease subset. Proc Annual Meeting Am Soc Clin Oncol. 11: A619.

[113] Bruchovsky N, Brown EM, Coppin CM, *et al.* The endocrinology and treatment of prostate tumour progression. In: Coffey DS, Bruchovsky N, Gardner WA, Eds. Current concepts and approaches to the study of prostate cancer: progress in clinical and biological research. New York: Alan R Liss 1987; Vol. 239: pp. 348-87.

[114] The Medical Research Council Prostate Cancer Working Party Investigators Group. Immediate *versus* deferred treatment for advanced prostatic cancer: initial results of the Medical Research Council Trial. Br J Urol 1997; 79(2): 235-46. [http://dx.doi.org/10.1046/j.1464-410X.1997.d01-6840.x] [PMID: 9052476]

[115] Messing EM, Manola J, Yao J, *et al.* Eastern Cooperative Oncology Group study EST 3886. Immediate versus deferred androgen deprivation treatment in patients with node-positive prostate cancer after radical prostatectomy and pelvic lymphadenectomy. Lancet Oncol 2006; 7(6): 472-9. [http://dx.doi.org/10.1016/S1470-2045(06)70700-8] [PMID: 16750497]

[116] Studer UE, Whelan P, Albrecht W, *et al.* Immediate or deferred androgen deprivation for patients with prostate cancer not suitable for local treatment with curative intent: European Organisation for Research and Treatment of Cancer (EORTC) Trial 30891. J Clin Oncol 2006; 24(12): 1868-76. [http://dx.doi.org/10.1200/JCO.2005.04.7423] [PMID: 16622261]

[117] Studer UE, Whelan P, Wimpissinger F, *et al.* EORTC Genitourinary Cancer Group. Differences in time to disease progression do not predict for cancer-specific survival in patients receiving immediate or deferred androgen-deprivation therapy for prostate cancer: final results of EORTC randomized trial 30891 with 12 years of follow-up. Eur Urol 2014; 66(5): 829-38. [http://dx.doi.org/10.1016/j.eururo.2013.07.024] [PMID: 23932338]

[118] Garcia-Albeniz X, Chan JM, Paciorek A, *et al.* Immediate *versus* deferred initiation of androgen deprivation therapy in prostate cancer patients with PSA-only relapse. An observational follow-up

study. Eur J Cancer 2015; 51(7): 817-24.
[http://dx.doi.org/10.1016/j.ejca.2015.03.003] [PMID: 25794605]

[119] Studer UE, Hauri D, Hanselmann S, *et al.* Immediate *versus* deferred hormonal treatment for patients with prostate cancer who are not suitable for curative local treatment: results of the randomized trial SAKK 08/88. J Clin Oncol 2004; 22(20): 4109-18.
[http://dx.doi.org/10.1200/JCO.2004.11.514] [PMID: 15483020]

[120] Walsh PC, DeWeese TL, Eisenberger MA. A structured debate: immediate *versus* deferred androgen suppression in prostate cancer-evidence for deferred treatment. J Urol 2001; 166(2): 508-15.
[http://dx.doi.org/10.1016/S0022-5347(05)65972-1] [PMID: 11458056]

[121] Alva A, Hussain M. Intermittent androgen deprivation therapy in advanced prostate cancer. Curr Treat Options Oncol 2014; 15(1): 127-36.
[http://dx.doi.org/10.1007/s11864-013-0272-2] [PMID: 24395278]

[122] Akakura K, Bruchovsky N, Goldenberg SL, *et al.* Effects of intermittent androgen suppression on androgen dependent tumours. Cancer 1993; 71: 2782-90.
[http://dx.doi.org/10.1002/1097-0142(19930501)71:9<2782::AID-CNCR2820710916>3.0.CO;2-Z] [PMID: 7682149]

[123] Noble RL. Hormonal control of growth and progression in tumors of Nb rats and a theory of action. Cancer Res 1977; 37(1): 82-94.
[PMID: 830424]

[124] Bruchovsky N, Rennie PS, Coldman AJ, Goldenberg SL, To M, Lawson D. Effects of androgen withdrawal on the stem cell composition of the Shionogi carcinoma. Cancer Res 1990; 50(8): 2275-82.
[PMID: 2317815]

[125] Klotz LH, Herr HW, Morse MJ, Whitmore WF Jr. Intermittent endocrine therapy for advanced prostate cancer. Cancer 1986; 58(11): 2546-50.
[http://dx.doi.org/10.1002/1097-0142(19861201)58:11<2546::AID-CNCR2820581131>3.0.CO;2-N] [PMID: 2429759]

[126] Bruchovsky N, Goldenberg SL, Akakura K, Rennie PS. Luteinizing hormone-releasing hormone agonists in prostate cancer. Elimination of flare reaction by pretreatment with cyproterone acetate and low-dose diethylstilbestrol. Cancer 1993; 72(5): 1685-91.
[http://dx.doi.org/10.1002/1097-0142(19930901)72:5<1685::AID-CNCR2820720532>3.0.CO;2-3] [PMID: 7688656]

[127] Matzkin H, Eber P, Todd B, van der Zwaag R, Soloway MS. Prognostic significance of changes in prostate-specific markers after endocrine treatment of stage D2 prostatic cancer. Cancer 1992; 70(9): 2302-9.
[http://dx.doi.org/10.1002/1097-0142(19921101)70:9<2302::AID-CNCR2820700915>3.0.CO;2-2] [PMID: 1382828]

[128] Miller JI, Ahmann FR, Drach GW, Emerson SS, Bottaccini MR. The clinical usefulness of serum prostate specific antigen after hormonal therapy of metastatic prostate cancer. J Urol 1992; 147(3 Pt 2): 956-61.
[PMID: 1371568]

[129] Crook JM, OCallaghan CJ, Duncan G, *et al.* Intermittent androgen suppression for rising PSA level after radiotherapy. N Engl J Med 2012; 367(10): 895-903.
[http://dx.doi.org/10.1056/NEJMoa1201546] [PMID: 22931259]

[130] Hussain M, Tangen CM, Berry DL, *et al.* Intermittent *versus* continuous androgen deprivation in prostate cancer. N Engl J Med 2013; 368(14): 1314-25.
[http://dx.doi.org/10.1056/NEJMoa1212299] [PMID: 23550669]

[131] Hussain M, Tangen CM, Higano C, *et al.* Southwest Oncology Group Trial 9346 (INT-0162). Absolute prostate-specific antigen value after androgen deprivation is a strong independent predictor of survival in new metastatic prostate cancer: data from Southwest Oncology Group Trial 9346 (INT-

0162). J Clin Oncol 2006; 24(24): 3984-90.
[http://dx.doi.org/10.1200/JCO.2006.06.4246] [PMID: 16921051]

[132] Gulley JL, Figg WD, Steinberg SM, *et al.* A prospective analysis of the time to normalization of serum androgens following 6 months of androgen deprivation therapy in patients on a randomized phase III clinical trial using limited hormonal therapy. J Urol 2005; 173(5): 1567-71.
[http://dx.doi.org/10.1097/01.ju.0000154780.72631.85] [PMID: 15821487]

[133] Hershman DL, Unger JM, Wright JD, *et al.* Adverse health events following intermittent and continuous androgen deprivation in patients with metastatic prostate cancer. JAMA Oncol 2016; 2(4): 453-61.
[http://dx.doi.org/10.1001/jamaoncol.2015.4655] [PMID: 26720308]

[134] Available at: www.UpToDate.com

[135] OBryant CL, Flaig TW, Utz KJ. Bicalutamide-associated fulminant hepatotoxicity. Pharmacotherapy 2008; 28(8): 1071-5.
[http://dx.doi.org/10.1592/phco.28.8.1071] [PMID: 18657023]

[136] Keating NL, OMalley AJ, Freedland SJ, Smith MR. Diabetes and cardiovascular disease during androgen deprivation therapy: observational study of veterans with prostate cancer. J Natl Cancer Inst 2010; 102(1): 39-46.
[http://dx.doi.org/10.1093/jnci/djp404] [PMID: 19996060]

[137] Gandaglia G, Sun M, Popa I, *et al.* Cardiovascular mortality in patients with metastatic prostate cancer exposed to androgen deprivation therapy: a population-based study. Clin Genitourin Cancer 2015; 13(3): e123-30.
[http://dx.doi.org/10.1016/j.clgc.2014.12.003] [PMID: 25547676]

[138] Fradet Y, Egerdie B, Andersen M, *et al.* Tamoxifen as prophylaxis for prevention of gynaecomastia and breast pain associated with bicalutamide 150 mg monotherapy in patients with prostate cancer: a randomised, placebo-controlled, dose-response study. Eur Urol 2007; 52(1): 106-14.
[http://dx.doi.org/10.1016/j.eururo.2007.01.031] [PMID: 17270340]

[139] [1 December 2016]; Available at: http://www.osteoporosis.ca/

[140] Dearnaley DP, Mason MD, Parmar MK, Sanders K, Sydes MR. Adjuvant therapy with oral sodium clodronate in locally advanced and metastatic prostate cancer: long-term overall survival results from the MRC PR04 and PR05 randomised controlled trials. Lancet Oncol 2009; 10(9): 872-6.
[http://dx.doi.org/10.1016/S1470-2045(09)70201-3] [PMID: 19674936]

[141] Vale CL, Burdett S, Rydzewska LH, *et al.* STOpCaP Steering Group. Addition of docetaxel or bisphosphonates to standard of care in men with localised or metastatic, hormone-sensitive prostate cancer: a systematic review and meta-analyses of aggregate data. Lancet Oncol 2016; 17(2): 243-56.
[http://dx.doi.org/10.1016/S1470-2045(15)00489-1] [PMID: 26718929]

[142] Denham JW, Nowitz M, Joseph D, *et al.* Impact of androgen suppression and zoledronic acid on bone mineral density and fractures in the Trans-Tasman Radiation Oncology Group (TROG) 03.04 Randomised Androgen Deprivation and Radiotherapy (RADAR) randomized controlled trial for locally advanced prostate cancer. BJU Int 2014; 114(3): 344-53.
[PMID: 24512527]

[143] Kachnic LA, Pugh SL, Tai P, *et al.* RTOG 0518: randomized phase III trial to evaluate zoledronic acid for prevention of osteoporosis and associated fractures in prostate cancer patients. Prostate Cancer Prostatic Dis 2013; 16(4): 382-6.
[http://dx.doi.org/10.1038/pcan.2013.35] [PMID: 24080992]

[144] Bhattacharya S, Hirmand M, Phung D, van Os S. Development of enzalutamide for metastatic castration-resistant prostate cancer. Ann N Y Acad Sci 2015; 1358: 13-27.
[http://dx.doi.org/10.1111/nyas.12846] [PMID: 26384731]

[145] White R, Khor R, Bressel M, *et al.* Efficacy of high-dose palliative radiotherapy for localised, castration-resistant prostate cancer. Clin Oncol (R Coll Radiol) 2015; 27(1): 16-21. [http://dx.doi.org/10.1016/j.clon.2014.09.013] [PMID: 25445554]

[146] de Bono JS, Oudard S, Ozguroglu M, *et al.* TROPIC Investigators. Prednisone plus cabazitaxel or mitoxantrone for metastatic castration-resistant prostate cancer progressing after docetaxel treatment: a randomised open-label trial. Lancet 2010; 376(9747): 1147-54. [http://dx.doi.org/10.1016/S0140-6736(10)61389-X] [PMID: 20888992]

[147] Antonarakis ES, Lu C, Wang H, *et al.* AR-V7 and resistance to enzalutamide and abiraterone in prostate cancer. N Engl J Med 2014; 371(11): 1028-38. [http://dx.doi.org/10.1056/NEJMoa1315815] [PMID: 25184630]

[148] Montgomery B, Eisenberger MA, Rettig MB, *et al.* Androgen Receptor Modulation Optimized for Response (ARMOR) Phase I and II Studies: Galeterone for the Treatment of Castration-Resistant Prostate Cancer. Clin Cancer Res 2016; 22(6): 1356-63. [http://dx.doi.org/10.1158/1078-0432.CCR-15-1432] [PMID: 26527750]

[149] [2 January 2017]; Available at: http://www.onclive.com/web-exclusives/galeterone-trial-closes-as-progressionfree-survival-rates-miss-mark

[150] [2 January 2017]; Available at: http://www.onclive.com/web-exclusives/galeterone-trial-closes-as-progressionfree-survival-rates-miss-mark

[151] Mateo J, Carreira S, Sandhu S, *et al.* DNA-Repair Defects and Olaparib in Metastatic Prostate Cancer. N Engl J Med 2015; 373(18): 1697-708. [http://dx.doi.org/10.1056/NEJMoa1506859] [PMID: 26510020]

[152] Vaishampayan UN. Sequences and combinations of multifaceted therapy in advanced prostate cancer. Curr Opin Oncol 2015; 27(3): 201-8. [http://dx.doi.org/10.1097/CCO.0000000000000187] [PMID: 25811344]

[153] Liu L, Dong X. Complex impacts of PI3K/AKT inhibitors to androgen receptor gene expression in prostate cancer cells. PLoS One 2014; 9(10): e108780. [http://dx.doi.org/10.1371/journal.pone.0108780] [PMID: 25360799]

CHAPTER 4

Cancer and its Treatment: Development of Anticancer Chemotherapeutic Agents from Natural Products

S.K. Mishra[1], S. Tiwari[2], A.A. Mahdi[3], S.K. Agarwal[3] and V. Lakshmi[1,3,*]

[1] *Medicinal and Process Chemistry Division, Central Drug Research Institute, Lucknow 226001, India*

[2] *Pesticide Toxicology Division, Indian Institute of Toxicology Research, Lucknow 226001, India*

[3] *Department of Biochemistry, King George's Medical University, Lucknow, 226003, India*

Abstract: Over the last 5 decades, biologically active compounds derived from natural resources have provided a number of useful cancer chemotherapeutic drugs. The search for natural product based drug candidates is growing rapidly with the advancements in drug discovery and development techniques in recent years, with the active fractions and isolates of marine organisms along with terrestrial plants. Microorganisms are also being explored for their anti-cancer activities. The present review highlights the information about occurrence, types, clinical features pathophysiology and etiology of cancer as well as conventional and recent advancements in anticancer drug development along with description of selected medicinal plants and compounds derived from natural sources or their derivatives with potential use as cancer chemotherapeutic agents. It is expected that such promising leads from natural origin tend to create extensive interest among researchers including medicinal chemists and pharmacologists working in anticancer drug research and therefore the availability of a given brief information about cancer and anticancer drug development focused on natural product may be proved useful to develop preliminary ideas of biochemical pathways and key enzymes regulating these pathways as well as new targets involved in different stages of the disease along with chemotherapeutic agents which selectively target a specific signaling pathway through structure-activity relationships and preclinical trials.

Keywords: Anticancer, Chemotherapy, Drug development, Grafts, Medicinal plants, Natural products.

[*] **Corresponding author V. Lakshmi:** Department of Biochemistry, King George's Medical University, Lucknow, India; Tel: 08005182248; E-mail: vijlakshmius@yahoo.com

Atta-ur-Rahman and M. Iqbal Choudhary (Eds.)

INTRODUCTION

Cancer is responsible for about 25% deaths caused due to diseases in the developed countries and is a major public health burden and challenge for world health organization and research organizations [1 - 3]. It is considered as an adversary of industrial revolution followed by advanced pattern of socio-cultural life dominated by excessive intake of exogenous chemicals and less physical activities. The number of incidences of different types of cancers is also increasing in developing countries, as the extensive technical advancements in the field of drug development and other areas allowed their populations live longer and make negative lifestyle changes leading to increased risk of cancer. Cancer is a broad group of diseases characterized primarily by uncontrolled cell division leading to increase in the number of malignant cells in a tissue, invasion of adjacent tissues by malignant cells, or spread of malignant cells through lymphatic or circulatory system to regional lymph nodes and distant tissues (metastasis). It develops through multi-step process that initiates with small preneoplastic changes, which may subsequently progress to neoplasia [4, 5]. Under certain conditions, neoplastic cells escape the host's immune surveillance that helps to develop the capacity of growth, invasion and metastasis. Cancer cells behave as independent cells and proliferate continuously without growth regulation, leading to tumor development through multistep process. An ideal anticancer drug would restore normal growth regulation and cell cycle control to cancer cells through restoring aberrant molecular signaling pathways and inducing apoptosis in these cells. It should selectively target different components of physiological and biochemical pathways related to different stages of cancer development without affecting the normal cells. The discovery of new compounds with novel mechanisms of action, contribute to improved and highly effective methods for cancer treatment.

A newer dimension in the anticancer drug research is the increasing awareness about natural product based chemotherapy. Several studies have demonstrated that different plant-based foods such as onion, grapes, garlic, ginger, soybean, turmeric, cabbage, cauliflower, broccoli and tomato can offer significant anticancer potential. Natural products have provided four important categories of antitumor agents: taxanes, camptothecins, bisindole alkaloids also known as vinca alkaloid and epipodophyllotoxins. Microorganisms have also provided several potent anticancer drugs in form of anticancer antibiotics such as doxorubicin, actinomycin and mitomycin C.

A natural product is a chemical compound or substance produced by a plant, animal or microorganism and usually has a pharmacological or biological activity which can be utilized in pharmaceutical drug discovery and drug design.

Chemically natural products are secondary metabolites, specifically produced by a particular group of organisms and have been postulated to play an important role in self defense against predators as well as in interspecies interactions. Their role is exceptionally pronounced in the field of anticancer drug research. Roughly 50% of the new chemical entities introduced during last three decades were either natural products or derived from natural products through structural modifications. Due to enormous advancement in the field of medicinal chemistry, design of natural product or natural product-mimetic scaffolds can be achieved readily in one-step with the help of multicomponent reactions. Usually, natural products are isolated only in minute amounts and thus subsequent techniques are required to scale-up of the biologically active molecules.

With reference to above facts, the review has been designed to cover the history of drug development from natural resources, anticancer compounds isolated from different natural resources along with brief view of occurrence, etiology, pathophysiology of cancer and mechanism of action of currently used anticancer agents.

CANCER

Cancer is recognized as the second most dangerous diseases of modern era and spreading continuously with increasing incidences [1 - 3]. It is caused due to series of intracellular molecular events leading to alteration of the fundamental properties of the cell including regulation of growth and cell cycle progression. These transformed cells develop new morphological and biochemical features and can grow and proliferate in absence of growth signals. These morphological and biochemical changes also promote angiogenesis and metastasis of tumors. It is well established that breast cancer, prostate cancer, lung cancer and colorectal cancer account for approximately 50% of all cancers. In the same way nearly half of the cancer mortality occurs due to these four types of cancers with lung cancer exceeding breast/prostate cancer as the main cause. Prostate cancer is the most commonly occurring cancer in males (about one fourth of new cases) while breast cancer is the most predominant cancer in females (also about one fourth). Other high incident types of cancer include lung, bronchial, colon and rectal cancers which occur equally in men and women. Consequently, the anticancer drug development is the major concern for the research organizations and pharmaceutical industries all over the world. Cancers are classified primarily on the basis of morphological appearance of the tumor, although it has serious limitations. For example tumors with similar histopathological appearance show significantly different clinical outcomes as well as show different responses to therapeutic agents because of significant different in nuclear morphology and molecular markers. Currently the classification of cancer is based on morphological characters, immunophenotyping through antibodies recognizing cell surface, enzyme-based histochemical analyses, and cytogenetic analysis. Recently DNA microarray has provided a powerful tool for cancer classification [6].

TYPES OF CANCER

Based on the histological characteristics hundreds of different cancers have been identified, which can be classified into six major groups.

1. Carcinomas

Cancers caused due to alteration in epithelial cells covering the surface of skin and internal organs are termed as carcinomas. It is the most common type of cancers, predominantly occurring in the old age, for example breast, prostate, lung, pancreas, and colon cancers. Carcinomas, account for 80 to 90 percent of all cancer cases. These can be further divided into two major subtypes: (i) Squamous cell carcinoma, which develops in the squamous epithelium and (ii) adenocarcinoma, which develops in an organ or gland.

2. Sarcomas

Cancers arising on different connective tissue including bone, cartilage and nervous system are termed as Sarcomas. These are known to develop from cells originating in mesenchyma outside the bone marrow. Most important examples of sarcoma include fibrosarcoma (fibrous tissue), rhabdomyosarcoma (skeletal muscle), angiosarcoma or hemangioendothelioma (blood vessels), glioma or astrocytoma (neurogenic connective tissue found in the brain) mesothelial sarcoma or mesothelioma (membranous lining of body cavities).

3. Myelomas

These include the cancers arising in the bone marrow plasma cells. These are also called cancers of antibody producing white blood cells.

4. Lymphomas

These are developed in the lymph glands and other organs of lymphatic system including tonsils, thymus gland and spleen playing active role in immune system. Lymphomas may also occur in some other organs including breast, stomach and brain. Lymphomas occurring in these organs are known as extranodal lymphomas. These can be further divided into two major subtypes: (i) Hodgkin lymphomas and (ii) non- Hodgkin lymphomas. Both of these subtypes can be differentiated on the basis of the presence of reed-sternberg cells in Hodgkin lymphoma.

5. Leukemias

The cancers occurring in bone marrow are termed as leukemia. It results in the overproduction of immature white blood cells (WBC) rendering the patients immunodeficient and susceptible to subsequent infections. In some cases it also affects red blood cells (RBC) and platelets leading to anemia as well as defective blood clotting. The important examples of leukemia include chronic myelocytic leukemia (CML) occurring in adults, acute myelocytic leukemia (AML) occurring in children, chronic lymphocytic, lymphatic, or lymphoblastic leukemia (CLL) common in adults, acute lymphocytic, lymphatic, or lymphoblastic leukemia (ALL) common in children and adults.

6. Mixed Types

These comprises of more than one component which may be within one category or from different categories. Examples of mixed type include adenosquamous carcinoma, mixed mesodermal tumor, carcinosarcoma and teratocarcinoma.

CLINICAL FEATURES/SYMPTOMS

Different types and stages of cancer can be identified based on potential signs and symptoms:

Appearance of blood in sputum along with shortness of breath, persistent cough and chest pain indicate lung cancer.

Prolonged bleeding in menstrual cycle for more than 10 days or bleeding between two menstrual cycles indicate the presence of uterine cancer.

Presence of a prolonged non-healing ulcer in mouth indicates the oral cancer.

Alternating diarrhea or constipation for a prolonged without any obvious reason followed by blood in stools indicates gastrointestinal cancer.

Appearance of reddish-color in urine with abdominal pain and fever indicate the renal cancer.

Persistent cough and hoarseness of voice could indicate cancer of the throat.

Presence of moles with size more than 7mm in diameter and asymmetrical shape or irregular border as well as multicolor (mosaic) itchy or bleeding moles indicates skin cancer (melanoma).

Presence of rapidly increasing lumps in breast in women above 35 years of age may be cancerous in some cases.

Unexpected continuous weight loss above two months unrelated to dietary changes, stress or exercise also indicate different types of cancer.

These symptoms can be further confirmed based on different tests such as a biopsy or X-ray and used to determine the appropriate treatment.

TUMOR CELL MARKERS

Cancer cells produce some specific markers which may be present on cell membranes or in cytoplasm. Immunological analysis of these markers in the blood, urine or spinal fluid may be used in diagnosis of the types of cancer as well as to identify the risk of cancer in individuals. These tumor cell markers are also used to analyze the clinical improvement in cancer patients undergoing cancer therapy as well as to evaluate the efficacy of anticancer treatment.

Tumor cell markers can be classified as antigens (such as carcinoembryonic antigen in adenocarcinomas, alfa fetoprotein in ovarian, testicular and hepatic carcinomas and squamous cell carcinoma antigen in epidermal cancers), enzymes (such as lactate dehydrogenase in leukaemias, acid phosphatase in prostate cancer, alkaline phosphatase in bone cancer, enolase in lung cancer and neuroblastoma and thymidine kinase in leukaemia and lymphomas) and hormones (such as Insulin and gastrin in pancreatic cancer human chorionic gonadotropin in trophoblastic cancers and calcitonin in thyroid and lung cancer).

PATHOPHYSIOLOGY

Cancer is a genetic disorder in which genetic alterations caused due to unrepaired mutations enable them to divide in the absence of growth signals through increasing the expression of growth factor receptors or through secreting specific growth factors. Activation of telomerase activity also contributes to maintain the length of telomere in cancerous cells resulting in continuous proliferation. Cancerous cells gain growth autonomy through activation of growth promoting oncogenes or inhibition of tumor suppressor genes (growth inhibiting genes), both of which are caused by multiple unrepaired genetic damages due to environmental factors or genetic inheritance. These multiple genetic damages may be subtle or large enough to be detected through the karyotype analysis.

Activation of protooncogenes is known to be caused by one of several processes including point mutation, translocation, gene amplification, enhancer insertion or promoter insertion. It is known to be developed through multistep carcinogenesis process involving three closely associated stages distinguishable from each other.

1. Initiation: it is the first stage of carcinogenesis in which a normal cell converts

in to transformed cell or initiated cell in response to exposure of carcinogenic factors. It is a rapid and irreversible process which induces changes in genome of the cells leading to mutation. In addition, chronic inflammation and oxidative stress may also lead to initiation.

2. Promotion: in this stage previously initiated cell undergo a sequence of changes to generate preneoplastic cell. Most of the chemical carcinogens are able to act as initiators and promoters. Deregulation of different cell signaling pathways also lead to carcinogenesis. These signaling pathways include mitogen activated protein kinase (MAPK), serine threonine kinase, nuclear factor kappa B (NF-□B), Akt kinase/protein kinase B (Akt/PKB), Raf/Ras, estrogen receptor, androgen receptor and activator protein 1(AP-1) pathways. These molecular changes ultimately result in inflammation, proliferation and avoidance of apoptosis.
3. Progression: it is the final step of carcinogenesis in which inflammatory changes and proliferation signals lead to excessive production and release of cytokines (angiogenic factors) which induce the preneoplastic cell for proliferation and promotion. Hypoxia is also considered as an important factor in carcinogenesis it is known to induce vascular endothelial growth factor (VEGF) in cancerous cells and induce the expression of matrix metalloproteinase (MMP) in endothelial cells.

CHARACTERISTIC FEATURES OF CANCER CELLS

There are three stringent properties of cancer cells which make them different from normal cells.

(i). Diminished regulation of cell cycle or uncontrolled growth
(ii). Capability of invasion of neighboring tissues and
(iii). Capability of spreading to distant parts of body through metastasis.

After transformation in to cancer cell these cells undergo a variety of morphological and biochemical changes which enable them to proliferate and spread in other locations.

Morphological Changes

The cancerous cells usually have round shape and show nuclear and cellular pleomorphism, hyperchromatism, altered nuclear: cytoplasm ratio and abundant mitosis. These cells often grow over one another forming multi layers and do not stop replication when come into contact with another cells as well as require low serum level of growth factors.

Cancer cells become able to grow without attachment to surface *in vitro*. An elevated level of telomerase enables these cells to maintain telomere length rendering them to divide continuously as immortal cells. Cancer cells can proliferate in a semisolid or liquid culture media as these do not require surface attachment and show anchorage-independent growth which result in clonal expansion of malignant cells [5]. Cancer cells undergo karyotypic changes characterized by an increase in the number of chromosomes resulting in increased expression of growth-promoting genes. These cells do not respond to the suboptimal growth conditions and refuse to enter in to G0 state. These cells also loss control of cell cycle check points and proceed to replicate the DNA with unrepaired damages leading to accumulation of mutations.

Biochemical Changes

Cancer cells show enhanced synthesis of Nucleic acids (DNA and RNA) and increased rate of glycolysis in both aerobic and anaerobic conditions. Change in composition of cell membrane results in alteration of permeability and surface charge. Different stages of cancer cells express different cell surface oligosaccharide characteristic to that stage. These surface oligosaccharides have binding specificity for different lectins and thus, can be used as probes to determine the glycoprotein and glycolipid composition as well as the stage of cancer. Change in composition of glycoprotein and glycosphingolipids on cell surface also results in appearance of new surface antigens, glycolipids and proteoglycans as well as altered cell-cell interactions and cell-extracellular microenvironment interactions. Cancer cells express some large glycopeptides containing N-linked oligosaccharides with lead to altered glycosylation patterns significantly different from normal cells [6]. Cancer cell express specific carbohydrate antigens which can be classified into three classes (1) epitopes expressed on glycolipids, epitopes expressed on glycoproteins and epitopes expressed equally on glycolipids and glycoproteins. These specific carbohydrate antigens arise due to incomplete synthesis or processing of carbohydrate chains or due to rearrangement of tumor cell membrane glycolipids or due to glycosyltransferases catalyzed *de novo* synthesis [7].

Cancer cells synthesize altered Proteoglycans which play a crucial role in cellular interactions with extracellular matrix through providing binding sites for components of extracellular matrix as well as act as cell adhesion factors and growth factor reservoir. These cells also secrete mucin with the altered glycosylation pattern which plays an important role in host immune response. The characteristic changes are represented in Fig. (**1**).

Cancer cells show an increased secretion of certain growth factors into surrounding medium as well as synthesize their own cytokines such as interleukin-6 and interleukin-1. In addition these secrete several lytic enzymes such as proteases, collagenases, and glycosidases which result in the degradation of extracellular Matrix Components including glycoproteins, proteoglycans, and collagen enabling metastatic cancer cells to invade through tissue barriers, lymphatic system and circulatory system. These cells also express altered integrins, cell surface receptors responsible for cell adhesion to the ECM. These receptor molecules act as a link between the extracellular matrix and intracellular actin cytoskeleton and control the expression of genes involved in cell differentiation and cell adhesion. It functions via a cascade involving ECM-bound integrins intracellular actin fibrils and signal transduction machinery [8].

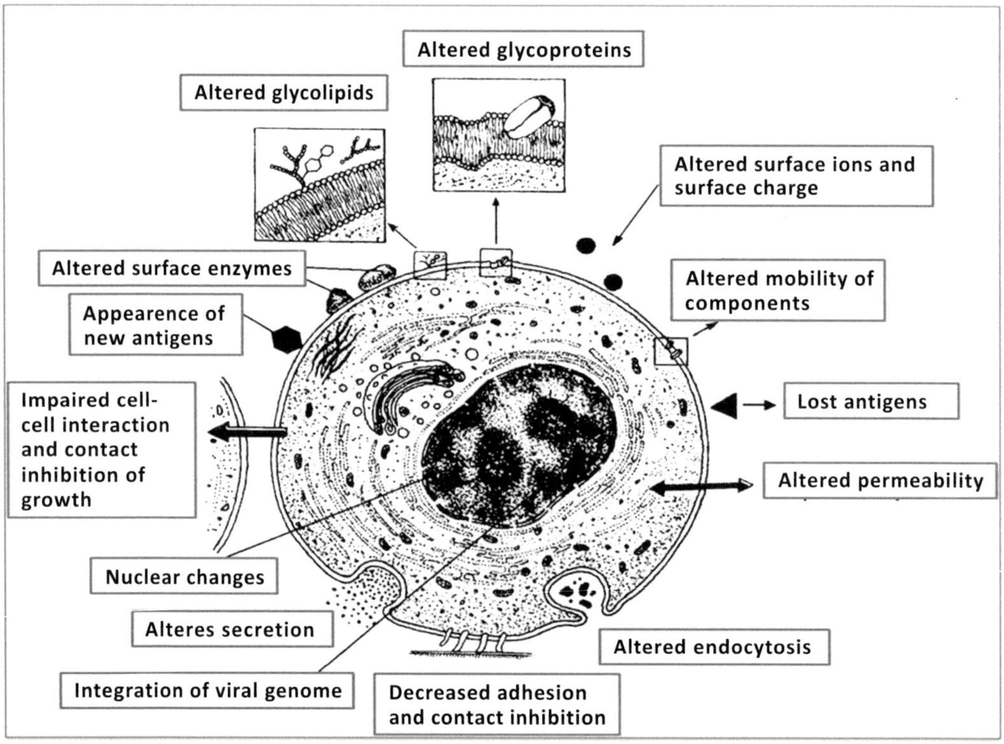

Fig. (1). Characteristic features of malignant cell.

Genetics of Cancer

Cancer is shown to be associated with mutations in three deferent types of genes proto-oncogenes, tumor suppressor genes and DNA repair genes, these three types of genes work together to maintain integrity of the genome and control the cell cycle. Proto-oncogenes code for different proteins which stimulate cell division through different signaling pathways.

More than half of the oncogenes act through protein tyrosine kinases. Remaining 50% oncogenes produce various other growth factors including GTP binding protein and DNA binding protein. These growth factors activate a cascade of signaling pathway as shown in Fig. (**2**).

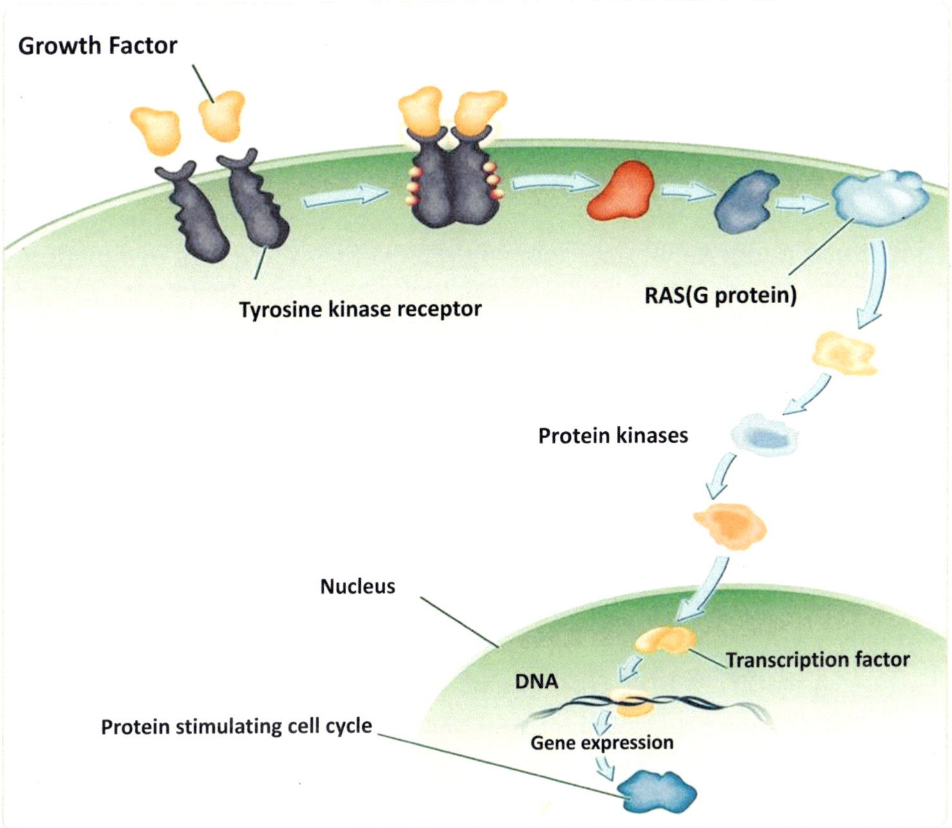

Fig. (2). Signal transduction pathway: a growth factor binds to a tyrosine kinase receptor on cell surface and activates the membrane protein which in turn activates cytoplasmic kinases ultimately activating the transcription factors which enter the nucleus and stimulate the expression of related genes.

This signaling pathway consists of a receptor molecule with a binding site for the growth factor, some intermediate molecules which transmit the effects produced by growth factor through the cytoplasm, and nuclear transcription factors which induce the gene activation leading to cell division. Followed by unrepaired mutations in genome, proto-oncogenes convert in to oncogenes which permanently activate the signaling pathway leading to an increased production of growth factors. Examples of oncogenic mutations include mutations in *ras gene* resulting in increased expression of adenylate cyclase and consequently increase in cAMP level leading to severe change in cellular metabolism and uncontrolled cell growth. Mutation in *ras* has been determined in approximately one third of tumors including thyroid, colon, lung and pancreatic cancers. Another example of oncogenic mutations include, *myc* encoding the DNA binding protein. Mutated *myc* gene is identified in seventy percent of cancers.

The tumor suppressor genes code for proteins which prevent tumor formation through inhibiting the growth of cell. These proteins may act in different targets present in cytoplasm, nucleus and cell membrane. Mutations in tumor suppressor genes lead to uncontrolled cell growth and proliferation.

The mutations in oncogenes are dominant mutations which results in a gain of function while tumor suppressor gene mutations result in a loss of function thus arise as recessive trait. Examples of cancers caused due to tumors suppressor genes include hereditary retinoblastoma, which occurs in retina in individuals carrying a mutated copy of the *RB* tumor suppressor gene when the second copy of the gene undergo mutation. Similarly familial adenomatous polyposis of the colon occurs through mutations in both copies of the *APC* gene. Hereditary breast cancer caused due to mutations in *BRCA2* and hereditary breast and ovarian cancer caused due to mutations in *BRCA1* also share same mechanism.

Mutations in DNA repair gene avoid the repair of DNA damages allowing the accumulation of further mutations and subsequently increasing the risk of cancer development. Mutation in a DNA repair gene Xeroderma pigmentosum (XP) increase the risk skin cancers caused due to exposure of UV radiation.

Cancer cells are shown to loss the genomic imprinting resulting in expression of both the maternal and paternal alleles leading to double dose of concerned growth factors. Deletion of genetic material is also frequently observed in several types of cancers leading to loss of heterozygosity, the tendency of the expression of only one allele of a gene. A mutation of a tumor suppressor gene followed by a deletion may results in loss of an important mechanism regulating cell growth.

Mutations in genes encoding proteins involved in histone acetylation, deacetylation and phosphorylation results in alterations in Chromatin structure and function and impaired transcription of DNA leading to malignant transformation. Point mutations of tumor-suppressor gene *rb* results in deregulation of the histone deacetylation through inhibition of transcription leading to cancer initiation [9]. Several types of cancer also exhibit altered methylation patterns in nuclear DNA it is postulated to be caused due to overexpression of DNA methyltransferase activity [10].

ETIOLOGY OF CANCER

1. Predisposing Factors

a. **Age:** Age is considered as a significant risk factor for cancer. Incidences of cancer are most common in elders over 55 years of age. After the industrial revolution incidence of cancer has drastically increased due to increased lifespan. Incidence of cancer is very rare in children and youngsters, with leukemia the most frequent. Neuroblastoma is reported to occur [REMOVED HYPERLINK FIELD]in the age of one year comprising 28% of infant cancer. Leukemia is second most common type of cancer in newly born children. Some other cancer types are also known to occur in the early age of life including teratoma, retinoblastoma.
b. **Genetic Factor:** Certain precancer conditions are inherited from one generation to next generation through inheritance of mutated genes. Susceptibility to childhood retinoblastoma is inherited as autosomal dominant trait and nearly half of these cases are of hereditary origin. Susceptibility to multiple colon poliposis is also inherited as autosomal dominant trait and approximately 40% are known to be caused through inheritance. Similarly Chromosomal DNA instability may be inherited as autosomal recessive trait defect in DNA repair. Xeroderma pigmentosa and skin cancer in UV exposed area are also considered as hereditary cancer.
c. **Environmental Factors**: 80% human cancers are known to be caused by environmental factors [11]. These include:

Life Style

Factors related to modernization of socioculture lifestyle, have increased the risk of cancer. These factors include-

i. Tobacco consumption and smoking: it is strongly associated with mouth cancer, lung cancer, throat cancer, bladder cancer and pancreatic cancer. Tobacco smoke contributes to as many as half of all deaths caused due to cancer
ii. Drinking Alcohol: it is associated with an increase in oral, esophageal, breast, and liver cancers.
iii. Excessive Energy Intake and Sedentary Lifestyles: in developed countries and most of the developing countries peoples have become habitual of excessive energy intake and sedentary lifestyles. These habits in association with other factors increase the risk of colon, breast, and other cancers.
iv. Obesity and Increased Body Mass Index: It is known to increase the risk of

colorectal, endometrial, thyroid, renal, gallbladder, pancreatic and ovarian cancers. Men are twice as likely as women to have susceptibility to these risk factors.

Dietary

A diet low in green vegetable and fruits is also shown to increase the risk of several types of cancer. Further some food products were shown to increase the cancer risk in some individuals for example groundnut infected with fungus like *Aspergilus* produce aflatoxin B1, a well known carcinogen [12]. Further some other lifestyle related and environmental factors are known to increase the risk of cancer these include the application of hormones as therapeutic agents, ultraviolet rays and ionizing radiation, and exposure to chemicals in work places.

Occupational

Currently, a large fraction of cancer related mortality in the developed world is known to be caused due to occupational risk factors. It is estimated that at least 200,000 workers involved in different industries die due to cancers related to their workplace all over the world every year. Several studies showed direct association between exposure to respiratory silica particle and lung cancer in workers engaged in ceramic, granite, refractory brick, and diatomaceous earth industries. Dyes, paints, rubber and aromatic amines induce bladder cancer in workers involved in these industries. Exposure to benzene at industrial sites increases the cancer risk in persons involved in these industries. Other examples of occupational carcinogenic agents include asbestos and naphthalamine. Use of organochlorine pesticides in agricultural practices has also been shown to increase the risk of liver and testis cancers [13 - 15]. Accidental exposure to nuclear radiation in persons working in nuclear reactors or uranium mines is established as risk factor for several types of cancers [16]. It also depends upon ecological and social status of a population for example incidence of liver cancer is very common in China and neighboring countries, probably due to the existence of hepatitis B and aflatoxin in that population. Similarly, incidences of lung cancer occur very frequently in several countries belonging to third world where tobacco smoking is very common.

Iatrogenic

Certain therapeutic drugs may act as carcinogens [17]. Tamoxifen used as an effective drug for the treatment of breast cancer is also recognized as a carcinogenetic agent. It has been reported in a recent study that the women who received tamoxifen in chemotherapy have shown to have increased risk for developing endometrial cancer as compare to normal women [18]. Psoralen ultraviolet A (PUVA) therapy, a combination treatment comprising administration of Psoralens followed by exposing the skin to UV-A (long wave ultraviolet radiation) used for the treatment of severe skin diseases is shown to be associated with an increased risk of skin cancers [19]. Chlornaphazine, used in treatment of polycythemia is shown to be associated with an increased risk of bladder cancer. Similarly, the use of tacrolimus and pimecrolimus as therapeutic agents is shown to increase the risk of Hodgkin's lymphomas and melanomas [20].

d. **Acquired Precancerous Disorders:** Certain clinical conditions are known to increase the risk of developing cancer such as Leukoplakia of oral and genital mucosa can develop in squamous cell carcinomas, some cases of untreated liver cirrhosis can develop in hepatic cancer, hepatoma.
   A gastrointestinal disorder known as ulcerative colitis can subsequently produce adenocarcinoma of colon, similarly carcinoma *in situ* of cervix can produce cervical squamous cell carcinoma. Human papiloma virus which causes cervical cancer and anal cancer is transmitted sexually from one person to other.

2. Carcinogenic Agents

Several carcinogenic agents including physical, chemical, and biological have been recognized which can cause cancer. The role of carcinogenic agents is represented in Fig. (**3**).

a. Physical Agents

Directly Effecting DNA

Excessive exposure of high frequency ionizing radiations with enough energy to remove an electron from a molecule, such as X rays, ϒ rays and ultra violet rays can directly induce mutagenesis through several ways: these can induce single strand or double strand break, formation of pyrimidine dimers in DNA, elimination of Pyrimidine or purine base from DNA or crosslinking between two DNA strands. There is a direct relationship between the effective radiation dose and cancer incidences caused due to these ionizing radiations [21]. Some tissues such as bone marrow and thyroid glands are highly sensitive and thus more affected by ionizing radiations. Examples of cancers caused due to ionizing radiations include leukemia, thyroid cancer, skin cancer, breast cancer, stomach cancer and lung cancer.

Indirectly Effecting DNA

Electromagnetic radiations such as X- rays and ϒ rays produce free radicals through randomly hitting intracellular macromolecules including proteins, lipids, and nucleic acids leading to molecular damage. These molecular damages in DNA lead to mutations and carcinogenesis. Examples of ultra violet radiation induced cancerous include carcinomas (basal cell and squamous cell cancers) and milanomas of exposed parts of skin prevalent in New Zealand and Australia.

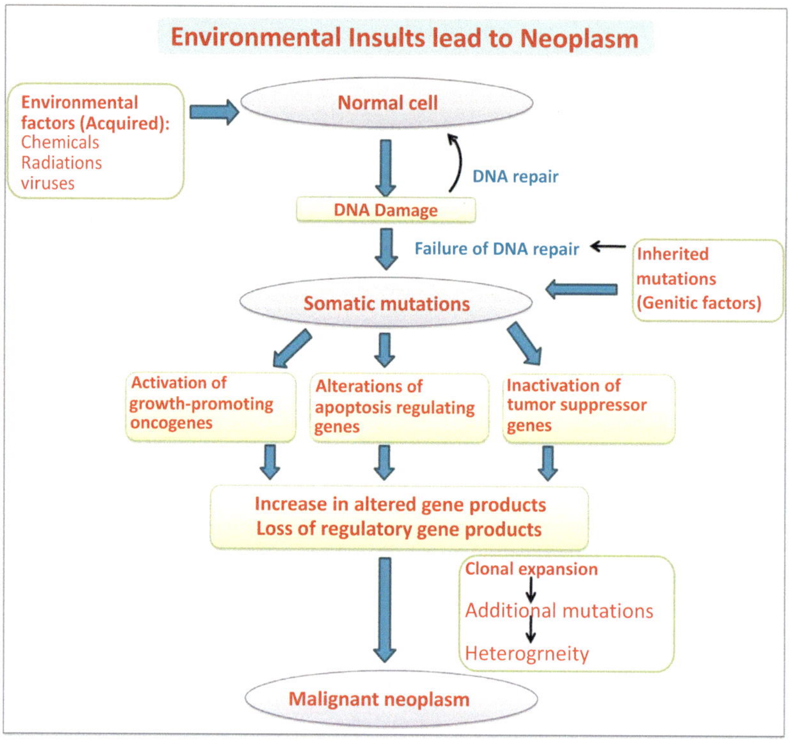

Fig. (3). The mechanism of cancer development and role of environmental carcinogenic agents in carcinogenesis.

b. Chemical Agents

These are the different chemical compounds which act as procarcinogen and after entering in the body get converted in to ultimate carcinogens.

c. Biological Factors

Some of the oncogenic viral infections leading to expression of viral oncogenes (v-onc) result in cancer development. These viruses either induce insertion of additional viral oncogenes into the host genome or activate the cellular oncogenes. Normal protooncogenes converted to oncogenes through transduction in to retrovirus or through changes *in situ* leading to alteration in expression and function and subsequently converting them into cellular oncogenes.

3. Major Classes of Virus Causing Cancer Involve

A. DNA Viruses

Following infection of host cell these viruses form a stable complex with the genome of host cell and transcribed with it. Insertion of the viral DNA near a gene involved in regulation of cell growth and division results in enhanced transcription of that gene and consequently transformation of the cell into cancerous cell. Viral genes transcribed early in the lifecycle of virus produce some specific proteins such as T antigens, E5 and E6 proteins which interfere with cell cycle and growth regulation leading to transformation of the host cell. Examples of cancer causing DNA viruses include

1. Herpes Virus/Epstein Barr Virus

It is the first identified human cancer virus which produces Burkitt lymphoma and nasopharyngeal carcinoma. It is endemic in Northern African and Asian countries and is associated with regular consumption of nitrosamines in diet.

2. Hepatitis B and Hepatitis C Viruses

In addition to causing hepatitis these are also shown to produce hepatocellular carcinoma.

3. Human Papiloma Virus

It induces transformation in host cells through modulating the activity of tumor suppressor genes such as p53 and RB protein rendering the host cell to proliferate and subsequently enabling the replication of viral genome. It is known to cause multiple warts, cervical cancer and anogenital carcinoma [22]. Human papiloma virus is considered as causative factor of genital warts (benign squamous papillomas) shown to be associated with diminished cell mediated immunity. In one third cases, warts may lead to malignant transformation. 99% of cervical cancers and high dose cervical cancer precursor lesions are caused due to Human papiloma virus infection. Some types of human papiloma virus are associated with increased risk of carcinoma *in situ* of cervix and cervical squamous cell carcinoma [23].

4. KSHV/HHV-8 (Kaposi Sarcoma Associated Herpes Virus)

it is known to causes AIDS-related Kaposi sarcoma, a skin cancer, some B cell lymphomas and some other cancers linked with HIV.

B. RNA Viruses

All oncogenic viruses are retroviruses which can be divided into two groups (i). Acute transforming retroviruses and (ii). Slow transforming retroviruses.

The acute transforming viruses include in its genome, a transforming sequence known as viral-oncogene (v-onc) which encodes overactive oncogene product leading to transformation of infected cell immediately after infection. Conversely, the slow transforming viruses do not contain transforming sequence and the virus genome is inserted adjacent to a proto-oncogene in the genome of host cell resulting in overexpression of that proto-oncogene subsequently leading to uncontrolled cell division. Since the chance of viral genome insertion near that proto-oncogene is very low, these viruses cause transformation of infected cell slowly as compared to acutely transforming viruses. Examples of cancer causing RNA viruses include:

1. Human T cell leukemia virus-1 (HTLV-1) it is the first identified human retrovirus which is associated with human leukemia/lymphoma and endemic in different regions of Japan.
2. Human T cell leukemia virus-2 (HTLV-2)
3. Rouse Sarcoma virus
4. Murine sarcoma virus
5. Murine leukemia virus
6. Avian leukemia and avian sarcoma

Some bacterial infections are also shown to be associated with some types of cancers such as *Helicobacter pylori* increase the risk of gastric cancer, *Opisthorchis viverrini* infection increase risk of cholangiocarcinoma, similarly *Schistosoma haematobium* is shown to be associated with bladder carcinoma.

Incidence of a Second Cancer in Survivors

Cancer survivors have increased risk to develop a new cancer. The usual lifetime probability of developing a primary cancer in cancer survivors is two in nine cases. This increased risk is thought to be mainly due to same risk factors which resulted in the first cancer, for example genetic factor, environmental factors and obesity, and in some cases the therapeutic agents used for the treatment of first cancer.

ROLE OF APOPTOSIS IN CANCER

Apoptosis is an essential intracellular process of program cell death that plays a crucial role as primary defense mechanism against the occurrence of cancer [24] and thus, loss of apoptosis can interfere with different stages of cancer including initiation, progression and metastasis.

Different genes and proteins involved in apoptosis are identified as potential drug targets. The recent advancements in cancer pharmacology and cancer genetics resulted increased understanding of molecular basis of apoptosis and its possible role in development of anticancer agents. It is well documented that some oncogenic mutations results in deregulation of apoptotic events which led to development of cancer. Different studies focused on pathways involving p53 and Bcl-2 postulated the key role of apoptosis in carcinogenesis [25, 26].

p53 play a crucial role as a checkpoint protein recognizing DNA damage and inducing cell-cycle arrest. Physiological conditions such as hypoxia as well as cellular stresses, including DNA damage and mitogenic oncogenes can activate the p53 and promote the apoptosis. Mutations in different components of the p53 pathway have been identified in different types of tumor these mutations are found to be responsible for deregulation of apoptosis. Another pathway involving Ras and PI-3 kinase is also disrupted in different types of cancer. Experimentally induced Bcl-2 overexpression in transgenic mice promoted the carcinogenesis. Similarly, p53 loss produced in transgenic mice promoted the carcinogenesis in several experiments [27]. Furthermore, disruption of p53 downstream components such as bax, caspase-9 and apaf-1 can induce oncogenic transformation and promote tumor progression in experimental animals [28]. Several apoptotic stimuli activate proapoptotic molecules while others act through alleviating the anti-apoptotic signal [29]. p53 induce apoptosis in response to different triggers such as excessive UV exposure, hypoxia or shortened telomeres and thus, loss of p53 function results in survival and clonal expansion of these cells.

Disturbance in apoptotic pathway may also promote metastasis of tumor. To spread in distant locations in the body, metastatic cancer cells should be able to survive in the blood circulation as well as to invade the other tissues. Normally, the epithelial cells are unable to survive in suspension and undergo apoptosis. The process is postulated to be governed by several factors, including focal adhesion kinase, p53 and Bcl-2 as well as different signaling pathways [30]. Thus, loss of apoptosis may contribute to tumor development through affecting different steps including initiation, progression and metastasis.

OXIDATIVE STRESS AND CANCER

Oxygen is the responsible factor for evolution of life in the existing form playing the central role in aerobic metabolic processes although about 5% of inhaled oxygen is converted to reactive oxygen species (ROS) such as superoxide or hydroxyl radicals during different steps of metabolic processes. These reactive oxygen species can also be generated through various exogenous sources. The production of these highly reactive molecules is markedly increased during some physiological conditions such as inflammatory response leading to oxidative injuries to cells through damaging the DNA, proteins, lipids, and cell membranes [31]. Superoxide radicals are primarily generated in mitochondria during the production of ATP which require a sequential flow of electrons along different components of the electron transport chain. During this process, some electrons escape and react with molecular oxygen to generate superoxide anions. It is further converted into other more damaging reactive oxygen species such as hydroxyl radical [32]. Some other enzymes such as nitric oxide synthases, NADPH oxidases, and lipoxygenases also produce reactive oxygen species. However, the increased oxidative stress followed by loss of the redox balance in a cellular metabolism results in oxidative damages in cellular membranes as well as in biomolecules through inducing sequential oxidation and fragmentation reactions as well as intermolecular cross-linking between the biomolecules.

Excessive accumulation of reactive oxygen species (ROS) followed by diminished efficiency of host antioxidant defense mechanisms can promote carcinogenesis [33, 34]. Reactive oxygen species may induce genotoxicity through inducing single-strand breaks and mutations in the DNA and are involved in various stages of cancer development [35, 36]. Similarly oxidation of lipid molecules may results in cytotoxicity and genotoxicity [37]. Lipid radical formed due to action of ROS, such as malondialdehyde and 4- hydroxynonenal can further induce DNA damage and mutations [38].

Primary Defense Against ROS: Catalytic Removal of ROS

Under normal conditions these oxidative damages are counteracted by antioxidant defense mechanism composed of different enzymes including superoxide dismutases, catalase, and glutathione peroxidases which reduce the reactive oxygen species and prevent the oxidative modifications of bio molecules and cell membranes. Most common intracellular ROS together with their source and the related antioxidant enzyme system involved in removal of these ROS molecules have been summarized in the Table **1**.

Superoxide Dismutases (SOD)

These are the first identified ROS metabolizing enzymes which reduce superoxide levels in the cell through catalyzing its conversion to molecular oxygen and hydrogen peroxide [39]. These comprise the first lines of defense against O_2^- produced in mitochondria or other cellular sources. Three isoforms of SOD have been identified in mammalian cells dimeric Cu/Zn SOD present in cytoplasm, tetrameric Mn SOD present in mitochondria, and extracellular SOD.

Table 1. Common Intracellular ROS, Their Source and the Related Antioxidant Enzyme System Involved in Removal of These ROS Molecules.

ROS Molecule	Source	Antioxidant enzyme
Superoxide (O_2^-)	Leakage of electron from etc. Xanthine oxidase Flavoenzymes Phagocyte activation	Superoxide dismutases (SOD)
Hydrogen peroxide(H_2O_2)	Action of SOD on O_2^- Xanthine oxidase Glucose oxidase NADPH oxidase	Glutathione peroxidases (GP_X) Catalase (CAT)
Hydroxyl radical (OH*)	From O_2^- and H_2O_2 through transition metals (Fe or Cu)	Glutathione (GSH)

Catalase (CAT)

These are tetrameric heme containing enzymes primarily located in the peroxisomes and convert H_2O_2, including those generated through SOD, into oxygen and water. It has the highest turnover rate converting 6 million substrate molecules into products in 1 minute. It efficiently removes the H_2O_2 produced in peroxisomes through β-oxidation, purine catabolism and photorespiration.

Glutathione Peroxidases (GPx)

Glutathione peroxidases can reduce peroxides (hydrogen peroxide as well as organic and lipid hydroperoxides) to water and alcohols. It use reduced glutathione (GSH) which is converted to glutathione disulphide.

$$ROOH/H_2O_2 + GSH = ROH/H_2O + GSSG$$

Eight isoforms of glutathione peroxidases have been identified which differ in tissue localization and substrate specificity GPx1 is the most abundant isoform which is responsible for much of the detoxification of H_2O_2 in the cytoplasm [32]. GPx4 is responsible for detoxification of lipid peroxides, such as hydroperoxides of phospholipid and cholesterol esters.

Peroxiredoxins (Prdx)

These are recently discovered class of antioxidants which reduce hydrogen peroxide, peroxynitrite, and different organic hydroperoxides [40]. Six isoforms of Peroxiredoxins have been identified which differ in cellular localization.

Secondary Defense Against ROS: Free Radical Scavengers

It comprises small molecules which react with free radicals to produce a less harmful radical. These are called antioxidants. Glutathione is an intracellular antioxidant present in all living aerobic cells in milimolar concentrations. It is essential to maintain the normal reduced environment of the cell and counteracting the oxidative effects of ROS. It is a potential scavenger of reactive oxygen species. Ascorbate, α- tocopherol and several polyphenolic compounds act as potent antioxidants and can be used to neutralize the effects of reactive oxygen species. Ascorbate quenches reactive oxygen species and inhibits oxidative consequences such as lipid peroxidation [41]. Sufficient dietary intake of ascorbate, Vitamin E and Vitamin A is directly related to decreased cancer risk [42, 43].

Several antioxidant enzymes act through repairing the oxidative damage from biomolecules. Thioredoxins and Methionine sulfoxide reductases can repair the proteins damaged by ROS. However overproduction of reactive oxygen species and impaired defense mechanisms results in oxidative stress which through a sequence of events lead to deregulation of normal cellular functions giving rise to various pathological conditions including neurodegenerative diseases, cardio-vascular disorders, gastrointestinal diseases, cancer and premature aging [44].

Genetic Landmarks in Cancer Research

Major achievements in the field of cancer research have been represented in Fig. (**4**).

DIAGNOSIS OF CANCER

Most cancers are initially diagnosed on the basis of signs or symptoms or during the diagnosis of other diseases. Both of these provide only intimation to the disease and further require the examination of a tissue sample to determine the type of proliferating cells, genetic abnormalities, its histological grade, and other morphological and biochemical characteristics of the cancer. Some other methods such as blood test, X-rays, CT scans and more recent tests involving Cytogenetics and immunohistochemistry can also be used to diagnose the cancer. Together, these examinations are used to predict the condition of disease and to decide the appropriate treatment. Cytogenetic and immunological tests are used to predict the molecular changes involved in cancer development including mutations, karyotypic changes and immunological changes leading to prediction of future pathological conditions of the cancer and to select the best treatment.

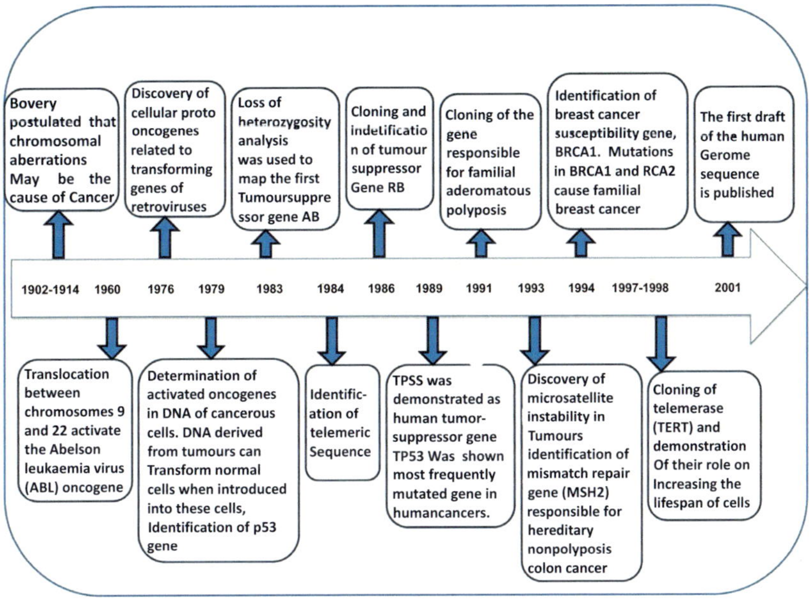

Fig. (4). Major landmarks in cancer research.

CANCER THERAPY

Different types of treatments are suggested for management of different cancer types depending on the type of cancer, its location in the body, and its state of advancement. The major therapeutic approaches involve surgery, chemotherapy radiation therapy, hormonal therapy, immunotherapy and targeted therapy. These different approaches can be applied alone or in combination depending upon type and stage of cancer.

Surgery

Surgery is the primary method applied to remove most isolated solid tumors. In localized cancer, surgery typically attempts to remove the entire mass along with the lymph nodes present in the surrounding area. For some types of cancer surgery can be successfully applied to completely eliminate the cancer. It is considered the successful treatment for several early stage cancers and benign tumors. Based on the outcome, various types of surgery are available such as diagnostic surgery- used to isolate a tissue sample for pathological evaluation to determine the type and stage of cancer, curative surgery- used to remove the cancer affected tissue from the specific part of the body, preventive surgery- applied to remove precancer tissue which may consequently develop into a cancer, staging surgery- used to determine the extent of cancer in the whole body. Debulking surgery- applied to removes a portion of a cancer affected tissue when removal of the entire tumor is harmful to the body. It may be followed by chemotherapy and radiation therapy. Palliative Surgery- used to treat advanced stages of cancer in order to minimize the effects of cancer.

Recently some specialized surgeries have been developed for cancer treatment such as cryosurgery in which extremely cold temperatures is used to kill cancer cells in this method, liquid nitrogen is applied directly or through a cryoprobe on the affected tissue.

Similarly laser surgery is applied to remove the small tumors without affecting the surrounding tissue using the beams of light energy in place of instruments. Another specialized surgery termed as electrosurgery kill the cancer cells by using electrical current.

Radiation Therapy

Radiation therapy through ionizing radiation is an effective approach to either cure or improve the symptoms of cancer. It kills cancer cells with high-energy radiation directly targeted to the tumor and is applied in nearly 50% of cancer cases. A constant dose of ionizing radiation is applied directly at the affected tissues which act primarily by damaging DNA and preventing its replication leading to the death of rapidly dividing cancer cells. It also kills some rapidly dividing normal cells and the radiation can be from either internal sources in the form of brachytherapy or external sources. Radiation therapy is often used in combination to surgery and or chemotherapy but for certain types of cancer for example early head and neck cancer the radiation therapy may be applied alone. It has been found to be effective in about 70% of cancer patients suffering from painful bone metastasis.

Chemotherapy

Chemotherapy deals with the treatment of cancer with the help of cytotoxic compounds that target rapidly growing cancerous cells. Unlike surgery and radiation therapy which are effective in treatment of cancer at a particular location, chemotherapy effectively kill cancer cells all over the body. Chemotherapy alone or in combination with surgery has proven useful in a number of different cancer types including: breast cancer, ovarian cancer, pancreatic cancer, testicular cancer, colorectal cancer, osteogenic sarcoma, and some lung cancers.

Chemotherapeutic agents primarily act through damaging DNA of the cancer cells, leading to apoptosis or through inhibiting DNA replication and thus, preventing cell division and blocking tumor growth. These agents selectively kill or inhibit rapidly dividing cancer cells. Cell cycle involves 4 phases:

1. G1 phase (Pre-synthetic phase):- It is the first stage in which cells make required preparations for replication of DNA. This phase is also characterized by the synthesis and accumulation of RNA and protein required for cell division.
2. S phase (Synthetic phase):- It involves the replication of nuclear DNA. Histone proteins are also synthesized in this phase, these proteins enter the nucleus and become associated with newly synthesized DNA. At the end of S phase the cell contains two copies of DNA.
3. G2 phase (Post-synthetic phase):- In this phase cell synthesizes several new proteins and complete all required preparations for cell division.
4. M Phase (Mitosis phase):- In this phase nucleus of the parent cell is dissolved, two pairs of chromosomes are pulled to opposite poles and each cell get completely divided into two daughter cells.

Some of these new cells enter the new cell cycle, while the others become non-proliferating cells. Many of the conventional chemotherapeutic agents interfere with the synthesis of DNA precursor molecules, the modulation of the synthesis of these precursor molecules interfere with the cell cycle through preventing the cell to complete the S phase. Several other drugs act through blocking mitosis through preventing the splitting of a cell at the end of mitosis into two daughter cells ultimately preventing the progression of cancer. The anticancer drugs targeting different stages of cell cycle have been shown in Fig. (**5**).

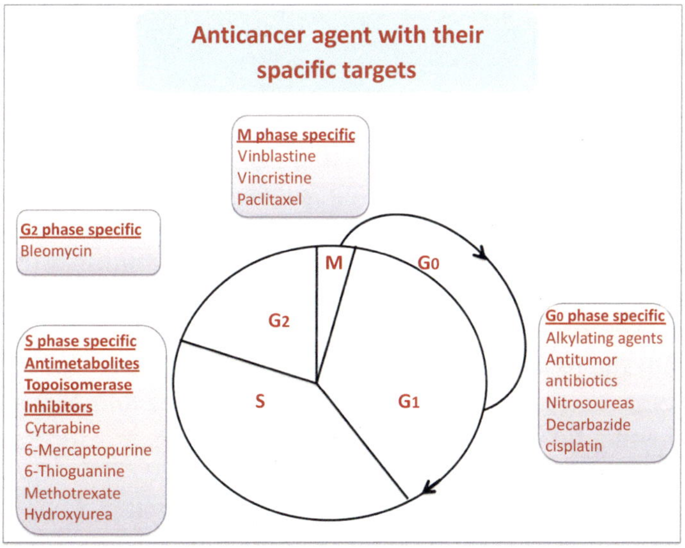

Fig. (5). Types of anticancer drugs targeting different stages of cell cycle with important examples.

DRUGS DAMAGING THE NUCLEAR DNA

This class of anticancer agents directly damage DNA in the nucleus. These are known to act through directly interrupting the DNA replication in cancerous cells and consequently arresting replication or synthesizing abnormal form of DNA or RNA which are not able to code for useful products. Important drugs of this class include antibiotics - daunorubicin, doxorubicin, cisplatin and etoposide.

DRUGS INHIBITING THE REPLICATION OF DNA

This type of drugs directly interferes with synthesis of DNA building blocks including nucleotides, folic acid, and nitrogen bases. These drugs interfere with different steps in synthesis of nucleotides or deoxyribonucleotides. This results in decrease in the cellular concentration of these building blocks preventing the synthesis of nucleic acids and ultimately leading to obstruction of replication. Important drugs of this class include methotrexate, mercaptopurine, hydroxyurea and fluorouracil.

DRUGS AFFECTING THE SYNTHESIS AND BREAKDOWN OF THE MITOTIC SPINDLES (ANTIMITOTIC AGENTS)

This type of drugs acts by inhibiting the function of microtubules through binding to their subunits and affecting the synthesis and breakdown of the mitotic spindles. Microtubules play central role in equal distribution of chromosome in daughter cells through formation of spindle apparatus during mitosis. Microtubules also play important role in cytokinesis. Thus the compounds targeting the microtubules can be used as potential anti-cancer agents. These compounds are also called antimitotic agents. Three different classes of drugs acting as antimitotic agents have been identified.

1. Taxanes

It is the first identified group of antimitotic drugs which include paclitaxel and docetaxel. These interfere with microtubules through binding to β-tubulin and preventing their disassembly after completion of cell division which results in the mitotic arrest and consequently lead to apoptosis and cell death. Paclitaxel has been isolated from the bark of the *Taxus brevifolia* (Western yew tree) [45]. It is used to treat breast cancer, ovarian cancer, lung cancer and Kaposi's sarcoma. Later on a semisynthetic analogue of paclitaxel known as Docetaxel has been synthesized from a compound isolated from *Taxus bacatta* (Himalayan yew tree) [46]. Docetaxel is more potent compound and has better toxicity profile as compare to paclitaxel. It is used to treat prostate cancer, breast cancer ovarian cancer and lung cancer.

2. Vinca Alkaloids

It is another class of antimitotic drugs which act through binding to the β-tubulin inhibiting it to bind with the α-tubulin thus inhibiting the synthesis of microtubules. These results in cell cycle arrest in metaphase and consequently lead to apoptosis. These include vinblastine, vincristine, vinorelbine, and vindesine isolated from a medicinal plant *Vinca rosea.*

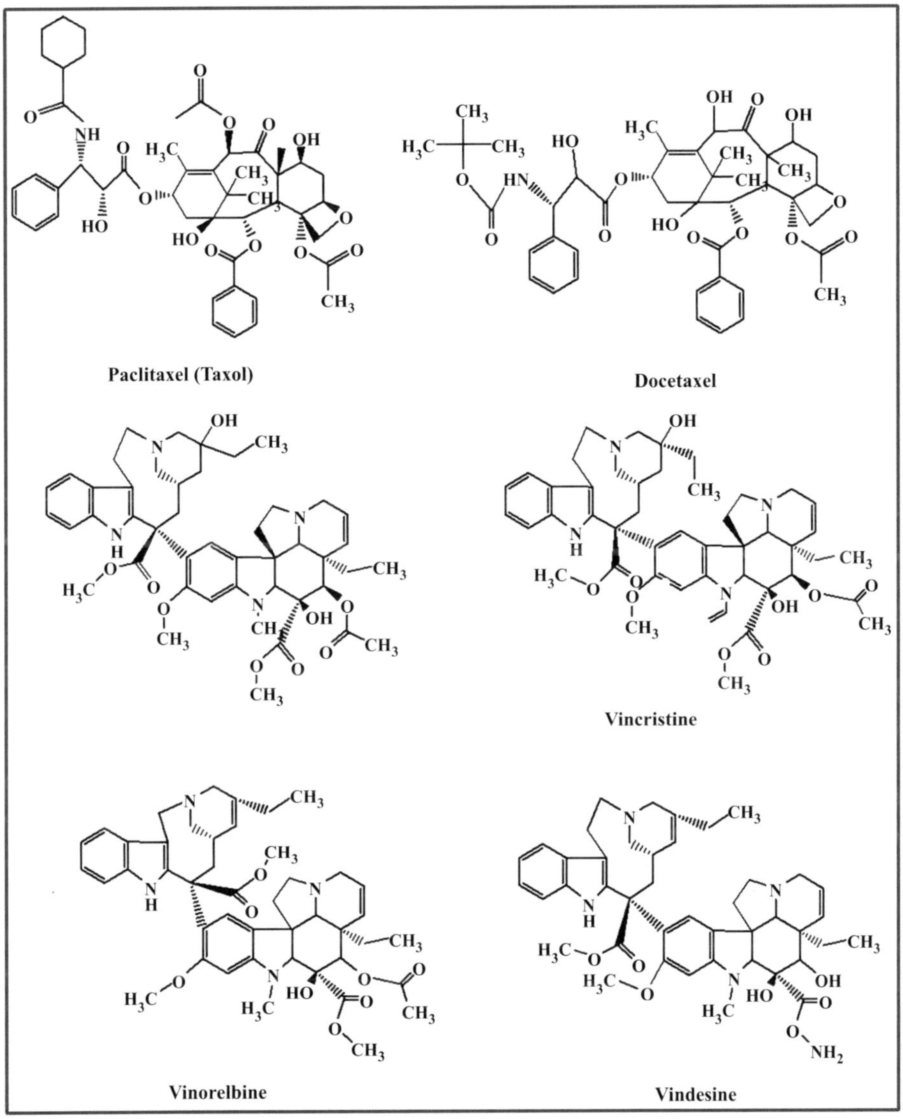

Structures of Taxanes and Vinca alkaloids.

Vinblastine is used in the treatment of bladder cancer, neuroblastoma, testicular cancers, Kaposi's sarcoma and Hodgkin's disease. Vincristine is used to treat leukemias and lymphomas of childhood, rhabdomyosarcoma, neuroblastoma and non Hodgkin's lymphoma. Vinorelbine is used for the treatment of breast cancer and lung cancer. Vindesine is effective in treatment of lung cancer breast cancer and leukemia.

3. Colchicine

It is small molecule isolated from *Colchicum autumnale* which act through binding with β-tubulin and promoting their polymerization eventually inducing apoptosis.

Although the efficiency of chemotherapeutic agents is often limited by its toxic effect on other tissues as these compounds also kill some normal noncancerous cells, particularly those that divide rapidly as part of their physiological roles such as bone marrow cells, germinal epithelium hair follicles and mucosal cells of gastrointestinal tract resulting in common side effects of chemotherapy including low white blood cell count, gastrointestinal disorders, anemia and hair loss. To overcome this problem target based chemotherapeutic agents are developed which selectively target a signaling pathway specific to cancerous cells and thus, showing selective toxicity. Considering on issue of toxicity development of chemotherapeutic agents the search for novel anticancer agents has been extended to compounds derived from natural resources.

On the basis of mechanism of action anticancer drugs are classified in following groups:

ALKYLATING AGENTS (NITROGEN MUSTARDS)

These drugs act through producing highly reactive carbonium ion species which can interact with a nucleophile (electron donor species such as hydroxyl, amine and sulfhydryl groups) present in biomolecule. The N7 of guanine, N1 and N3 of adenine, and N3 of cytosine are all act as nucleophiles to react with carbonium ion produced by alkylating agents. Most of the drugs of this class have two alkylating groups and may react with two different nucleophilic groups leading to the cross linking of DNA. These drugs act by interfering with transcription as well as replication of DNA causing cytotoxic effect. Examples of alkylating drugs include mechlorethamines, Cyclophosphamide, ifosfamide, chlorambucil, melphalan, ethylenimine and thio-TEPA. Other alkylating agents include busulfan, nitrosoureas, carmustine, lomustine, triazine and dacarbazine.

ANTIMETABOLITES

These drugs have structural similarity with DNA constituents or with coenzymes involved in the synthesis of nucleotides. These inhibit the synthesis of purine or pyrimidine or compete with them in synthesis of DNA or RNA. For example methotrexate inhibits the enzyme folate reductase, an enzyme involved in conversion of folic acid to tetrahydrofolic acid. It irreversibly binds with folate reductase, thus inhibiting the synthesis of tetrahydrofolic acid which lead to inhibition of DNA synthesis and subsequently arrest of cell cycle in S phase. Similarly purine and pyrimidine antagonists act through interfering with the synthesis of purines and pyrimidines. Examples of antimetabolites include:

a. Folate antagonists such as methotrexate
b. Purine antagonists such as 6-mercaptopurine (6-MP), 6-thioguanine (6-TG) and azathioprine
c. Pyrimidine antagonists such as 5-Fluorouracil (5-FU) and Cytarabine (cytosine arabinoside)

PLANT ALKALOIDS

Vinca Alkaloids

These are the alkaloids obtained from the plant *Vinca rosea*. These drugs prevent the spindle formation through binding with tubulin and cause mitotic arrest. Examples: vincristine (Oncovin), vinblastine (Velban) and vindesine.

Taxanes

They form stable non-functioning microtubule by promoting polymerization through binding with tubulin, thus resulting in mitotic arrest. Examples- Paclitaxel (taxol), Docetaxel (taxotere).

Podophyllotoxin

Podophyllotoxin and deoxypodophyllotoxin, the active constituents isolated from the roots of *Podophyllum peltatum* Linnaeus have been found active against different types of cancer, acting through inhibiting the assembly of microtubules and inducing cell cycle arrests in metaphase. Epipodophyllotoxin, an isomer of podophyllotoxin has been shown to be more effective and less toxic against different cancer cell lines. Semi-synthetic analogues of epipodophyllotoxin termed as etoposide and teniposide were found very effective against different human cancers including lymphomas, bronchial cancer and testicular cancer.

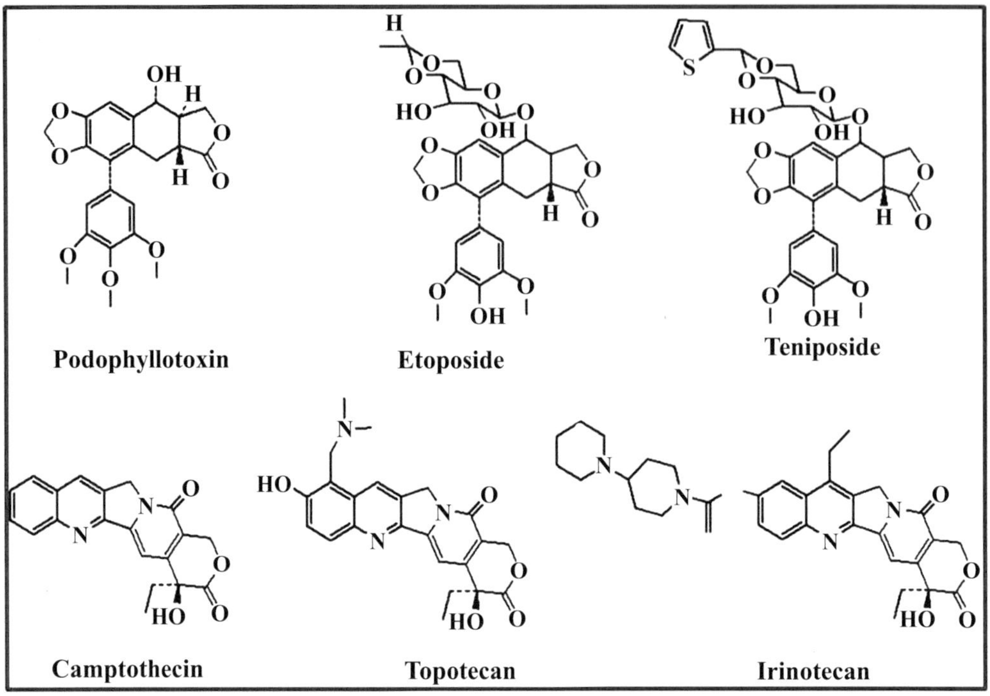

Structures of Podophyllotoxin Camptothecin and their analogues.

Camptothecin Analogues

Camptothecin is a cytotoxic alkaloid isolated from, *Camptotheca acuminate* which is known to act through inhibiting DNA Topoisomerase I. In order to increase its solubility and improve toxicity profile, certain analogues have been synthesized such as topotecan (hycamtin), irinotecan (camptosar), exatecan, rubitecan, lurtotecan and 9- aminocamptothecin (9-AC). Topotecan is found very effective in patients with epithelial ovarian cancer and small cell lung cancer as a second-line treatment. Similarly, irinotecan acts as first- and second-line treatment for metastatic colorectal cancer.

Antibiotics anthracyclines such as doxorubicin (adriamycin), daunorubicin (rubidomycin), actinomycin (dactinomycin) mitoxantrone, bleomycins (blenoxane), mitomycin (mutamycin), mithramycin (plicamycin), dactinomycin (cosmegen). Different targets of anticancer drugs interfering with the synthesis of nucleic acids have been represented in Fig. (**6**).

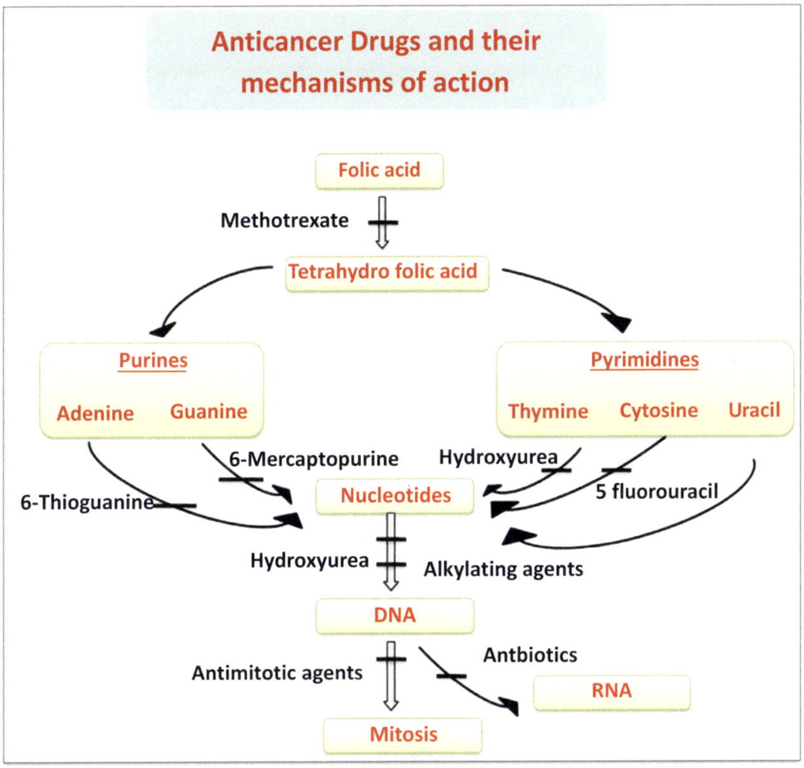

Fig. (6). Different targets of anticancer drugs interfering with the synthesis of nucleic acids with important examples.

DRUGS INHIBITING ANGIOGENESIS

These drugs specifically target the pathways involved in development of vasculature in a tumor preventing blood supply to the tumor. 5, 6-dimethylxanthenone-4-acetic acid is postulated to exert anticancer activity through obstructing the development of vascular system in tumors and also showed prominent cancer inhibition when given in combination with other cytotoxic drugs [47]. Angiogenesis inhibitors are known to possess less toxic effect in comparison to other anticancer drugs.

HORMONAL AGENTS

These drugs act through restoring the hormonal balance and are useful in treatment of breast cancer, prostate cancer, ovarian cancer and endometrial cancer for example tamoxifen (nolvadex), flutamide (eulexin) and gonadotropin-releasing hormone agonists.

MISCELLANEOUS AGENTS

These include hydroxyurea, L-asparaginase, cisplatin, mitoxantrone (Novantrone), derivatives of retinoic acid and bone marrow growth factors *etc*.

Enzyme L-asparaginase act through interfering with the metabolism of asparagines. Cancerous cells, particularly lymphatic cancer cells, need continuous supply of asparagines and for this requirement they mainly depend upon dietary asparagines. Recent studies revealed that leukemia cells are unable to synthesize asparagine while normal cells can synthesize it in normal circumstances. This metabolic difference between cancerous and normal cells can be exploited in treatment of leukemia. The enzyme L-asparaginase is recognized as useful agent for the treatment of different types of leukemia. Administration of L-asparaginase degrades the extracellular asparagines through converting into aspartic acid. Cancerous cells become deficient of asparagine and die while normal cells synthesize the required quantity of asparagine internally thus remain unaffected. L-asparaginase was isolated from *E. coli* as well as some rodent animals and was shown to exert significant activity against different types of human leukemias.

DEVELOPMENT OF ANTICANCER DRUGS

Historical Background

Most of the conventional anticancer molecules were discovered by serendipity or through random screening of compounds through evaluation of their effect on inhibition of cell division. An important example of coincident discovery of anticancer agent include the findings that nitrogen mustard significantly suppressed the lymphoma and myeloma in the soldiers accidentally exposed to this gas during the World War II.

This finding lead to the development of several related alkylating agents, including chlorambucil and cyclophosphamide. In the similar way, the anticancer potential of platinum containing anticancer drugs came into existence coincidently during another study demonstrating the inhibition of bacterial growth after putting them in influence of an electric field. During the experiment, it was observed that multiplication of bacterial cells blocked due to accumulation of the electrolysis product of the platinum electrode which is thought to contaminate the growth medium. This serendipitous discovery has provided valuable anticancer drugs such as cisplatin. Folate antagonists, including aminopterin and amethopterin, came in to existence in 1948. A brief history of development of anticancer drugs is summarized in Fig. (**7**).

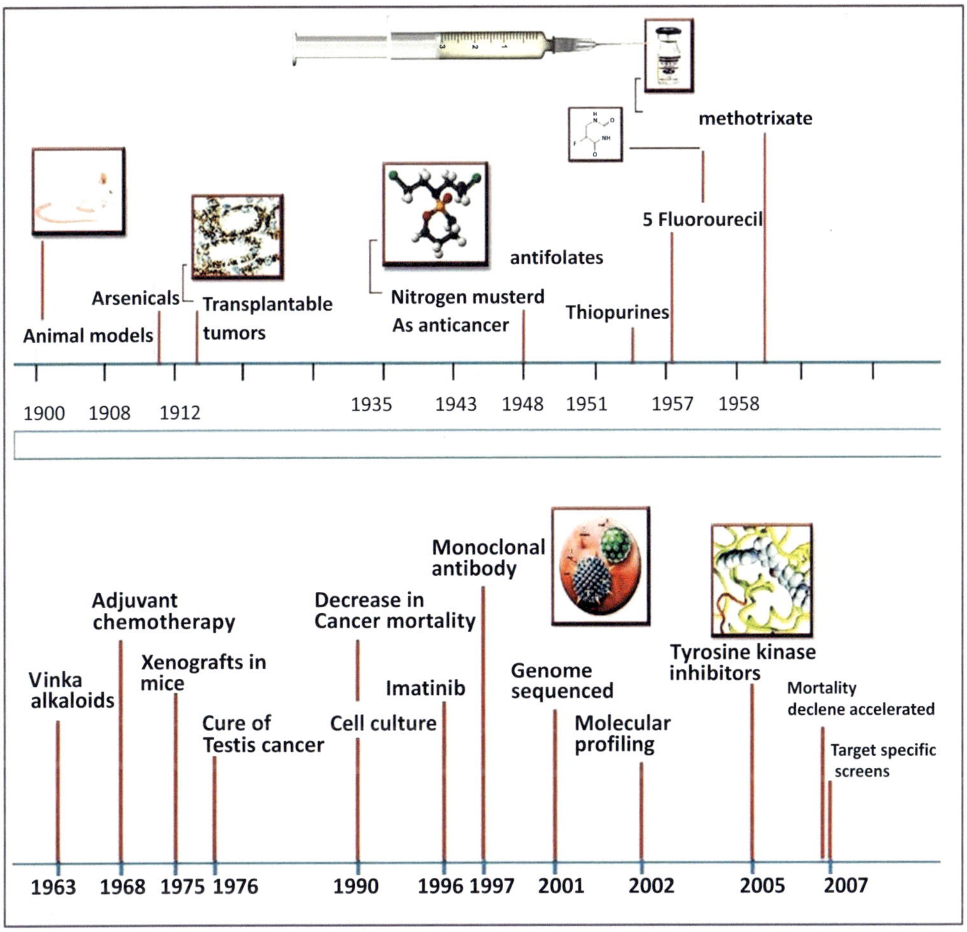

Fig. (7). Key advances in the history of anticancer drug development.

Cancer was recognized as a disease caused due to uncontrolled and excessive cell division. Thus, to develop anticancer agents, attempts were focused in the identification of cytostatic and antiproliferative molecules. Anticancer compounds are initially screened in cell lines derived from different types of cancer possessing characteristic molecular markers and other relevant features related to cell cycle regulation and differentiation. Since an anticancer compound specifically target some molecular pathways, these compounds are evaluated against a panel of different cancer cell lines belonging to different cancer types to determine exact mechanism of action.

Drug found active in *in vitro* screening are evaluated in *in vitro* murine models. Initially developed murine models include L1210 mouse leukemia model and P388 murine leukemia allograft, Murine models of cancer are used for *in vivo* experiments as rapidly growing tumor models provide a more relevant condition in preliminary evaluation of the anticancer potential. Compounds showing significant activity in murine model are further evaluated in other *in vivo* model. *In vivo* study provides more accurate information about activity profile and mechanism of action. In addition to determining the specificity and extent of activity, the *in vivo* studies also provide valuable information on toxicity profile and maximum tolerable doses. Compounds significantly reducing the size of tumor and increasing the life span of the mice are identified as potential agents and recommended for further studies.

National Cancer Institute introduced an advanced *in vivo* model, human tumor xenografts in nude mice. After a detailed analysis and considering all aspects of molecular mechanism related to different types of cancer, NCI recently introduced an *in vitro* system of evaluation of anticancer activity using 60 different tumor cell lines (NCI-60 screen) derived from different types of human cancers including leukemia, breast cancer, prostate cancer, small-cell and non-small-cell lung cancers, and others.

Anticancer drugs development has fundamental difference from other drug development. It need fine selectivity of therapeutic compounds to rapidly dividing cancerous cells without affecting remaining normal cells of whole body. This fact can be easily understood from the fact that out of 600,000 molecules evaluated for anticancer potential, only 38 have reached in clinical trials to be used as drugs.

Development of conventional chemotherapeutic agents is based on the antiproliferative potential of compounds. The screening of molecules is performed to select the compounds with significant cytotoxic or cytostatic effect on different cancer cell lines. The anticancer potential of compounds is further validated through evaluating the effect of these compounds on regression of tumors in murine tumor xenografts or allografts. The anticancer agents were discovered basically through randomly screening the compounds for cytotoxic potential or evaluating their potential to modulated metabolic pathways related to cell division.

The recent advancements in the field of molecular biology and an understanding of the biochemical basis of cancer have provided new way to develop target-based potent anticancer drugs. After the identification of biochemical pathways and key enzymes regulating these pathways it become easy to develop a therapeutic agent which selectively target a pathway involved in different stages of the disease including growth, metastasis or angiogenesis. A number of target-based anticancer agents have been developed following these developments.

ANTICANCER DRUGS ACTING THROUGH FACILITATING THE APOPTOSIS

Different cytotoxic drugs exert their activity through triggering the apoptosis. Most of the currently used anticancer drugs were developed based on evaluation of their potential to selectively kill tumor cells. These can modulate the activity of genes and proteins controlling apoptosis [48, 49]. Many of these are known to act through activating the p53 or inhibiting Bcl-2 activity [50].

Several molecules inhibiting the activity of NF-κB or proteosome or different enzymes involved in kinase/Akt pathway are shown to be potentially inducing cell death in cancerous cells [51]. Molecules modulating the function of Ras and its activator farnysltransferase are also used as potential anticancer agents. The compounds modulating the activity of any of these signaling molecules can restore the apoptosis in cancerous cells or facilitate the other anticancer agents to induce cell death. These drugs induce the damaging effect in the nuclear DNA subsequently resulting in the activation and release of the pro-apoptotic factors from mitochondrial intermembrane space or upregulation of expression of pro-apoptotic receptors (Fas/CD95, TNF-R1 and TRAIL receptors) on cancerous cells, which subsequently interact with pro-apoptotic proteins to initiate apoptotic signaling pathways [52]. Several natural products including flavones and alkaloids have been shown to act through selectively inducing the apoptosis in cancer cells [53, 54]. Similarly, luteolin and apigenin have been shown to induce apoptosis selectively in myeloid leukemia and prostate cancer respectively [55, 56]. Some flavones such as fisetin and wogonin as well as red wine polyphenolic extract have been shown to induce apoptosis mediated by cascade involving caspase 3 [57].

ANTICANCER DRUG DEVELOPMENT BASED ON MOLECULAR TARGETS

Anticancer agents are developed based on *in vitro* screening of cytotoxic activity using different cancer cell lines followed by *in vivo* screening using animal models. To determining the non toxic dose of these drugs, the preclinical study is followed by early phase of human clinical trials.

Anticancer agents show toxic effect when their concentration exceeds the limiting dose hence it become essential to determine tolerable maximum doses with no detectable toxic effect. In case of anticancer agents based on molecular targets, the possibilities of toxic effect get reduced considerably as these agents are postulated to be directly targeting a specific pathway. Molecular target based agents usually act through targeting key enzymes of different intracellular and extracellular processes with reduce toxicity and less chance of drug resistance.

Examples of these key enzymes include topoisomerase, farnesyltransferase, receptor tyrosine kinases, dihydrofolate reductase and matrix metalloproteinase. The development of anticancer agents with molecular targets is an intricate process requiring well understanding of several related intracellular and extracellular processes. Beyond all these obstacles research efforts are focused on development of molecular targets based anticancer agents which involve the identification of a potent target molecule followed by development and validation of a molecular assay specific to that target and the relationship between the molecular target and the cancer type.

Since these anticancer drugs are developed with a pre-determined target and mechanism of action, some modifications are needed in preclinical and clinical studies. Determination of the effects of these drugs on a particular target is not enough to demonstrate therapeutic effect, it should be authenticated through several other studies determining their effects on other related processes.

Furthermore, toxicity profile is the major factor in development of molecularly targeted anticancer drugs. It includes the adverse effects of these drugs on other metabolic pathways and general toxicity. To overcome these effects the compounds should be chemically modified to enhance the activity and consequently to decrease the toxicity.

The combination therapy is another way to overcome these effects as it require comparatively low dose of drugs eventually minimizing the toxic effects. In combination therapy the effects of molecular targets based drugs are enhanced by other chemotherapeutic agents that may act through sensitizing the cancerous cells to these agents.

ANTICANCER DRUGS ACTING THROUGH INHIBITION OF METASTASIS

The spread of the cancer from its origin site to other parts of the body is known as metastasis. It is attributed to the movement of cancer cells to distant locations in the body. The mechanism of translocation of cancerous cell involves cellular movement together with the extracellular matrix remodeling (ECM remodeling) which facilitates physical entrapment of the cells and ultimately determines the shape of a tissue at both the site of initial as well as the site of metastasis. Several enzymes including plasminogen activators (Pas), proteases and matrix metalloproteinases (MMPs) have been shown to be associated with the extracellular matrix remodeling facilitating the invasion and propagation of cancerous cells to distant parts of the body. Consequently, the compounds modulating the activity of plasminogen activators, proteases and matrix metalloproteinases may act as potential anticancer agents. Some recent studies postulated that p53 mutations and Bcl-2 overexpression also influence the metastasis [58, 59].

ANTICANCER DRUGS ACTING THROUGH INHIBITION OF ANGIOGENESIS

The development of new blood vessels in cancerous tissues to maintain the blood supply to all the cells in growing tumor is known as angiogenesis. It is an essential step to fulfill the requirement of oxygen and nutrients for the cells present in the center of tumor to grow as well as its spread to other parts of the body. Consequently, the drug candidates preventing the supply of oxygen and nutrients through blocking the angiogenesis may be applied as anticancer agents.

Tumor cells secrete some angiogenic factors which induce the blood vessel cells to divide and develop new blood vessels in tumor. Different studies have shown that some oncogenes such as bcl2 increase the expression of genes encoding different angiogenic factors.

The process of angiogenesis is postulated to be regulated through intricate network of signal transduction cascade and can be divided in three closely associated steps (i) initiation of angiogenesis, (ii) development of blood vessel lining through proliferation and migration of endothelial cells, and (iii) remodeling of the extracellular matrix.

Recent advancement in the understanding of tumor angiogenesis has led to the identification of several novel drug targets including platelet-derived growth factor (PDGF), fibroblast growth factor (FGF), vascular endothelial growth factor (VEGF) and receptor tyrosine kinases related to these growth factors. Some other validated targets include matrix metalloproteinases, cell adhesion molecules and plasminogen activators. Compounds modulating the activities of these targets lead to the inhibition of endothelial cell proliferation and subsequent inhibition of angiogenesis. The inhibitory potential may be used in the development of potential anticancer drugs. Taxanes have been postulated to act through disrupting the microvessel mediated by inhibition of VEGF and MMP and enhanced expression of E-cadherin [60, 61].

DEVELOPMENT OF ANTIBODIES AGAINST TUMOR-SPECIFIC ANTIGENS

Development of antibodies against tumor-specific and tumor associated antigens is used as powerful strategy to find new anticancer drugs. These antibodies are used to induce antitumor immune responses in cancer patients it is considered to be free of toxic effects. These specific antibodies can be designed to be conjugated with tumor specific drugs, radioisotopes or prodrug specific enzymes and used against different types of tumors. Furthermore different tumor specific antibodies can itself induce tumor regression through stimulation of antibody-dependent cellular toxicity (ADCC) or targeting the complement system. Antibody-dependent cellular toxicity is demonstrated to be mediated through monocytes, granulocytes and natural killer cells. Tumor specific antibodies can also be used to induce the expression of tumor-specific antigens on the antigen-presenting cells/dendritic cells to activate the T-cell immune response against cancer.

ROLE OF METABOLOMICS AND PHARMACOGENETICS IN TREATMENT OF CANCER

These are relatively new techniques came in to existence due to advancement in molecular biology. These used to predict the drug response and toxicity profile in individual patents. Cytotoxic drugs exhibit toxic effect in normal cells at higher doses, considering this fact it become essential to determine the safe dose for a patent. Pharmacogenetics is used to determine the nontoxic dose through monitoring of drug response and toxicity using the genetic constitution of the individual patient to recognize the key factors involved in drug response and toxic effect. It primarily considers the drug-metabolizing enzymes cytochrome P450 (CYP) superfamily several of which are found to be responsible for the inactivation of anticancer drugs. Variations in drug targets such as thymidylate synthase and epidermal growth factor receptor (EGFR) are also considered. Person to person difference in drug–response can be minimized through it. Quantification of metabolites through metabolite profiling (analyses of all the metabolites in a sample to identify the characteristic metabolite profile of that sample) and target analysis (quantification of metabolites specific to a particular drug or pathway) provide useful information about cellular metabolism. It can be achieved through isotopic labeling of selected metabolites and monitoring their movement through diverse pathways followed by different assays such as NMR, mass spectroscopy, liquid chromatography – tandem MS (LC-MS/MS) and gas chromatography – tandem MS GC-MS/MS). Metabolic profiling can be used as a marker to determine the disease state and to differentiate the normal tissues from different states of the disease [62].

OTHER ANTICANCER AGENTS ACTING THROUGH INDIRECT MECHANISMS

Several drugs acting through indirect mechanisms other than cytotoxic and molecularly targeted are used in the cancer treatment. The important examples of these drugs include the drugs reversing the multidrug resistance, drugs modulating immune response, chemoprotective agents, drugs restoring hormonal balance, photosensitizers, and Supportive cancer-care agents.

Drugs Reversing the Multidrug Resistance

Multi-drug resistance (MDR) is a major concern in the anticancer drug development. The upregulation of the membrane efflux protein, P-glycoprotein (P-gp) and failure of therapeutic agents to induce apoptosis result in multi-drug resistance. Consequently the inhibitors of the membrane efflux protein may be used to potentiate the activity of anticancer drugs. Several P-glycoprotein inhibitors including zosuquidar, tariquidar, and laniquidar, have showed potential anticancer potential when used in combination with other cytotoxic agents [63].

Vaccines or Immunomodulators

It is a group of drugs which act through improving the immune response to tumor cells. Tumor-specific antigens are used to generate humoral and/or T-cell mediated immunity. Immune-mediated anticancer activity can be attain through a number of approaches such as through potentiating immune interaction by increasing the activity of antigen presenting cells (APC) or directly increasing the immune response by cytokines [64].

Chemoprotective Agents

These are known to alleviate the toxic effects of anticancer drugs. Nephrotoxicity caused by nitrogen mustard ifosfamide can be neutralized by sodium---sulfanylethanesulfonate when administered as combination therapy. Similarly amifostine act as a chemoprotective agent through effectively minimizing the nephrotoxicity caused by anticancer drug cisplatin.

Drugs Restoring Hormonal Balance

Another effective non-cytotoxic anticancer therapeutic approach include the hormonal therapy which can be effectively used for the treatment of some particular types of cancer which are known to be influenced by hormonal imbalance such as breast cancer, prostate cancer, ovarian cancer and endometrial cancer. Steroids such as antiandrogens and antiestrogens are used for the treatment of these cancer types without showing any toxic effect. Recent studies showed that the breast cancers can be treated through removal of the ovaries [65]. Similarly prostate cancer can be treated by removal of testis or by administration of the estrogen [66].

Photosensitizers

These are the biologically inactive compounds but become active when irradiated by light. Administration of photosensitizers followed by laser irradiation of cancer affected tissue results in the generation of free radicals in that portion of the body, leading to destruction of the tumor. Precaution should be taken in determination of concentration of the photosensitizer and focused irradiation. 5-Aminolaevulinic acid, a porphyrin precursor is postulated to be effective photosensitizing agent [67].

Supportive Cancer-Care Agents

These are the drugs used to reduce the side effects caused by chemotherapeutic agents aiming to enhance their therapeutic efficacy as well as improve the quality of life after chemotherapy. Painkillers such as opiates, anti-emetic drugs such as butyrophenones, and growth factors such as granulocyte colony stimulating factor and monocyte colony stimulating factor are some important drugs of this class [68].

PROCESS OF ANTICANCER DRUG DEVELOPMENT

The development of anticancer drug is primarily based on the identification of cytostatic or cytotoxic compounds which act through reducing the growth of tumor or demolishing the tumor. The process of anticancer drug development has been extended to exploit target specificity of drug candidates to identify the molecular targets as well as to develop molecules selectively acting on these targets. Several other drug types including immunomodulators, chemoprotective agents, Multi-drug resistance-reversing agents, drugs based on hormonal therapy and photosensitizers are in progress with the potential to be used in combination with conventional cytotoxic agents. Moreover the application of recent technologies such as pharmacogenetics and metabolomics is known to improve the process of development of novel anticancer agents. The development of new drug usually consists of following steps:

1. Identification of Biologically Active Compounds

New bioactive compounds can be identified through activity directed fractionation of different extracts from natural resources or by chemical synthesis. This step is supported by several analytical techniques to characterize and purify these compounds as well as to determine their bioavailability and stability under physiological conditions. Different types of chromatography together with spectroscopic techniques are used to purify and characterize the compound. Their physicochemical properties including solubility, melting point, and stability are determined through different techniques. Method is developed and validated to ensure large scale isolation or synthesis of compound as it progresses in the drug development pathway.

2. Screening of Biological Activity and Preclinical Pharmacology

The possible drug structure is determined through pharmacophore mapping and docking analysis and comparing their structures to those of existing drugs. Selected compounds are screened using different cancer cell lines to determine the extent and specificity of anticancer activity. Toxicity of these compounds is determined using normal cell lines. These compounds were finally evaluated in animal models to validate their efficacy and toxicity, preclinical study provide sufficient information about efficacy, toxicity and pharmacokinetics of drug candidate.

3. Clinical Development

It is the final step of drug development process which encompasses three major steps termed as phase I, phase II and phase III clinical trials. In phase I clinical trials these drugs are evaluated in healthy human volunteers to determine the maximum tolerable dose as well as the toxic effects. The gradually increased doses of the drug candidates are administered to a small group (usually, 20 to 100 persons) of closely supervised healthy volunteers. Subsequently, in phase II clinical trials the drugs are evaluated and their effects are studied in detail in a small group of carefully observed and continuously assessed patients (usually, 100 to 300 patients) suffering from selected types of cancer to determine the efficacy of drug, the method of delivery, effective dosage and the dosing interval as well as to reconfirm the maximum tolerable dosage. To confirm findings of phase I and II trials, the drugs are evaluated in long duration (usually 2 to 10 years) phase III clinical trials in a larger population involving thousands of patients in multiple locations These studies are designed to compare the therapeutic potential of these newly developed drug candidates with that of the existing most potent therapeutic agent as well as to further confirm the efficacy and maximum tolerable dosage The drug found successful in Phases I, II, and III clinical trials can be approved by national drug regulatory authority.

NATURAL PRODUCTS AS SOURCE OF THERAPEUTIC AGENTS

The Mother Nature has been continuously serving the mankind as most efficient arsenal, playing an important role in health care and prevention of diseases. Natural products have traditionally been used in form of plant extracts, dry powders, infusions, or other therapeutic preparations to treat several diseases over centuries and continue to play a highly significant role in the modern drug discovery and development process providing a diverse and unique source of medicinally active molecules. Medicinal plants play a major role and constitute the backbone of almost all the traditional systems of medicine. Ayurveda, known as the science of life is one of the oldest system of medicines. This system of using natural resources for betterment of health was originated in India long ago in the pre-Vedic period through day by day experiences and experimentations with the aim of maintaining health and treatment of various diseases. Several other systems of complementary and alternative medicines including Siddha and Unani are also developed from plant based formulations through experience and interactions with natural resources. The earliest written evidence related to use of plant products as therapeutic agents is available on *Atharvaveda,* one of the four most ancient books of knowledge and culture related to Hindu religion showing the strength of Indian wisdom. As many as 114 different therapeutic formulations have been described for the treatment of different diseases. The therapeutic importance of Indian medicinal plants has been exposed thoroughly in the *Susruta samhita* and C*haraka samhita* during the Vedic period. Indian Materia medica has description of more than 2000 drugs derived from natural resources most of which are originated from different systems of traditional and folk practices. 80% of these drugs are of plant origin whereas the rest are minerals or animal products.

Indian medicinal plants possess enormous therapeutic potential but only a small proportion of it has been explored by mankind leaving the great opportunity to discover novel drugs from natural origin. Numerous therapeutic preparations have been developed by traditional healers and Ayurvedic practitioners for the treatment of various disorders and diseases. Subsequently after the emergence of natural product chemistry thousands of new medicinal plant were identified with immense therapeutic potential. Natural Product chemistry together with analytical chemistry, spectroscopy, pharmacology, biochemistry and other related disciplines demonstrated its value for drug development. It has not only enriched modern medicine with novel bio-active molecules but also provided valuable leads for drug designing. Since the isolation of morphine from *Papaver somniferum* in 1806, extensive efforts are being done to isolate therapeutically active molecules from medicinal plants. Some important examples include emetine, c_olchicines, atropine, cocaine, ephedrine and quinidine.

Natural products are continuously providing new leads in terms of structural novelty as well as novel mechanism of action. Compounds isolated from natural product are shown to have chiral centers, complex ring systems, and in some cases heterocyclic rings, and thus have the potential to exhibit diverse biological activities [69]. Natural products serve as established template for the development of new scaffolds of drugs [70]. An important example of natural product based drug development include the synthesis of the anti-inflammatory drug, acetylsalicyclic acid (aspirin), a derivative of natural product, salicin. Similarly, pilocarpine isolated from *Pilocarpus jaborandi* has been used as therapeutic agent for the treatment of several diseases for more than 100 years. Morphine isolated from *Papaver somniferum* L. has provided strong basis for the development of anticancer agents. A representative process for the development of natural product based drug has been illustrated in Fig. (**8**).

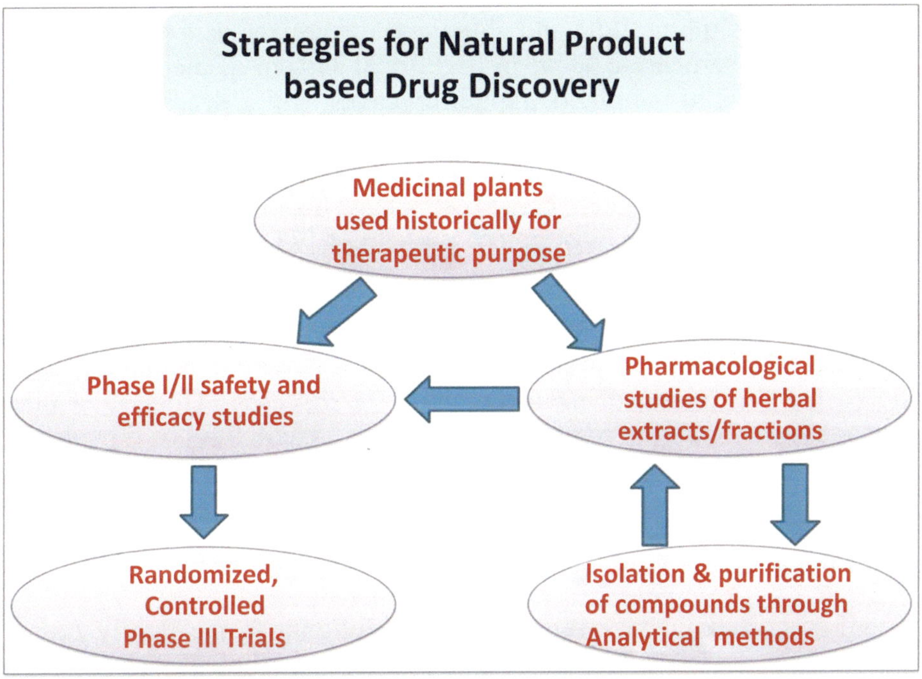

Fig. (8). Procedure of the development of therapeutic agents from natural resources.

At present time research interest has extremely focused on medicinal plants to find novel bioactive compounds as these could provide relatively simple but promising lead, since it is much easier to identify an active constituent from therapeutically active herbal preparation than to find a new drug from a large group of new synthetic molecules [71]. Furthermore, the molecules obtained from natural resources are relatively more compatible to living system as these are synthesized in living organisms to perform biological functions. These may have biologically relevant structures and can be easily metabolized in living system, hence lesser side effects. Flavonoids and other polyphenolic compounds taken with diet may prevent the development of cancer in alimentary canal. Sufficient intake of green vegetables and fruits rich in these compounds may also reduce the risk of many other types of cancer [72].

Several terrestrial plant species and marine organisms possessing diverse biological activities have been used as source of therapeutic agents. Some important examples include:

Azadirachta Indica Juss (Neem)

It is a large tree belonging to the family *Meliaceae* widely distributed in the tropical countries including India and china and recognized as a potential source of multidirectional therapeutic agent in traditional system of medicine since the Vedic times. All parts of the plants including leaves, fruits, seeds and stem bark have been used as traditional medicine against a variety of human ailments from ancient times. Several researchers have been working in medicinal aspects of *Azadirachta indica.* Several active constituents have been isolated from this plant out of which azadiractin is the most potent constituent [73 - 75].

Thymus Vulgaris (Ajowan)

It possesses significant antimicrobial potential and it is used in traditional system of medicine for the treatment of some parasitic diseases. Thymol, a phenol compound is the major active constituent present in essential oil of this plant and is found to be responsible for the activity. It exhibit antiseptic and anti diarrheal activities.

Ocimum Sanctum Linn (Tulsi)

It is a small erect herbaceous aromatic plant belonging to the family *Labiatae* commonly known as Tulsi. It is widely distributed in tropical and subtropical regions of India. The leaves of *Ocimum sanctum* are commonly used to treat a number of diseases including constipation, postnatal disorders, cough, fever, vomiting, cholera, edema, hydrosarca, septicemia, antiulcer, dog bite and many other ailments [76]. It has also been shown to possess significant anticancer activity in mice model [77]. Leaves are very rich source of essential oils. A wide range of active compounds with diverse biological activities have been isolated from the leaves of *Ocimum sanctum*, out of these compounds eugenol is identified as the major active constituent of the oily fraction of the leaves. Several other components have also been identified including caryophyllene, eugenol methyl ester, terpinene-4-ol, decyladehyde, cervacrol and camphor.

Garlic

It is the edible bulb belonging to the family liliaceae. Garlic and other species of the genus like onion, leek, scallion and shallot are used as house hold remedy. These are termed as allium vegetables. Garlic is a rich source of natural sulfur and iodine and has several therapeutic effects. Consumption of garlic and other allium vegetables in diet provide several enzymes which are capable of neutralizing the effects of some carcinogenic substances. It is traditionally used to treat several diseases including tuberculosis, heart disease, arthritis, hay fever and cancer [78 - 81]. Several studies showed that different extracts of garlic showed significant antiatherosclerosis and antidyslipidemic potential. Phytochemical investigation of garlic provided several sulfur compounds as well as glutathione precursors, which are known to acts as potential antioxidants and also display anticarcinogenic properties. S-allyl-L-cysteine sulfoxide and diallyldisulfide S-oxide (allicin) isolated from bulbs of garlic have shown antimicrobial property. Allyl sulfur and other several compounds isolated from different extracts of garlic inhibited the growth of cancerous cells. Recent studies have established that different allyl sulfur compounds, naturally occurring in garlic and onions, increase the susceptibility of cells to the stress created by products of cell division.

Natural products have provided the inspiration for most of the existing drugs. 28% of drugs developed in last two decades were directly based on compounds isolated from natural resources or their semisynthetic derivatives, with another 25% created around a pharmacophore obtained from natural products. Currently, medicinal chemists are involved in synthesis of novel active molecules inspired from natural products [82, 83]. The recent advancement in medicinal chemistry and analytical techniques allowed the medicinal chemists to synthesize the natural products in lab as well as modify their structure to improve the activity and other qualities such as solubility or stability in the human body [84].

In the field of infectious disease several antibacterial agent have been isolated from natural resources belonging to different classes including β-lactams, tetracyclines, glycopeptides, macrolides and spectinomycins. Similarly a number of antifungal drugs have also been obtained from natural products including nikkomycin Z, amphotericin B and nystatin analogues. Some important drugs in this class including streptogramins have also been produced through genetically modified strains of *Streptomyces*. A potential combination of antibiotic has been prepared by combination of two different water soluble semisynthetic antibiotics namely dalfopristin and quinupristin in ratio of 7:3. It has promising activity against multi drug resistant *Staphylococcus aureus* and *Staphylococcus epidermidis*, and is used for treatment of a variety of microbial Infections. It is known to act through interfering bacterial cell wall synthesis and is effective against a broad range of pathogenic strains. Other potential antibiotics obtained from natural resources or derived from natural products include Ziracin, LY-303, L-743, GR-135402, and GM-237354 [85]. A series of lipopeptide antibiotics has been isolated from *Streptomyces roseosporus* exhibiting potential activity against Gram-positive bacteria. A semisynthetic analogue daptomycin prepared by reacylation of the N-terminus with n-decanol was found most effective without any toxicity [86 - 88]. Different plant-derived flavonoids belonging to different structural groups were evaluated against a wide range of pathogenic bacteria some of these compounds exhibited prominent activity [89]. Several semisynthetic flavones were also showed significant antibacterial activity [90]. *Calophyllum lanigerum* yielded a potent anti HIV molecule Calanolide A which is known to act through inhibiting reverse-transcriptase. Pre clinical studies have showed that Calanolide A is effective against AZT resistant strains HIV- 1 [91]. A potent antiparasitic drug, ivermectin is isolated from a *Streptomyces* sp. It is a WHO recognized drug used in vector born disease prevalent in several parts of Africa and America. It is also used in treatment and control of parasitic diseases in animals. Considering the neurological disease dopamine receptor agonism remains the focus of most of researchers. Aporphine, a large group of naturally occurring compound isolated from a wide range of plant species is known to exhibit significant activity against neuronal disorders. Apomorphine, a semisynthetic analogue with dopamine (DA) receptor agonist activity is used in treatment of Parkinson's disease [92, 93]. Similarly, varenicline, a semisynthetic molecule obtained through the modification of cytosine is known to activate nicotinic acetylcholine receptor (nAChR) [94]. Several natural products including pure compounds, plant extracts and other herbal preparations have been explored for their therapeutic potentials in neurodegenerative disorders and some of these have shown considerable neuroprotective potential.

Stem of *Baeckea frutescens* L. is used in traditional Chinese medicine for treatment of rheumatism and snake-bite. Bioactivity directed fractionation of its crude extract yielded a chromone derivative 5-hydroxy-2-isoprop-l-7-methoxychromone as active ingredient [95]. In the current era attention has also been given to microbial fermentations leading to the discovery of many clinically useful drugs. A significant number of natural product derived drugs are known to be produced directly by microbes or interactions of microbial with the host plant. In this regard, endophytic fungi have been recognized as a possible alternative source of natural products primarily obtained from plants. Different medicinally active natural products of plant origin including camptothecin, taxol, taxane, hypericin, rohitukine and hypercin have been reported to be produced in significant amount by different species of endophytic fungi obtained from these plants [96 - 100].

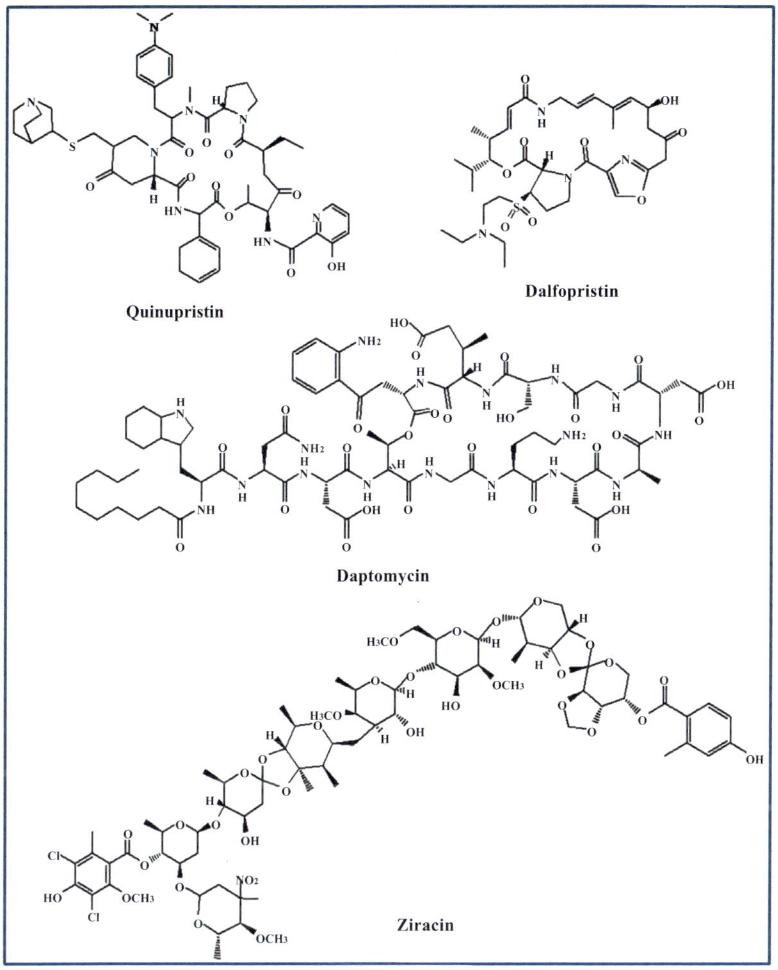

Structures of Quinupristin, Dalfopristin, Daptomycin and Ziracin.

BIOASSAY GUIDED DRUG DISCOVERY

Bioassay-directed fractionation supported by several recent techniques is extensively used to identify the active principles/pure compounds present in crude natural products preparations. This approach can be used systematically to reduce the complexity of the extracts/fractions in order to locate the biological activities of complex materials. It resolves the complex mixtures to more simple and pure form [101, 102]. Considering on therapeutic preparation obtained from crude extracts, only a specific portion of the extract-the active principles/bioactive molecules with specific biological targets is of interest. In view of this fact, a biomolecular interaction step should be included into analytical methods to achieve bio-selectivity and to purify the compounds with specific therapeutic activity.

The technique has been extensively used for very long period. Two different studies have been carried out by Durston and Ames 1974 and Commoner *et al.* 1974 for detection of metabolic carcinogen intermediates in urine samples [103, 104]. Some other research groups also performed similar studies based on bioassay guided fractionation [105, 106]. Several aspects of activity-guided analysis and the potential role of these analytical techniques in drug development together with different new approaches related to screening of biological activities have been studied in details recently [107 - 109]. The bioassay-directed fractionation can be divided in to three main steps namely biological assay, fractionation and detection. The biological assay (pharmacological or biochemical) is the basic and major part, which deals with determination of the active principles or compounds responsible for biological activity.

Biological activities of different plant extracts, fractions and pure compounds isolated from these fractions are determined through several biological assays. The choice of biological assay depends on the type of activity present in plant extracts and compounds. The selected biological assay should be highly sensitive and specific for the activity. It should also be cost effective and easy to handle. Two major types of biological assays are applied- the mechanism-based assays and cell-based assays.

MECHANISM-BASED ASSAYS

These assays evaluate the effect of the compounds or plant extracts and fractions on a specific target such as enzyme, DNA or receptor involved in a molecular signaling cascade. These include *in vitro* assays performed using several methods. Since *in vitro* conditions significantly differ from normal physiological conditions, it should be standardized as well as supported by additional experiments. *In vitro* assays can accurately determine the biological activity of the compounds or extract at very low concentrations. The major limitation of Mechanism-based assays is that they have significant difference from normal physiological conditions as these assays focus particularly on only target pathway thus overlooking the influence of several other related pathways on that particular pathway. Moreover, several other molecules present in active fractions may show their effects through a different mechanism, modulating the effect of the target molecule on specific signaling pathway. This may result in a misinterpretation of the effect produced by active extract or fractions. In addition, molecules or plant extracts found active on *in vitro* assay may be inactive in normal physiological conditions when evaluated in animal models due to their poor water solubility and less bioavailability.

CELL-BASED ASSAYS

These assays involve the assessment of drug-cell interactions with the whole intact cell rather than just isolated systems. These assays are able to determine the activity of wide range of active compounds in small time. Although the exact mode of action of compound cannot be determined through these assays, they can provide the initial information about the possible mechanisms. Compounds that cannot pass through the cell membrane can also be evaluated through this method. These assays have many advantages as compare to mechanism-based assays since a broad range of compounds can be screened with a much higher hit rate through cell based assays. Although the *in vitro* study can provide valuable information related to their anticancer potential including mechanism of action but before clinical evaluation, it should be validated through *in vivo* experiments for example evaluation of anticancer activity in human tumor xenograft in an immunodeficient mouse. Large amount of pure compound is required for *in vivo* study that can be achieved through re-isolating the compound by repeated collection of the source organism or by additional fermentation if the compound is of terrestrial microbial origin or by production of the compound through total synthesis in a synthetic laboratory. Since these procedures may be quite time consuming, steps can be taken to decide that whether a given lead compound has the potential for further development as an anticancer agent. Recently some rapid *in vivo* assays such as hollow fiber assay have been developed which requires very less time to predict the activity and also need relatively small quantity of compound. In hollow fiber assay cancer cells are cultured inside fibers which are subsequently implanted in immunodeficient mice [110, 111]. A 60-cell line panel developed by U.S. National Cancer Institute (NCI) is used to test different molecules against different types of human cancers and to determine the mechanism of action of these molecules [112].

The second step is the fractionation step which is performed in order to increase the purity of active ingredients and simultaneously avoiding the presence of undesired compounds. It can be a very simple procedure encompassing partition of the extract into a few fractions through column chromatography or it can be a complex method involving sophisticated techniques like high-performance liquid chromatography [HPLC] and electrophoresis. The third step (detection) comprises different techniques related to structural elucidation, including mass spectrometry (ESIMS, MALDI-TOF), NMR (1H, 13C, COSEY, NOESY, HMBC, HSQC), IR, X Ray crystallography and alimental analysis. Over the time several novel analytical approaches have been introduced which facilitated the field of drug development through increasing the efficiency and sensitivity as well as reducing the time requirement [113 - 115]. With the help of recent version of liquid chromatography equipped with biochemical detectors different biochemical interactions can be detected online. Complex mixtures can be resolved in relatively simple and more active fractions as well as the active constituents of the complex natural extracts can be purified and characterized with the help of different types of chromatography including conventional Column chromatography, HPLC, counter current chromatography, UPLC and molecular exclusion chromatography. Although the different organic solvents used as solvents in liquid chromatography may exert their own effects and interfere with actual results of biological assays, these effects can be reduced through evaporation of the fractions to be evaluated. Molecular exclusion chromatography is used for separating the molecules of similar polarity but different molecular weights.

POTENTIAL ANTICANCER AGENTS OBTAINED FROM NATURAL PRODUCTS

Citrus fruits and green vegetables provide a rich source of vitamins, flavonoids and other polyphenolic compounds, adequate consumption of these plant products reduce the risk of cancer. More than 1,000 non-nutritive plant derived compounds are known to have cancer-preventive activity. More than 400 plant derived compounds with anticancer potential are under investigation. . Most of the species of higher plants, microorganisms, arthropods, and marine invertebrates are still not studied and thus these diverse natural resources can be explored to provide novel anticancer agents. Recent studies have identified new species of bacteria, algae, fungi, and vertebrates which are able to provide new anticancer molecules. Some important medicinal plants possessing anticancer potential are listed in following Table **2**.

Table 2. Some Important Medicinal Plants Possessing Anticancer Activity.

Plant name	Family	Active part	Plant name	Family	Active part
Acacia xanthophloea	Leguminosae	Fruit	*Ipomea batata*	Convolvulaceae	Rhizome
Adenium obesum	Apocynaceae	Leaf	*Juncus acutus*	Juncaceae	Leaf
Adiantum macrophyllum	Pteridaceae	Entire	*Lannea stuhlmannii*	Anacardiaceae	Root
Aeonium arboretum	Crassulaceae	Leaf	*Lavandula angustifolia*	Meliaceae	Leaves
Aglaia foveolata	Meliaceae	Fruit	*Leptadenia hastate*	Asclepiadaceae	Bark
Alnus japonica	Betulaceae	Wood	*Ligustrum lucidum*	Oleaceae	Seed
Aphanamixis polystachya	Meliaceae	Stem bark	*Maytenus canariensis*	Celastraceae	Fruit juice

(Table 2) contd.....

Plant name	Family	Active part	Plant name	Family	Active part
Arisaema erubescens	Araceae	Root	*Maytenus macrocarpa*	Celastraceae	Stem bark
Aster amellus	Compositae	Entire	*Maytenus serrata*	Celastraceae	Seed
Azadirachta indica	Meliaceae	Leaf	*Monnina obtusifolia*	Polygalaceae	Aerial parts
Begonia glabra	Begoniaceae	Entire	*Morinda citrifolia*	Rubiaceae	Root
Carapa guianensis	Meliaceae	Seed oil	*Ocotea foetens*	Lauraceae	Branchlets
Cassia quinquangulata	Caesalpiniaceae	Root	*Pinus parviflora*	Pinaceae	Strobilus
Celastrus orbiculatus	Celastraceae	Entire	*Piper latifolium*	Piperaceae	Leaf
Crassocephalum bojeri	Compositae	Entire	*Plantago asiatica*	Plantaginaceae	Leaf
Combretum caffrum	Combretaceae	Bark	*Pleione bulbocodioides*	Orchidaceae	Tuber
Cyathea fauriei	Cyatheaceae	Shoot	*Pratia nummularia*	Campanulaceae	Entire
Dillenia suffruticosa	Dilleniaceae	Fruit	*Phymatosorus diversifolium*	Polydiaceae	Root
Dioscorea collettii	Dioscoreaceae	Rhizome	*Phytolacca esculenta*	Phytolaccaceae	Root
Dysosma pleiantha	Berberidaceae	Root	*Rabdosia rubescens*	Labiatae	Leaf
Caragana cuneata	Leguminosae	Leaf	*Ruellia tuberose*	Acanthaceae	Bark
Croton flavens	Euphorbiacaeae	Leaf	*Salvia chinensis*	Labiatae	Entire
Croton lechleri	Euphorbiacaeae	Latex	*Salvia officinalis*	Labiatae	Leaves
Cynanchum hancoekianum	Asclepiadaceae	Entire	*Scirpus holoschoenus*	Cyperaceae	Inflorescence
Deeringia amaranthoides	Amaranthaceae	Fruit	*Scutellaria barbata*	Labiatae	Entire
Echinops grijisii	Compositae	Root	*Scutellaria indica*	Labiatae	Root
Echinops latifolius	Compositae	Root	*Sempervivum armenum*	Crassulaceae	Leaf
Echites vucatanensis	Apocynaceae	Latex	*Sempervivum arvense*	Crassulaceae	Leaf
Epilobium hirsutum	Onagraceae	Entire	*Swietenia humilis*	Meliaceae	Seed
Euphorbia ebracteolata	Euphorbiacaeae	Aerial parts	*Tabebuia impetiginosa*	Bignoniaceae	Stem bark and wood
Euphorbia heterophylla	Euphorbiacaea	Stem	*Tabebuia rosea*	Bignoniaceae	Stem bark and wood

(Table 2) contd.....

Plant name	Family	Active part	Plant name	Family	Active part
Euphorbia marginata	Euphorbiacaeae	Entire	*Tabebuia serratifolia*	Bignoniaceae	Stem bark and wood
Euphorbia kansui	Euphorbiacaeae	Root	*Thalictrum fabri*	Ranunculaceae	Root
Euphorbia prolifera	Euphorbiacaeae	Latex	*Thevetia ahouia*	Apocynaceae	Leaf and Stem
Ficus pretoiae	Moraceae	Sap	*Thevetia gaumeri*	Apocynaceae	Leaf and Stem
Hedyotis chrysotricha	Rubiaceae	Entire	*Thevetia peruciana*	Apocynaceae	Leaf and Stem
Hippophae salicifolia	Elaeagnaceae	Fruit	*Uncaria tomentosa*	Rubiaceae	Bark
Hypoxis nyasica	Hypoxiaceae	Rhizome	*Virola bicuhyba*	Myristicaceae	Seed
Hypoxis rooperii	Hypoxiaceae	Tuber	*Viscum album*	Loranthaceae	Leaves
Inula linariaefolia	Compositae	Flowers	*Viscum calcaratum*	Loranthaceae	Entire

Compounds obtained from natural resources tend to be in only one stereoisomeric form since the active sites of enzymes catalyzing the synthesis of these compounds are asymmetric, allowing them to catalyze a steriospesific reaction. This specific feature of natural products allows them to exhibit biological activity which can be exploited in development of therapeutic agents.

The positive and negative effects of secondary metabolites obtained from plants insects and microorganisms were experienced by mankind in ancient time during their quest for food and survival. Secondary metabolites produced in any species have been proposed to facilitate its survival through repelling or attracting other organisms. Various toxic compounds produced by plants, mollusks, insects and reptiles were postulated to be used as defense mechanism by which they avoided being eaten by other animals [116]. Antitumor antibiotics from micro organisms include the anthracyclines (such as doxorubicin), bleomycin, dactinomycin (actinomycin), and mitomycin C. Moreover, four classes of plant derived anticancer drugs are being used for the treatment of different types of cancers these include vinca alkaloids (bisindole alkaloids), taxanes, epipodophyllotoxins and camptothecins. At present time, several potential natural product-derived anticancer agents are in the market and several another are in advanced clinical trials [117, 118]. Compounds with anticancer activity have been discovered from various skeleton types, mainly from plants, but also from other organisms such as fungi and marine organisms [119]. Marine organisms uniquely synthesize halogen atom (mostly) chlorine and bromine containing secondary metabolites, apparently due to their excessive availability in that environment. In addition to plant derived and microorganism derived antineoplastic agents, several natural products of marine origin have also reached in advanced stage of clinical development. Some important anticancer natural products isolated from marine and terrestrial resources have been described bellow and some others are listed in Table **3**.

Table 3. Some Important Anticancer Compounds Obtained from Natural Resources

S.N.	Compound	Organism	Mechanism of action
1	Anethole	*Foeniculum vulgare*	NF-kB, AP-1, JNK, MAPK
2	Aaptamine	Sponge	p21, cyclins
3	Bastadine 6	Sponge	Inhibition of angiogenesis *in vitro* and *in vivo* involves apoptosis
4	Boswellic acids	*Salai guggul*	NF-kB, p42 MAPK, p38 MAPK, 5-LOX, surviving,cyclin D1, Bcl-2, Bcl-xL, CIAP
5	Capsaicin	*Capsicum annum*	NF-kB, urviving, cyclin D1, Bcl-2, Bcl-xL,CIAP, Cdc25, Cdk1, Bcl-2, Bcl-xL
6	Camptothecin Topotecan Irinotecan	*Camptotheca acuminata*	topoisomerase I
7	Cephaiostatin	Worm	Apoptosis and increased mitochondrial matrix density
8	Cortistatin A	Sponge	regulators of angiogenesis
9	Curcumin, Curcuminoids	*Curcuma longa*	Egr1, STAT-1,3,5, PPARγ, EGFR, HER2, TYK2, JNK, PKA, PKC, Bcl-2, IL-6, Bcl-XL, p53, GSH-px, cyclin D1, 5-LOX, COX-2, INOS, MMP-9, TNF, IL-8, IL-12 NF-kB, AP-1, Akt,Src, JAK2
10	Dibenzoylmethane	*Glycyrrhiza echinata*	COX2, LOX, HIF, VEGF
11	Dictyostatin	Sponge	tubulin polymerization
12	Ellagic acid	*Punica granatum*	NF-kB, COX-2, cyclin D1, MMP-9, PDGF, VEGF, p21/WAF1, p53
13	Emodin	*Rheum emodi*	NF-kB, HER-2/neu, caspase-3, AR, MMP-9, CYP1A1, CYP1B1
14	Etoposide	*Podophyllum peltatum*	topoisomerase II
15	Eugenol, isoeugenol	*Eugenia caryophyllus*	NF-kB
16	Flavonoids, Catechins	*Camellia sinensis*	NF-kB,AP-1,JNK,COX-2,cyclinD1, MMP-9, HO-1, IL-6, VEGF,IGF,p53,Bcl-2
17	Fostriecin	*Streptomcyces sp.*	Topoisomerase II
18	Garcinol	*Garcinia indica*	NF-kB, COX-2, iNOS, HAT
19	Genistein	*Glycine max*	NF-kB, caspase-12,p21/WAF1, glutathione peroxidase
20	Gingerol, paradol	*Zingiber officinale*	TNF, NF-kB, AP-1, COX-2, ODC, iNOS,,p38MAPK, HIF, VEGF, caspase-3, Bcl2

(Table 3) contd.....

S.N.	Compound	Organism	Mechanism of action
21	Guggulsterone	*Commiphora mukul*	NF-kB, IAP1, XIAP, Bfl-1/A1, Bcl-2, cFLIP, survivin, cyclin D1,c-Myc, MMP-9, COX-2, VEGF, BAR, CYP7A1, FXR, CYP3A, Cyp2b10
22	Ingenol	*Euphorbia ingens*	protein kinase C
23	Laxaphycins A and B	Bacterium	topoisomerase II
24	Leptosins C and F	Fungus	DNA topoisomerase I and II
25	Limonene	*Elettaria cardamomum*	COX-2, iNOS
26	Linalool, monoterpenes	*Coriandrum sativum*	NF-kB, AP-1, JNK, MAPK
27	Neoamphimedine	Sponge	Induction of topoisomerase II α-mediated
28	Paclitaxel Docetaxel	*Taxus brevifolia*	tubulin
29	parthenolides	*Tanacetum parthenium*	NF-kB, p53, reactive oxygen species
30	Pentostatin	*Streptomyces sp.*	adenosine deaminase
31	Podophyllotoxin Etopophos NK-611	*Podophyllum peltatum*	topoisomerase I and II
32	Protopanaxadiol	*Pana quinquefolium*	caspase 3, 8 and 9
33	Quercetin	*Citrus sp.*	NF-kB, Bax, Bcl-2, cyclin D1, caspase, PARP, Gadd 45
34	Resveratrol	*Vitis vinifera*	COX-2, iNOS, JNK, MEK, AP-1, NF-kB, P21Cip1/WAF1, p53, Bax, caspases, survivin, cyclin D1, cyclin E, Bcl-2, Bcl-xL, CIAP, Egr-1, PKC, PKD, VEGF, IL-1, IL-6, IL-8, AR, Cdc2-tyr15a, endothelin-1
35	Squalamine (aminosterol antibiotic)	shark	Inhibits angiogenesis, prevents growth factor-induced endothelial cell proliferation
36	Sulforaphane, indole-3-carbinol	*Brassica sp.*	NF-kB, survivin, cyclin D1, Bcl-2, Bcl-xL, CIAP, Cdc25, Cdk1, Bcl-2, Bcl-xL
37	Tecogalan	*Arthrobacter* sp.	Angiogenesis
38	Taxol	*Taxus brevifolia*	tubulin
39	Variolin B	Sponge	cyclin-dependent kinases
40	Vinblastine	*Vinca rosea*	tubulin
41	Vincristine	*Vinca rosea*	tubulin
42	Withonalide	*Withania somnifera*	NF-kB, COX-2, cyclin D1, MMP-9, survivin,cyclin E, Bcl-2, Bcl-xL, CIAP

Alvaradoin E

It is an anthracenone *C*-glycoside which has been isolated from leaves of *Alvaradoa haitiensis* Urb belonging to family picramniaceae through bioactivity-guided fractionation of the extract showing anticancer activity. It showed potent antiproliferative activity against KB, LNCaP, and Col2 cell lines [120]. Cytotoxic activity of Alvaradoin E has been demonstrated to be mediated through apoptosis. Treatment with Alvaradoin E initiated the chromatin condensation and mitochondrial membrane depolarization leading to apoptosis in LNCaP prostate cancer cell line. Its antiproliferative activity has been further validated through several other studies. It showed potential decrease in cell viability as well as increased the DNA cleavage within 36 hours of exposure [120]. Several other compounds belonging to this series including alvaradoin A and alvaradoin B have also showed significant anticancer potential [121].

Psammaplin A

It is a bromotyrosine metabolite isolated from different marine sponges which is shown to possess antiproliferative activity against P388 cells [122]. Since then several other psammaplin compounds have been identified including psammaplins B-L and biprasin [123]. These molecules showed potent antimicrobial activity. Psammaplin A and biprasin were found to have significant DNA methyltransferase as well as histone deacetylase inhibitory activities. In addition, Psammaplin A has been shown to inhibit the aminopeptidase N as well as topoisomerase II activities.

Psammaplin F, showed elective histone deacetylase inhibitory activity while psammaplin G, showed selective DNA methyltransferase inhibitory potential. A synthetic analogue NVP-LAQ824 showed significant *in vitro* anticancer potential with low toxicity and high tolerance in human xenografts. It has been shown to induce apoptosis at smaller concentrations [124].

Pancratistatin

It is a phenanthridine alkaloid isolated from bulbs of the *Pancratium littorale* Jacq (Amaryllidaceae) as a major active constituent [125]. Later on, in order to increase the water solubility and bioavailability of parent compound, Pancratistatin 3,4-*O*-cyclic phosphate sodium salt has been prepared which showed considerable anticancer potential in P338 murine cancer cell line. It also showed significant activity against *in vivo* ovary sarcoma tumor model. Pancratistatin has also been prepared in lab through total synthesis. Recent studies have demonstrated that Pancratistatin induce apoptosis through activation of caspase-3 and flipping of phosphatidyl serine to the outer phase of plasma membrane [126]. It induced the caspase-3 activity in the Jurkat cell line and shown to activate the Fas receptor within lipid rafts in plasma membrane. One of its derivative pancratistatin 3, 4-O-cyclic phosphate sodium salt also showed antiproliferative activity in different cancer cell lines.

Didemnin B

Didemnin B is a cyclic depsipeptide isolated from *Trididemnum solidum, a* Caribbean tunicate which showed significant anticancer potential and is currently in phase II clinical trials for the treatment of breast cancer, ovarian cancer, lung cancer, myeloma, glioblastoma/astrocytoma, and cervical cancers [127]. It is postulated to act through inhibiting the synthesis of nucleic acids, and proteins as well as through binding to thioesterase [128]. Aplidine a synthetic analogue of didemnin B is shown to act as a potent anticancer agent through interfering with the synthesis of DNA and proteins and inducing cell cycle arrest. It also uniquely inhibits the ornithine decarboxylase, an enzyme involved in the growth of tumor and angiogenesis. Antiangiogenic effect is shown to be mediated by decreased secretion of VEGF as well as diminished expression of the VEGF-r1 receptor [129]. Aplidine showed prominent activity against different solid tumor models. It showed low toxicity and high tolerance with the most common adverse events being vomiting, nausea, asthenia, and hypersensitivity. It is currently in phase II clinical trials against a wide range of solid tumors.

Neopeltolide

It is a potential anticancer compound of marine origin isolated from a sponge belonging to family Neopeltidae collected from the coastal regions of Jamaica [130]. It has been reported to possess potential cytotoxic activity in the concentration of nM range against various cancer cell lines. It also induced cell cycle arrest at the G1 stage in A549 lung cancer cell lines. Recent studies have showed that it exhibit the anticancer potential through targeting cytochrome bc1 complex.

Bryostatin 1

It has been isolated from marine bryozoans through the bioactivity guided fractionation of active extracts. It showed significant anticancer activity mediated through protein kinase C.

Palmerolide A

It is an important anticancer compound obtained from marine organism *Synoicum adareanum*, a tunicate distributed in the shallow waters around the Antarctic

Peninsula [131]. It was found to possess anticancer potential against a panel of cell lines. Several follow-up studies revealed that it inhibit different vacuolar-ATPase. Several stereoisomers of palmerolide have been synthesize and evaluated for biological activities [132].

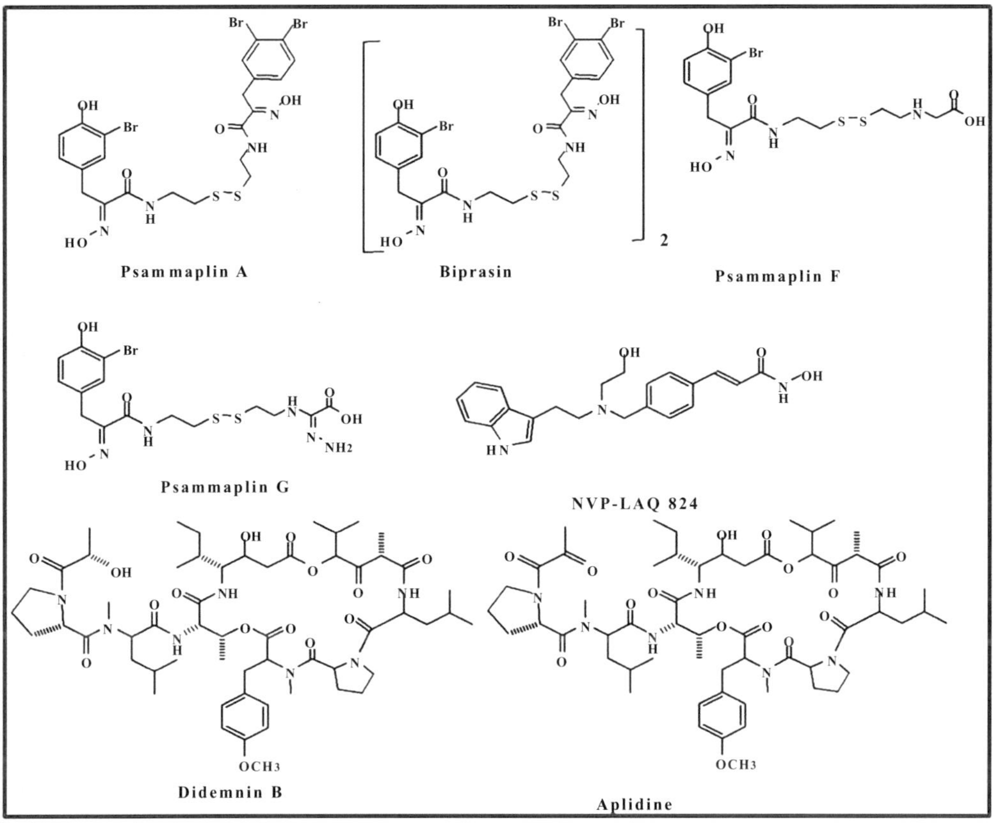

Structures of different Psammaplins, Didemnin B and their synthetic analogues.

Dolastatin 10

Dolastatin 10 has been isolated through the bioactivity guided fractionation of active extracts of *Dolabella auricularia* (sea hare). It is a pentapeptide having four structurally unique amino acids including dolaproline, dolavaline, dolaisoleucine, and dolaphenine. It is thought to be synthesized by cyanobacteria which serve as primary diet of *Dolabella auricularia* [133]. It has been shown to exhibit potent antiproliferative activity against murine PS leukemia cells. It also inhibited the binding of *Vinca* alkaloid to tubulin as well as affected the tubulin-dependent hydrolysis of guanosine triphosphate leading to the arrest of cell cycle in metaphase. During the clinical studies, dolastatin 10 has been shown to develop moderate peripheral neuropathy so it was dropped from clinical trials. It provided the basis for a synthetic analogue Soblidotin (TZT-1027) with potent anticancer activity and reduced toxicity [134]. Administration of TZT-1027 in experimental animals significantly inhibited the growth of P388 leukemia and solid tumor cell lines with better activity profile. It has been shown to exhibit the activity irrespective of the presence of functional p53 gene. Furthermore, it showed significant activity in human xenograft models of lung carcinoma and breast carcinoma. It also interferes with angiogenesis through interacting with VEGF leading to the necrosis of tumor [135].

Pericosine A

It is a cyclohexenoid derivative, isolated from a fungal strain *Periconia byssoides* found in the gut of *Aplysia kurodai* [136]. It has been shown to possess selective cytotoxic activity against a wide range of cancer cell lines. It also showed promising anticancer potential *in vivo.* It is shown to act through inhibiting protein kinase, EGFR and topoisomerase II [137].

Dolastatin 15

Dolastatin 15 was isolated from *D. auricularia* (sea hare). It is a depsipeptide having seven amino acid or hydroxyl acid residues. It showed potent anticancer activity against P388 lymphocytic leukemia cell line [138]. It directly binds to the *Vinca* domain of tubulin. In order to enhance the water solubility and therapeutic efficacy synthetic analogues including cemadotin and synthadotin, have been developed based on Dolastatin 15. Cematodin is shown to act through interfering with tubulin polymerization as well as inducing the depolymerization of microtubules leading to mitotic arrest. Synthadotin is shown to be active against non-small cell lung cancer and prostate cancer.

Silvestrol

It has been isolated from ethanolic extract of the fruits and leaves of *Aglaia foveolata* (Meliaceae) [139], later on it has been isolated from another plant *Aglaia leptantha.* It is a rocaglate derivative containing benzofuran ring. It is shown to exert selective cytotoxicity against different cancerous cell lines. Several studies demonstrated that this class of compounds exerts anticancer activity through modulating the protein synthesis and arresting the cell cycle in G2/M-stage. These are also known to act through inhibiting the activity of NF-κB and tumor necrosis factor alpha (TNFα) [140]. Furthermore it exhibited potential anticancer activity in different *x*enograft models with no obvious toxic effect. Mechanistic Studies revealed that it act through modulating different genes involved in apoptosis and cell cycle regulation. It is shown to act through upregulating p21 and p300 and downregulating p53 and MDM2 at transcription and translation levels leading to cell cycle arrest. It also induced cytochrome c release through modulating the mitochondrial membrane potential ultimately leading to apoptosis. Silvestrol was also shown to be effective in combination therapy.

Ecteinascidin-743

It is a tetrahydroisoquinolones alkaloid isolated as major active constituent from aqueous extracts of the *Ecteinascidia turbinata,* a tunicate [141]. It has also been prepared semisynthetically from cyanosafracin B, an abundant natural product obtained from *Pseudomonas fluorescens*. A recent study has shown that it interferes with nucleotide excision repair during the transcription and induces p53 independent apoptosis. It also interacts with the minor groove of DNA and subsequently induces bending in the DNA helix. Furthermore, it showed significant effect on different types of cancers pretreated with platinum/taxanes in phase I clinical trials [142].

Symplocamide A

It is a depsipeptide with having two unusual amino acid constituents. It was isolated from *Symploca,* a cyanobacterium of marine origin. It was found to be an effective anticancer agent, showing significant antiproliferative activity against different cancer cell lines.

Spiruchostatin A

It is a bicyclic depsipeptide with potential anticancer activity isolated from a *Pseudomonas* extract together with another compound spiruchostatin B. It showed potent antiproliferative activity in different cancer cell lines. It has shown to act through inhibiting histone deacetylase activity leading to increase in acetylated histones and ultimately cell death. It also showed significant activity in different *in vivo* models [143].

Halichondrin B

It has been isolated from *Halichondria okadai*. Its anticancer potential is postulated to be mediated by inhibition of tubulin polymerization leading to breakdown of the mitotic spindle and cell cycle arrest in G2/M-stage [144].

The structural complexity and potential anticancer activity of halichondrins led the development of semisynthetic and total synthetic analogues. Some of these analogues have shown potent anticancer activity. For example E-7389 act through modulating the function of microtubules as well as inducing the phosphorylation of p27 and Bcl2 without involvement of p53 and subsequently leading to apoptosis and cytotoxic effect [145].

Flavopiridol

It is a semisynthetic analogue of a natural chromone alkaloid that exhibit anticancer potential through inhibiting different cyclin-dependent kinases which regulate the cell cycle [146]. Moreover, it selectively induces apoptosis and exhibit anti-angiogenic properties. During the several recent *in vitro* and *in vivo* studies, it was shown to inhibit the proliferation of a broad range of human cancer cells and is currently under Phase II and Phase III clinical trials, both as a single agent and in combination with other anticancer drugs [147 - 150].

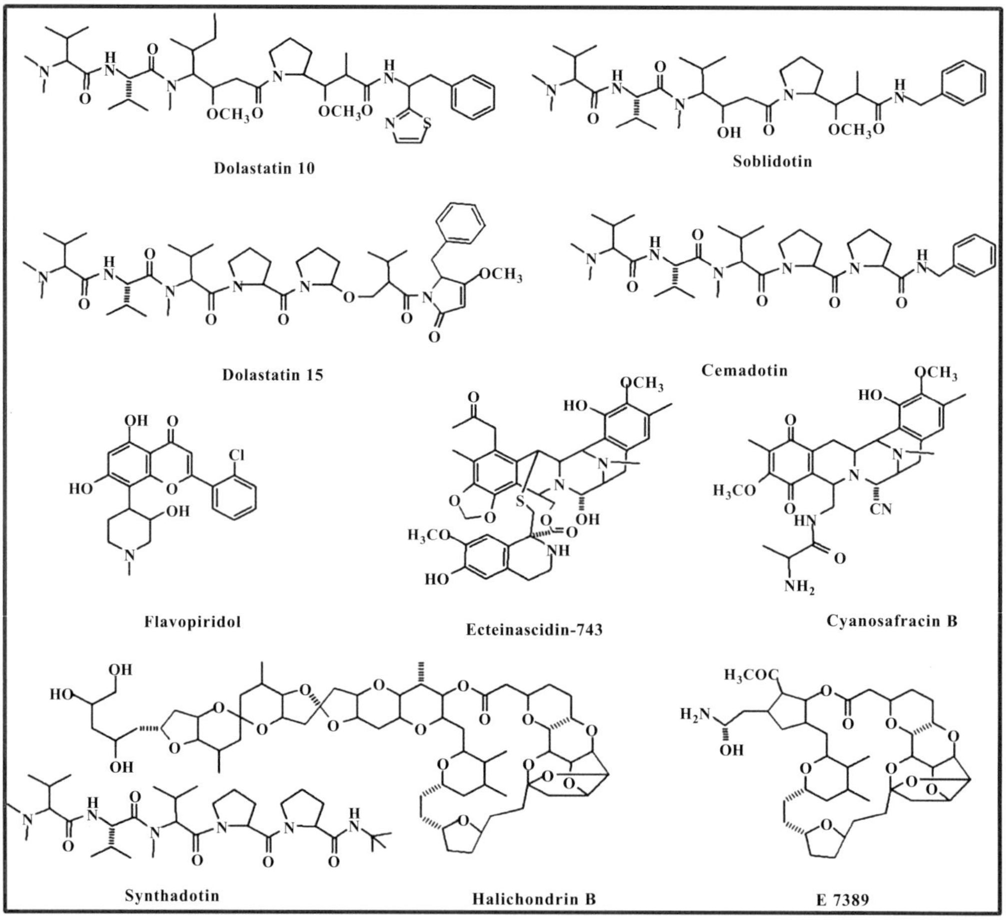

Structures of Dolastatins, flavopiridol, Ecteinascidin-743, Cyanosafracin B, Halichondrin B and their synthetic analogues.

CONCLUSION

Research work done up to date has showed the importance of medicinal plants in the field of different human diseases including cancer, intense efforts and multiple approaches have fruitified in form of number of anticancer drugs in the area but the main problem associated with these drugs is the toxicity, solubility and lack of specificity as healthy cells are also become the target, most of the modern anticancer drugs available are either inspired from natural product or their analogues, efforts are still required to keep the delicate balance between toxicity, bioavailability and efficacy, drugs available are not good enough to treat cancer at advance stage though may prolong the life span of person, other drawback is the cost of anticancer drugs which must also be taken into account for the countries like India, a lot need to be done and nature has given the direction. More clinical trials are also needed to validate the usefulness of these agents either alone or in combination with existing therapy.

CONFLICT OF INTEREST

The authors confirm that they have no conflict of interest to declare for this publication.

ACKNOWLEDGEMENTS

The authors are grateful to the Director CSIR-CDRI, Lucknow, India for excellent library facility and CSIR, New Delhi for providing financial support in the form of senior research fellowships to Sunil Kumar Mishra.

REFERENCES

[1] American Cancer Society. Cancer Facts and Figures American Cancer Society Inc 250 Williams Street, NW. Atlanta, GA: American Cancer Society 2012.

[2] Stewart BW, Kleihues P, Eds. World Cancer Report (World Health Organization, International Agency for Cancer Research). Lyon, France: IARC Press 2003; pp. 11-20.

[3] Golub TR, Slonim DK, Tamayo P, *et al.* Molecular classification of cancer: class discovery and class prediction by gene expression monitoring. Science 1999; 286(5439): 531-7. [http://dx.doi.org/10.1126/science.286.5439.531] [PMID: 10521349]

[4] Hakomori S. Aberrant glycosylation in cancer cell membranes as focused on glycolipids: overview and perspectives. Cancer Res 1985; 45(6): 2405-14. [PMID: 3886132]

[5] Ogata SI, Muramatsu T, Kobata A. New structural characteristic of the large glycopeptides from transformed cells. Nature 1976; 259(5544): 580-2. [http://dx.doi.org/10.1038/259580a0] [PMID: 175288]

[6] Sanders FK, Burford BO. Ascites tumours from BHK 21 cells transformed *in vitro* by polyoma virus. Nature 1964; 201: 786-9. [http://dx.doi.org/10.1038/201786a0] [PMID: 14161203]

[7] Giancotti FG, Ruoslahti E. Integrin Science 1999; 1028-32.

[8] DePinho RA. Transcriptional repression. The cancer-chromatin connection. Nature 1998; 391(6667): 533-536, 535-536.
[http://dx.doi.org/10.1038/35257] [PMID: 9468130]

[9] Feinberg AP, Gehrke CW, Kuo KC, Ehrlich M. Reduced genomic 5-methylcytosine content in human colonic neoplasia. Cancer Res 1988; 48(5): 1159-61.
[PMID: 3342396]

[10] Wenk J, Brenneisen P, Meewes C, *et al.* UV-induced oxidative stress and photoaging. Curr Probl Dermatol 2001; 29: 83-94.
[http://dx.doi.org/10.1159/000060656] [PMID: 11225204]

[11] Shukla Y, Pal S. Dietary Cancer Chemoprevention. Int J Hum Genet 2004; 4: 265-76.

[12] Davies D, Bradlow HL. Can environmental estrogen cause breast cancer. Sci Am 1995; 273: 166-72.
[http://dx.doi.org/10.1038/scientificamerican1095-166]

[13] Cocco P, Blair A, Congia P, *et al.* Proportional mortality of dichloro-diphenyl-trichloroethane (DDT) workers: a preliminary report. Arch Environ Health 1997; 52(4): 299-303.
[http://dx.doi.org/10.1080/00039899709602202] [PMID: 9210731]

[14] Stefanie S, Ulrike B, Dennis N. Quantification of ETS expose in hospitality workers who have never smoked. Environ Health 2010; 49: 1096-9.

[15] Turai I, Veress K. Radiation accidents: occurrence, types, consequences, medical management, and the lessons to be learned. Cent Eur. J Occup Environ Med 2001; 7: 3-14.

[16] Klein-Szanto AJ. Carcinogenic effects of chemotherapeutic compounds. Prog Clin Biol Res 1992; 374: 167-74.
[PMID: 1620702]

[17] Mignotte H, Lasset C, Bonadona V, *et al.* Fédération Nationale des Centres de Lutte Contre le Cancer (FNCLCC). Iatrogenic risks of endometrial carcinoma after treatment for breast cancer in a large French case-control study. Int J Cancer 1998; 76(3): 325-30.
[http://dx.doi.org/10.1002/(SICI)1097-0215(19980504)76:3<325::AID-IJC7>3.0.CO;2-X] [PMID: 9579567]

[18] Stern RS, Lange R. Non-melanoma skin cancer occurring in patients treated with PUVA five to ten years after first treatment. J Invest Dermatol 1988; 91(2): 120-4.
[http://dx.doi.org/10.1111/1523-1747.ep12464137] [PMID: 3397587]

[19] Patel TS, Greer SC, Skinner RB Jr. Cancer concerns with topical immunomodulators in atopic dermatitis: overview of data and recommendations to clinicians. Am J Clin Dermatol 2007; 8(4): 189-94.
[http://dx.doi.org/10.2165/00128071-200708040-00001] [PMID: 17645374]

[20] Muller HJ. Artificial mutation of the genes. Science 1927; 66(1699): 84-7.
[http://dx.doi.org/10.1126/science.66.1699.84] [PMID: 17802387]

[21] Scheffner M, Werness BA, Huibregtse JM, Levine AJ, Howley PM. The E6 oncoprotein encoded by human papillomavirus types 16 and 18 promotes the degradation of p53. Cell 1990; 63(6): 1129-36.
[http://dx.doi.org/10.1016/0092-8674(90)90409-8] [PMID: 2175676]

[22] Schiffman M, Castle PE, Jeronimo J, Rodriguez AC, Wacholder S. Human papillomavirus and cervical cancer. Lancet 2007; 370(9590): 890-907.
[http://dx.doi.org/10.1016/S0140-6736(07)61416-0] [PMID: 17826171]

[23] Martin KR. Targeting apoptosis with dietary bioactive agents. Exp Biol Med (Maywood) 2006; 231(2): 117-29.
[PMID: 16446487]

[24] Hockenbery D, Nuñez G, Milliman C, Schreiber RD, Korsmeyer SJ. Bcl-2 is an inner mitochondrial membrane protein that blocks programmed cell death. Nature 1990; 348(6299): 334-6. [http://dx.doi.org/10.1038/348334a0] [PMID: 2250705]

[25] Clarke AR, Purdie CA, Harrison DJ, *et al.* Thymocyte apoptosis induced by p53-dependent and independent pathways. Nature 1993; 362(6423): 849-52. [http://dx.doi.org/10.1038/362849a0] [PMID: 8479523]

[26] Strasser A, Harris AW, Bath ML, Cory S. Novel primitive lymphoid tumours induced in transgenic mice by cooperation between myc and bcl-2. Nature 1990; 348(6299): 331-3. [http://dx.doi.org/10.1038/348331a0] [PMID: 2250704]

[27] Soengas MS, Alarcón RM, Yoshida H, *et al.* Apaf-1 and caspase-9 in p53-dependent apoptosis and tumor inhibition. Science 1999; 284(5411): 156-9. [http://dx.doi.org/10.1126/science.284.5411.156] [PMID: 10102818]

[28] Miyashita T, Reed JC. Tumor suppressor p53 is a direct transcriptional activator of the human bax gene. Cell 1995; 80(2): 293-9. [http://dx.doi.org/10.1016/0092-8674(95)90412-3] [PMID: 7834749]

[29] Giancotti FG, Ruoslahti E. Integrin signaling. Science 1999; 285(5430): 1028-32. [http://dx.doi.org/10.1126/science.285.5430.1028] [PMID: 10446041]

[30] Sierra A, Castellsagué X, Tórtola S, *et al.* Apoptosis loss and bcl-2 expression: key determinants of lymph node metastases in T1 breast cancer. Clin Cancer Res 1996; 2(11): 1887-94. [PMID: 9816145]

[31] Halliwell B, Gutteridge JM. Free Radicals, ageing and disease. In: Halliwell B, Gutteridge JM, Eds. Free Radicals in Biology and Medicine. Oxford, UK: Oxford University Press 1989; pp. 416-08.

[32] Finkel T, Holbrook NJ. Oxidants, oxidative stress and the biology of ageing. Nature 2000; 408(6809): 239-47. [http://dx.doi.org/10.1038/35041687] [PMID: 11089981]

[33] Allen RG, Tresini M. Oxidative stress and gene regulation. Free Radic Biol Med 2000; 28(3): 463-99. [http://dx.doi.org/10.1016/S0891-5849(99)00242-7] [PMID: 10699758]

[34] Oberley LW, Oberley TD. Free radicals, cancer and aging. In: York N, Ed. Free Radicals, Aging and Degenerative Diseases, Johnson J, Walford R, Harman D, Miquel J. New York: Alan R Liss Inc 1986; pp. 325-71.

[35] Troll W, Frenkel K, Teebor G. Free oxygen radical necessary contributions to tumor promotion and cocarcinogenesis. In: Fujiki H, Ed. Cellular Interactions by EnvironmentalTumor Promoters. Utrech: VNU Scientific Press 1983; pp. 207-10.

[36] Cerutti PA. Prooxidant states and tumor promotion. Science 1985; 227(4685): 375-81. [http://dx.doi.org/10.1126/science.2981433] [PMID: 2981433]

[37] Esterbauer H. Cytotoxicity and genotoxicity of lipid-oxidation products. Am J Clin Nutr 1993; 57(5) (Suppl.): 779S-85S. [PMID: 8475896]

[38] Hartley DP, Kroll DJ, Petersen DR. Prooxidant-initiated lipid peroxidation in isolated rat hepatocytes: detection of 4-hydroxynonenal- and malondialdehyde-protein adducts. Chem Res Toxicol 1997; 10(8): 895-905. [http://dx.doi.org/10.1021/tx960181b] [PMID: 9282839]

[39] Fridovich I. Biological effects of the superoxide radical. Arch Biochem Biophys 1986; 247(1): 1-11. [http://dx.doi.org/10.1016/0003-9861(86)90526-6] [PMID: 3010872]

[40] Wood ZA, Schröder E, Robin Harris J, Poole LB. Structure, mechanism and regulation of peroxiredoxins. Trends Biochem Sci 2003; 28(1): 32-40. [http://dx.doi.org/10.1016/S0968-0004(02)00003-8] [PMID: 12517450]

[41] Kalka K, Mukhtar H, Turowski-Wanke A, Merk H. Biomelanin antioxidants in cosmetics: assessment based on inhibition of lipid peroxidation. Skin Pharmacol Appl Skin Physiol 2000; 13(3-4): 143-9. [http://dx.doi.org/10.1159/000029919] [PMID: 10859532]

[42] Rahman S, Bhatia K, Khan AQ, *et al.* Topically applied vitamin E prevents massive cutaneous inflammatory and oxidative stress responses induced by double application of 12--tetradecanoylphorbol-13-acetate (TPA) in mice. Chem Biol Interact 2008; 172(3): 195-205. [http://dx.doi.org/10.1016/j.cbi.2007.11.017] [PMID: 18262176]

[43] Niles RM. Recent advances in the use of vitamin A (retinoids) in the prevention and treatment of cancer. Nutrition 2000; 16(11-12): 1084-9. [http://dx.doi.org/10.1016/S0899-9007(00)00436-6] [PMID: 11118831]

[44] Halliwell B. Introduction: Free Radicals and human disease- trick or treat. In: Kalyanaraman B, Ed. Oxygen Radicals and the disease process, The Netherlands Hardwood academic publishers. Thomas, CE 1997; pp. 1-14.

[45] Wani MC, Taylor HL, Wall ME, Coggon P, McPhail AT. Plant antitumor agents. VI. The isolation and structure of taxol, a novel antileukemic and antitumor agent from *Taxus brevifolia.* J Am Chem Soc 1971; 93(9): 2325-7. [http://dx.doi.org/10.1021/ja00738a045] [PMID: 5553076]

[46] Bissery MC, Guénard D, Guéritte-Voegelein F, Lavelle F. Experimental antitumor activity of taxotere (RP 56976, NSC 628503), a taxol analogue. Cancer Res 1991; 51(18): 4845-52. [PMID: 1680023]

[47] McKeage MJ. The potential of DMXAA (ASA404) in combination with docetaxel in advanced prostate cancer. Expert Opin Investig Drugs 2008; 17(1): 23-9. [http://dx.doi.org/10.1517/13543784.17.1.23] [PMID: 18095916]

[48] Myrick D, Blackinton D, Klostergaard J, *et al.* Paclitaxel-induced apoptosis in Jurkat, a leukemic T cell line, is enhanced by ceramide. Leuk Res 1999; 23(6): 569-78. [http://dx.doi.org/10.1016/S0145-2126(99)00048-X] [PMID: 10374850]

[49] Sharif T, Auger C, Alhosin M, *et al.* Red wine polyphenols cause growth inhibition and apoptosis in acute lymphoblastic leukaemia cells by inducing a redox-sensitive up-regulation of p73 and down-regulation of UHRF1. Eur J Cancer 2010; 46(5): 983-94. [http://dx.doi.org/10.1016/j.ejca.2009.12.029] [PMID: 20074931]

[50] Searle J, Lawson TA, Abbott PJ, Harmon B, Kerr JF. An electron-microscope study of the mode of cell death induced by cancer-chemotherapeutic agents in populations of proliferating normal and neoplastic cells. J Pathol 1975; 116(3): 129-38. [http://dx.doi.org/10.1002/path.1711160302] [PMID: 1195050]

[51] Heimbrook DC, Oliff A. Therapeutic intervention and signaling. Curr Opin Cell Biol 1998; 10(2): 284-8. [http://dx.doi.org/10.1016/S0955-0674(98)80152-X] [PMID: 9561854]

[52] Eastman A. Activation of programmed cell death by anticancer agents: cisplatin as a model system. Cancer Cells 1990; 2(8-9): 275-80. [PMID: 2223389]

[53] Spinozzi F, Pagliacci MC, Migliorati G, *et al.* The natural tyrosine kinase inhibitor genistein produces cell cycle arrest and apoptosis in Jurkat T-leukemia cells. Leuk Res 1994; 18(6): 431-9. [http://dx.doi.org/10.1016/0145-2126(94)90079-5] [PMID: 8207961]

[54] Jee SH, Shen SC, Tseng CR, Chiu HC, Kuo ML. Curcumin induces a p53-dependent apoptosis in human basal cell carcinoma cells. J Invest Dermatol 1998; 111(4): 656-61. [http://dx.doi.org/10.1046/j.1523-1747.1998.00352.x] [PMID: 9764849]

[55] Ko WG, Kang TH, Lee SJ, Kim YC, Lee BH. Effects of luteolin on the inhibition of proliferation and induction of apoptosis in human myeloid leukaemia cells. Phytother Res 2002; 16(3): 295-8.

[http://dx.doi.org/10.1002/ptr.871] [PMID: 12164283]

[56] Gupta S, Afaq F, Mukhtar H. Involvement of nuclear factor-kappa B, Bax and Bcl-2 in induction of cell cycle arrest and apoptosis by apigenin in human prostate carcinoma cells. Oncogene 2002; 21(23): 3727-38.
[http://dx.doi.org/10.1038/sj.onc.1205474] [PMID: 12032841]

[57] Lee WR, Shen SC, Lin HY, Hou WC, Yang LL, Chen YC. Wogonin and fisetin induce apoptosis in human promyeloleukemic cells, accompanied by a decrease of reactive oxygen species, and activation of caspase 3 and $Ca^{(2+)}$-dependent endonuclease. Biochem Pharmacol 2002; 63(2): 225-36.
[http://dx.doi.org/10.1016/S0006-2952(01)00876-0] [PMID: 11841797]

[58] Chang BD, Xuan Y, Broude EV, *et al.* Role of p53 and p21waf1/cip1 in senescence-like terminal proliferation arrest induced in human tumor cells by chemotherapeutic drugs. Oncogene 1999; 18(34): 4808-18.
[http://dx.doi.org/10.1038/sj.onc.1203078] [PMID: 10490814]

[59] Chang BD, Broude EV, Dokmanovic M, *et al.* A senescence-like phenotype distinguishes tumor cells that undergo terminal proliferation arrest after exposure to anticancer agents. Cancer Res 1999; 59(15): 3761-7.
[PMID: 10446993]

[60] Wang J, Lou P, Lesniewski R, Henkin J. Paclitaxel at ultra low concentrations inhibits angiogenesis without affecting cellular microtubule assembly. Anticancer Drugs 2003; 14(1): 13-9.
[http://dx.doi.org/10.1097/00001813-200301000-00003] [PMID: 12544254]

[61] Inoue K, Chikazawa M, Fukata S, Yoshikawa C, Shuin T. Docetaxel enhances the therapeutic effect of the angiogenesis inhibitor TNP-470 (AGM-1470) in metastatic human transitional cell carcinoma. Clin Cancer Res 2003; 9(2): 886-99.
[PMID: 12576464]

[62] Kim YS, Maruvada P. Frontiers in metabolomics for cancer research: Proceedings of a National Cancer Institute workshop. Metabolomics 2008; 4: 105-13.
[http://dx.doi.org/10.1007/s11306-008-0109-3]

[63] Ross DD. Modulation of drug resistance transporters as a strategy for treating myelodysplastic syndrome. Best Pract Res Clin Haematol 2004; 17(4): 641-51.
[http://dx.doi.org/10.1016/S1521-6926(04)00080-5] [PMID: 15494300]

[64] Berinstein NL. Enhancing cancer vaccines with immunomodulators. Vaccine 2007; 25 (Suppl. 2): B72-88.
[http://dx.doi.org/10.1016/j.vaccine.2007.06.043] [PMID: 17916464]

[65] Beaston G. On the treatment of inoperable cases of carcinoma of the mamma: Suggestions for a new method of treatment, with illustrative cases. Lancet 1896; 2: 104-7.

[66] Huggins C, Clark PJ. Quantitative studies of prostatic secretions. II. The effect of castration and of estrogen injection on the normal and on the hyperplastic prostate glands of dogs. J Exp Med 1940; 72(6): 747-62.
[http://dx.doi.org/10.1084/jem.72.6.747] [PMID: 19871058]

[67] Wainwright M. Photodynamic therapy: the development of new photosensitisers. Anticancer Agents Med Chem 2008; 8(3): 280-91.
[http://dx.doi.org/10.2174/187152008783961888] [PMID: 18393787]

[68] Houston D. Supportive therapies for cancer chemotherapy patients and the role of the oncology nurse. Cancer Nurs 1997; 20(6): 409-13.
[http://dx.doi.org/10.1097/00002820-199712000-00004] [PMID: 9409062]

[69] Feher M, Schmidt JM. Property distributions: differences between drugs, natural products, and molecules from combinatorial chemistry. J Chem Inf Comput Sci 2003; 43(1): 218-27.
[http://dx.doi.org/10.1021/ci0200467] [PMID: 12546556]

[70] Newman DJ, Cragg GM, Snader KM. The influence of natural products upon drug discovery. Nat Prod Rep 2000; 17(3): 215-34.
[http://dx.doi.org/10.1039/a902202c] [PMID: 10888010]

[71] Cragg GM, Newman DJ, Snader KM. Natural products in drug discovery and development. J Nat Prod 1997; 60(1): 52-60.
[http://dx.doi.org/10.1021/np9604893] [PMID: 9014353]

[72] Knekt P, Kumpulainen J, Jarvinen R, *et al.* Flavonoid intake and risk of chronic diseases1,2. Natural Products in Drug Discovery and Development. J Nat Prod Am J Clin Nutr 2002; 76: 560-8.

[73] Kraus W, Bokel M, Klenk A, Pohnl H. The structure of azadirachtin and 22, 23-dihydro-23 β-methoxy azadirachtin. Tetrahedron Lett 1985; 26: 6435-8.
[http://dx.doi.org/10.1016/S0040-4039(00)99020-8]

[74] Kraus W, Bokel M, Bruhn A, *et al.* Structure determination by NMR of azadirachtin and related Compounds from *Azadirachta indica* A. Juss (Meliaceae). Tetrahedron 1987; 43: 2817-30.
[http://dx.doi.org/10.1016/S0040-4020(01)86887-3]

[75] Lee SM, Klocke JA, Balandrin MF. The structure of 1- cinnamoylmelianolone, a new insecticidal tetranortriterpenoid, from. *Melia azedarach* L. (Meliaceae). Tetrahedron 1987; 28: 3543-6.
[http://dx.doi.org/10.1016/S0040-4039(00)95530-8]

[76] Dharmani P, Kuchibhotla VK, Maurya R, Srivastava S, Sharma S, Palit G. Evaluation of anti-ulcerogenic and ulcer-healing properties of Ocimum sanctum Linn. J Ethnopharmacol 2004; 93(2-3): 197-206.
[http://dx.doi.org/10.1016/j.jep.2004.02.029] [PMID: 15234753]

[77] Prashar R, Kumar A. Chemopreventive action of *Ocimum sanctum* on DMBA -Induced pappilloma genesis in the skin of mice. Int J Pharmacol 1994; 33: 181-7.
[http://dx.doi.org/10.3109/13880209509065360]

[78] Dubick MA. Dietary supplements and health aids. A critical evaluation. Part Natural and miscellaneous products. J Nutr Educ 1983; 15: 123-9.
[http://dx.doi.org/10.1016/S0022-3182(83)80127-7]

[79] Chang ML, Johnson MA. Effect of garlic on carbohydrate metabolism and lipid synthesis in rats. J Nutr 1980; 110(5): 931-6.
[PMID: 6989965]

[80] Bordia A, Bansal HC, Arora SK, Singh SV. Effect of the essential oils of garlic and onion on alimentary hyperlipemia. Atherosclerosis 1975; 21(1): 15-9.
[http://dx.doi.org/10.1016/0021-9150(75)90091-X] [PMID: 1131298]

[81] Bordia A. Effect of garlic on blood lipids in patients with coronary heart disease. Am J Clin Nutr 1981; 34(10): 2100-3.
[PMID: 7293938]

[82] Newman DJ, Cragg GM, Snader KM. Natural products as sources of new drugs over the period 19812002. J Nat Prod 2003; 66(7): 1022-37.
[http://dx.doi.org/10.1021/np030096l] [PMID: 12880330]

[83] Beghyn T, Deprez-Poulain R, Willand N, Folleas B, Deprez B. Natural compounds: leads or ideas? Bioinspired molecules for drug discovery. Chem Biol Drug Des 2008; 72(1): 3-15.
[http://dx.doi.org/10.1111/j.1747-0285.2008.00673.x] [PMID: 18554253]

[84] Hunter P. Harnessing Natures wisdom. Turning to Nature for inspiration and avoiding her follies. EMBO Rep 2008; 9(9): 838-40.
[http://dx.doi.org/10.1038/embor.2008.160] [PMID: 18762775]

[85] Nicas TI, Zeckel ML, Braun DK. Beyond vancomycin: new therapies to meet the challenge of glycopeptide resistance. Trends Microbiol 1997; 5(6): 240-9.

[http://dx.doi.org/10.1016/S0966-842X(97)01051-2] [PMID: 9211645]

[86] Canepari P, Boaretti M, Lleó MM, Satta G. Lipoteichoic acid *as a* new target for activity of antibiotics: mode of action of daptomycin (LY146032). Antimicrob Agents Chemother 1990; 34(6): 1220-6. [http://dx.doi.org/10.1128/AAC.34.6.1220] [PMID: 2168145]

[87] Denning DW. Echinocandins and pneumocandinsa new antifungal class with a novel mode of action. J Antimicrob Chemother 1997; 40(5): 611-4. [http://dx.doi.org/10.1093/jac/40.5.611] [PMID: 9421307]

[88] Kinsman OS, Chalk PA, Jackson HC, *et al.* Isolation and characterisation of an antifungal antibiotic (GR135402) with protein synthesis inhibition. J Antibiot 1998; 51(1): 41-9. [http://dx.doi.org/10.7164/antibiotics.51.41] [PMID: 9531986]

[89] Xu HX, Lee SF. Activity of plant flavonoids against antibiotic-resistant bacteria. Phytother Res 2001; 15(1): 39-43. [http://dx.doi.org/10.1002/1099-1573(200102)15:1<39::AID-PTR684>3.0.CO;2-R] [PMID: 11180521]

[90] Ohemeng KA, Schwender CF, Fu KP, Barret JF. DNA gyrase inhibitory and antibacterial activity of some flavones (1). Bioorg Med Chem Lett 1993; 3: 225-30. [http://dx.doi.org/10.1016/S0960-894X(01)80881-7]

[91] Kashman Y, Gustafson KR, Fuller RW, *et al.* HIV inhibitory natural products. Part 7.The calanolides, a novel HIV-inhibitory class of coumarin derivative from the tropical rainforest tree, *Calophyllum lanigerum.* J Med Chem 1992; 35: 2735-43. [http://dx.doi.org/10.1021/jm00093a004] [PMID: 1379639]

[92] Mathiessen A, Wright CR. Researches into the chemical constitution of narcotine and of its products of decomposition. Proceed Royal Soc B 1869; 17: 455-62.

[93] Goldman ME, Kebabian JW. Aporphine enantiomers. Interactions with D-1 and D-2 dopamine receptors. Mol Pharmacol 1984; 25(1): 18-23. [PMID: 6231468]

[94] Coe JW, Brooks PR, Vetelino MG, *et al.* Varenicline: an α4β2 nicotinic receptor partial agonist for smoking cessation. J Med Chem 2005; 48(10): 3474-7. [http://dx.doi.org/10.1021/jm050069n] [PMID: 15887955]

[95] Tsui WY, Brown G. Chromones and chromanones from baeckea-frutescens. Phytochemistry 1996; 43: 871-6. [http://dx.doi.org/10.1016/0031-9422(96)00360-3]

[96] Aly AH, Debbab A, Kjer J, Proksch P. Fungal endophytes from higher plants: a prolific source of phytochemicals and other bioactive natural products. Fungal Divers 2010; 41: 1-16. [http://dx.doi.org/10.1007/s13225-010-0034-4]

[97] Puri SC, Verma V, Amna T, Qazi GN, Spiteller M. An endophytic fungus from *Nothapodytes foetida* that produces camptothecin. J Nat Prod 2005; 68(12): 1717-9. [http://dx.doi.org/10.1021/np0502802] [PMID: 16378360]

[98] Patel MK, Sebastian Z, Vaidyanathan P, *et al. Fusarium proliferatum*, an endophytic fungus from *Dysoxylum binacteriferum* Hook.f, produces rohitukine, a chromane alkaloid possessing anti-cancer activity. Antvan Leeuwen 2012; 101: 323-9. [http://dx.doi.org/10.1007/s10482-011-9638-2]

[99] Kusari S, Lamshöft M, Zühlke S, Spiteller M. An endophytic fungus from *Hypericum perforatum* that produces hypericin. J Nat Prod 2008; 71(2): 159-62. [http://dx.doi.org/10.1021/np070669k] [PMID: 18220354]

[100] Stierle A, Strobel G, Stierle D. Taxol and taxane production by *Taxomyces andreanae,* an endophytic fungus of Pacific yew. Science 1993; 260(5105): 214-6.

[http://dx.doi.org/10.1126/science.8097061] [PMID: 8097061]

[101] Altenburger R, Backhaus T, Boedeker W, Faust M, Scholze M, Grimme LH. Predictability of the toxicity of multiple chemical mixtures to *Vibrio fischeri*: Mixtures composed of similarly acting chemicals. Environ Toxicol Chem 2000; 19: 2341-7. [http://dx.doi.org/10.1002/etc.5620190926]

[102] Warne MS, Hawker DW. The number of components in a mixture determines whether synergistic and antagonistic or additive toxicity predominate: the funnel hypothesis. Ecotoxicol Environ Saf 1995; 31(1): 23-8. [http://dx.doi.org/10.1006/eesa.1995.1039] [PMID: 7544261]

[103] Commoner B, Vithayathil AJ, Henry JI. Detection of metabolic carcinogen intermediates in urine of carcinogen-fed rats by means of bacterial mutagenesis. Nature 1974; 249(460): 850-2. [http://dx.doi.org/10.1038/249850a0] [PMID: 4209968]

[104] Durston WE, Ames BN. A simple method for the detection of mutagens in urine: studies with the carcinogen 2-acetylaminofluorene. Proc Natl Acad Sci USA 1974; 71(3): 737-41. [http://dx.doi.org/10.1073/pnas.71.3.737] [PMID: 4522788]

[105] Ames BN. Citation classic-Methods for detecting carcinogens and mutagens with the salmonella mammalian-microsome mutagenicity test. Curr Cont Life Sci 1984; 12: 18-9.

[106] Potterat O, Hamburger M. Natural products in drug discovery-Concepts and approaches for tracking bioactivity. Curr Org Chem 2006; 10: 899-20. [http://dx.doi.org/10.2174/138527206776894401]

[107] Marston A. Thin-layer chromatography with biological detection in phytochemistry. J Chromatogr A 2011; 1218(19): 2676-83. [http://dx.doi.org/10.1016/j.chroma.2010.12.068] [PMID: 21236438]

[108] Effects-related analysis of xenoestrogens: Hyphenation of receptor assays with LC-MS. Fresenius J Anal Chem 1999; 363: 767-70. [http://dx.doi.org/10.1007/s002160051288]

[109] Weins C. Overview of bioactivity-based analysis by HPTLC. bridging the gap between cause and effect-HPTLC. detection of bioactive compounds in the environment and in food. J Planar Chromatog 2008; 21: 405-10. [http://dx.doi.org/10.1556/JPC.21.2008.6.2]

[110] Casciari JJ, Hollingshead MG, Alley MC, *et al.* Growth and chemotherapeutic response of cells in a hollow-fiber *in vitro* solid tumor model. J Natl Cancer Inst 1994; 86(24): 1846-52. [http://dx.doi.org/10.1093/jnci/86.24.1846] [PMID: 7990159]

[111] Kinghorn AD, Farnsworth NR, Soejarto DD, *et al.* Novel strategies for the discovery of plant-derived anticancer agents. Pharm Biol 2003; 41: 53-67. [http://dx.doi.org/10.1080/1388020039051744]

[112] Shoemaker RH. The NCI60 human tumour cell line anticancer drug screen. Nat Rev Cancer 2006; 6(10): 813-23. [http://dx.doi.org/10.1038/nrc1951] [PMID: 16990858]

[113] Schenk T, Breel GJ, Koevoets P, *et al.* Screening of natural products extracts for the presence of phosphodiesterase inhibitors using liquid chromatography coupled online to parallel biochemical detection and chemical characterization. J Biomol Screen 2003; 8(4): 421-9. [http://dx.doi.org/10.1177/1087057103255973] [PMID: 14567794]

[114] de Boer AR, Bruyneel B, Krabbe JG, Lingeman H, Niessen WM, Irth H. A microfluidic-based enzymatic assay for bioactivity screening combined with capillary liquid chromatography and mass spectrometry. Lab Chip 2005; 5(11): 1286-92. [http://dx.doi.org/10.1039/b506559c] [PMID: 16234953]

[115] Schebb NH, Faber H, Maul R, *et al.* Analysis of glutathione adducts of patulin by means of liquid

chromatography (HPLC) with biochemical detection (BCD) and electrospray ionization tandem mass spectrometry (ESI-MS/MS). Anal Bioanal Chem 2009; 394(5): 1361-73. [http://dx.doi.org/10.1007/s00216-009-2765-1] [PMID: 19390846]

[116] Tan G, Gyllenhaal C, Soejarto DD. Biodiversity as a source of anticancer drugs. Curr Drug Targets 2006; 7(3): 265-77. [http://dx.doi.org/10.2174/138945006776054942] [PMID: 16515527]

[117] Williams DH, Stone MJ, Hauck PR, Rahman SK. Why are secondary metabolites (natural products) biosynthesized? J Nat Prod 1989; 52(6): 1189-208. [http://dx.doi.org/10.1021/np50066a001] [PMID: 2693613]

[118] Cragg GM, Newman DJ. A tale of two tumor targets: topoisomerase I and tubulin. The Wall and Wani contribution to cancer chemotherapy. J Nat Prod 2004; 67(2): 232-44. [http://dx.doi.org/10.1021/np030420c] [PMID: 14987065]

[119] Butler MS, Newman DJ. Mother Nature's gifts to diseases of man: the impact of natural products on anti-infective, anticholestemics and anticancer drug discovery. 2008. [http://dx.doi.org/10.1007/978-3-7643-8117-2_1]

[120] Mi Q, Lantvit D, Reyes-Lim E, *et al.* Apoptotic anticancer effect of alvaradoin E isolated from *Alvaradoa haitiensis.* Anticancer Res 2005; 25(2A): 779-87. [PMID: 15868909]

[121] Harding WW, Henry GE, Lewis PA, Jacobs H, McLean S, Reynolds WF. Alvaradoins A-D. Anthracenone C arabinosides from *alvaradoa jamaicensis.* J Nat Prod 1999; 62(1): 98-101. [http://dx.doi.org/10.1021/np980300i] [PMID: 9917291]

[122] Arabshahi L, Schmitz FJ. Brominated tyrosine metabolites from an unidentified sponge. J Org Chem 1987; 52: 3584-6. [http://dx.doi.org/10.1021/jo00392a016]

[123] Rodriguez AD, Akee R, Scheuer P. Two bromotyrosine-cysteine derived metabolites from a sponge. Tetrahedron Lett 1987; 28: 4989-92. [http://dx.doi.org/10.1016/S0040-4039(00)96677-2]

[124] Remiszewski SW. The discovery of NVP-LAQ824: from concept to clinic. Curr Med Chem 2003; 10(22): 2393-402. [http://dx.doi.org/10.2174/0929867033456675] [PMID: 14529481]

[125] Pettit GR, Gaddamidi V, Herald DL, *et al.* Antineoplastic agents, 120. Pancratium littorale. J Nat Prod 1986; 49(6): 995-1002. [http://dx.doi.org/10.1021/np50048a005] [PMID: 3572427]

[126] Kekre N, Griffin C, McNulty J, Pandey S. Pancratistatin causes early activation of caspase-3 and the flipping of phosphatidyl serine followed by rapid apoptosis specifically in human lymphoma cells. Cancer Chemother Pharmacol 2005; 56(1): 29-38. [http://dx.doi.org/10.1007/s00280-004-0941-8] [PMID: 15726366]

[127] Nuijen B, Bouma M, Manada C, *et al.* Pharmaceutical development of anticancer agents derived from marine sources. Anticancer Drugs 2000; 11(10): 793-811. [http://dx.doi.org/10.1097/00001813-200011000-00003] [PMID: 11142687]

[128] Vera MD, Joullié MM. Natural products as probes of cell biology: 20 years of didemnin research. Med Res Rev 2002; 22(2): 102-45. [http://dx.doi.org/10.1002/med.10003] [PMID: 11857636]

[129] Broggini M, Marchini SV, Galliera E, *et al.* Aplidine, a new anticancer agent of marine origin, inhibits vascular endothelial growth factor (VEGF) secretion and blocks VEGF-VEGFR-1 (flt-1) autocrine loop in human leukemia cells MOLT-4. Leukemia 2003; 17(1): 52-9. [http://dx.doi.org/10.1038/sj.leu.2402788] [PMID: 12529660]

[130] Wright AE, Botelho JC, Guzmán E, *et al.* Neopeltolide, a macrolide from a lithistid sponge of the

family Neopeltidae. J Nat Prod 2007; 70(3): 412-6.
[http://dx.doi.org/10.1021/np060597h] [PMID: 17309301]

[131] Diyabalanage T, Amsler CD, McClintock JB, Baker BJ. Palmerolide A, a cytotoxic macrolide from the antarctic tunicate *Synoicum adareanum.* J Am Chem Soc 2006; 128(17): 5630-1. [http://dx.doi.org/10.1021/ja0588508] [PMID: 16637618]

[132] Nicolaou KC, Sun YP, Guduru R, Banerji B, Chen DY. Total synthesis of the originally proposed and revised structures of palmerolide A and isomers thereof. J Am Chem Soc 2008; 130(11): 3633-44. [http://dx.doi.org/10.1021/ja710485n] [PMID: 18298117]

[133] Luesch H, Moore RE, Paul VJ, Mooberry SL, Corbett TH. Isolation of dolastatin 10 from the marine *cyanobacterium Symploca* species VP642 and total stereochemistry and biological evaluation of its analogue symplostatin 1. J Nat Prod 2001; 64(7): 907-10. [http://dx.doi.org/10.1021/np010049y] [PMID: 11473421]

[134] Miyazaki K, Kobayashi M, Natsume T, *et al.* 1995; 43: 1706-18.

[135] Kobayashi M, Natsume T, Tamaoki S, *et al.* Antitumor activity of TZT-1027, a novel dolastatin 10 derivative. Jpn J Cancer Res 1997; 88(3): 316-27. [http://dx.doi.org/10.1111/j.1349-7006.1997.tb00383.x] [PMID: 9140117]

[136] Numata A, Iritani M, Yamada T, *et al.* Novel antitumor metabolites produced by a fungal strain from a sea hare. Tetrahedron Lett 1997; 38: 8215-8. [http://dx.doi.org/10.1016/S0040-4039(97)10198-8]

[137] Yamada T, Iritani M, Ohishi H, *et al.* Pericosines, antitumour metabolites from the sea hare-derived fungus *Periconia byssoides*. Structures and biological activities. Org Biomol Chem 2007; 5(24): 3979-86. [http://dx.doi.org/10.1039/b713060k] [PMID: 18043803]

[138] Pettit GR, Kamano Y, Dufresne C, Cerny RL, Herald CL, Schmidt JM. Isolation and structure of the cytostatic linear depsipeptide dolastatin 15. J Org Chem 1989; 54: 6005-6. [http://dx.doi.org/10.1021/jo00287a003]

[139] Hwang BY, Su BN, Chai H, *et al.* Silvestrol and episilvestrol, potential anticancer rocaglate derivatives from *Aglaia silvestris.* J Org Chem 2004; 69(10): 3350-8. [http://dx.doi.org/10.1021/jo040120f] [PMID: 15132542]

[140] Baumann B, Bohnenstengel F, Siegmund D, *et al.* Rocaglamide derivatives are potent inhibitors of NF-kappa B activation in T-cells. J Biol Chem 2002; 277(47): 44791-800. [http://dx.doi.org/10.1074/jbc.M208003200] [PMID: 12237314]

[141] Wright A, Forleo D, Gunawardana G, Gunasekera S, Koehn F, McConnell O. Antitumor tetrahydroisoquinoline alkaloids from the colonial ascidian *Ecteinascidia turbinata*'. J Org Chem 1990; 55: 4508-12. [http://dx.doi.org/10.1021/jo00302a006]

[142] Amador ML, Jimeno J, Paz-Ares L, Cortes-Funes H, Hidalgo M. Progress in the development and acquisition of anticancer agents from marine sources. Ann Oncol 2003; 14(11): 1607-15. [http://dx.doi.org/10.1093/annonc/mdg443] [PMID: 14581267]

[143] Masuoka Y, Nagai A, Shin-ya K, *et al.* Spiruchostatins A and B, novel gene expression-enhancing substances produced by *Pseudomonas sp.* Tetrahedron Lett 2001; 42: 41-4. [http://dx.doi.org/10.1016/S0040-4039(00)01874-8]

[144] Bai RL, Paull KD, Herald CL, Malspeis L, Pettit GR, Hamel E. Halichondrin B and homohalichondrin B, marine natural products binding in the vinca domain of tubulin. Discovery of tubulin-based mechanism of action by analysis of differential cytotoxicity data. J Biol Chem 1991; 266(24): 15882-9. [PMID: 1874739]

[145] Wang Y, Habgood GJ, Christ WJ, Kishi Y, Littlefield BA, Yu MJ. Structure-activity relationships of

halichondrin B analogues: modifications at C.30-C.38. Bioorg Med Chem Lett 2000; 10(10): 1029-32. [http://dx.doi.org/10.1016/S0960-894X(00)00150-5] [PMID: 10843209]

[146] Senderowicz AM, Headlee D, Stinson SF, *et al.* Phase I trial of continuous infusion flavopiridol, a novel cyclin-dependent kinase inhibitor, in patients with refractory neoplasms. J Clin Oncol 1998; 16(9): 2986-99.
[PMID: 9738567]

[147] Senderowicz AM, Sausville EA. Preclinical and clinical development of cyclin-dependent kinase modulators. J Natl Cancer Inst 2000; 92(5): 376-87.
[http://dx.doi.org/10.1093/jnci/92.5.376] [PMID: 10699068]

[148] Senderowicz AM, Headlee D, Stinson SF, *et al.* Phase I trial of continuous infusion flavopiridol, a novel cyclin-dependent kinase inhibitor, in patients with refractory neoplasms. J Clin Oncol 1998; 16(9): 2986-99.
[PMID: 9738567]

[149] Thomas JP, Tutsch KD, Cleary JF, *et al.* Phase I clinical and pharmacokinetic trial of the cyclin-dependent kinase inhibitor flavopiridol. Cancer Chemother Pharmacol 2002; 50(6): 465-72.
[http://dx.doi.org/10.1007/s00280-002-0527-2] [PMID: 12451473]

[150] Chao SH, Fujinaga K, Marion JE, *et al.* Flavopiridol inhibits P-TEFb and blocks HIV-1 replication. J Biol Chem 2000; 275(37): 28345-8.
[http://dx.doi.org/10.1074/jbc.C000446200] [PMID: 10906320]

CHAPTER 5

Polyhydroxyalkanoates as Promising Materials in Biomedical Systems

Michał Michalak[1], Sebastian Jurczyk[2], Katarzyna Jelonek[1], Minna Hakkarainen[3] and Piotr Kurcok[1,4,*]

[1] *Centre of Polymer and Carbon Materials, Polish Academy of Sciences, 34, M. Curie-Skłodowskiej St., 41-819 Zabrze, Poland*

[2] *Paint and Plastics Department in Gliwice, Institute for Engineering of Polymer Materials and Dyes, 50A, Chorzowska St., 44-100 Gliwice, Poland*

[3] *Department of Fibre and Polymer Technology, KTH Royal Institute of Technology, Stockholm, Sweden*

[4] *Institute of Chemistry, Environment Protection and Biotechnology, Jan Długosz Academy, 13/15 Armii Krajowej Ave., 42-200 Czestochowa, Poland*

Abstract: Polyhydroxyalkanoates (PHAs) are the natural polymers that have been a subject of a significant research interest in the past few decades. The PHAs (natural as well as their synthetic analogs) as biodegradable and biocompatible polymers were studied intensively for biomedical applications, that is, scaffolds for tissue engineering. Drug-loaded implants or scaffolds based on these polyesters were also used in the drug release systems. Drug delivery systems should provide an optimal release profile of an active compound that allows to increase therapeutic effect, decrease side effects, and improve patient convenience and compliance. Therefore, recently, the increasing interest is focused on the use of PHA as drug carriers because of significant improvement in the bioavailability of bioactive substances. Recent developments introduced such strategies as conjugation of the drug with low-molecular-weight poly(3-hydroxybutyrate) or preparation of PHA particles loaded with the drug. On the contrary, there is a growing interest in functionalized PHA technology. The advancement of these strategies allows to obtain the targeting systems based on the chemical modification, for example, by folic acid attachment or biosynthesis of targeting proteins on the PHA particle surface. In addition, the PHAs were presented as materials that could be used in transdermal administration of bioactive substances for medical or cosmetic purposes. The development of novel functionalized PHAs has opened new possibilities to combine good biocompatibility of PHA-based drug delivery systems with improved drug loading and release properties, targeting, or imaging possibilities. Further progress in PHA-based drug delivery systems is expected because of the combination of excellent biocompatibility of these biopolymers and strong beneficial effect on drug administration.

* **Corresponding author Piotr Kurcok:** Centre of Polymer and Carbon Materials, Polish Academy of Sciences, 34 M. Curie-Skłodowskiej St., 41-819 Zabrze, Poland; E-mail: pkurcok@cmpw-pan.edu.pl

Atta-ur-Rahman and M. Iqbal Choudhary (Eds.)

Keywords: Polyhydroxyalkanoates, Poly(3-hydroxybutyrate), Drug delivery systems, Implants, Polymeric nanoparticles, Conjugate.

INTRODUCTION

A large number of biodegradable polymers have been explored to be used as drug delivery systems such as scaffolds and implants releasing drugs or micro- and nanoparticles. The most commonly used synthetic polymers include (co)polymers of lactic acid, poly(ε-caprolactone), poly(anhydrides), and so on. However, natural polymers have also been utilized for the formulation of drug delivery systems. Among many natural polymers such as chitosan, hyaluronic acid, dextran, starch, collagen, and others, polyhydroxyalkanoates are an interesting and versatile option.

Polyhydroxyalkanoates (PHAs) are a family of biopolyesters, homo- or copolymers, mainly consisting of 3-hydroxyalkanoate units; however, sometimes copolymers also contain 4-hydroxybutyrate (4HB) or other hydroxyalkanoate units. PHAs with high molar mass are produced by many bacteria under nutrient-limited conditions as a carbon and energy storage source in the form of granules within the microorganisms [1, 2]. For example the simplest PHA homolog poly(3-hydroxybutyrate) (P(3HB)) is presented in Fig. (**1**) [3, 4].

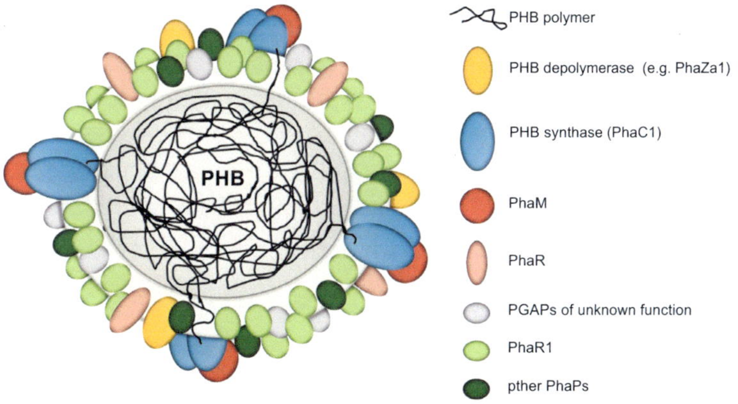

Fig. (1). Model of an *in vivo* PHB granule in *Ralstonia eutropha* H16. The surface layer is free of phospholipids and consists of only proteins. The presently known PHB granule–associated proteins (PGAPs) are symbolized by differentially colored globules (PhaP, PhaM, PhaR – phasin proteins; phasins are PHB granule–associated proteins with putative structural function). Reprinted with permission from Bresan *et al.* [4].

Low molar mass P(3HB), the so-called complexed P(3HB) (cPHB), includes polyesters of chain lengths in the range from several to 100 repeating units. Such cPHB, associated with other biological polymers including proteins and polyphosphates [5, 6], has been found in all living organisms, suggesting that it may have an important biological role [7 - 10].

Based on the monomeric unit chain length, the high molar mass PHAs are divided into two groups. The first group consists of short chain length 3-hydroxyalkanoate constitution units (scl-PHAs), composed of units with 3–5 carbon atoms, and the second group consists of medium chain length PHAs (mcl-PHAs), with 6–14 carbon atoms in the repeating unit [11].

In 1926, Lemoigne [12] identified poly(3-hydroxybutyrate) (P(3HB)); however, the biosynthetic pathway for its production from sugar was proposed many years later. It involves three enzymatic reactions catalyzed by three different enzymes, respectively. Biosynthetic pathways from fatty acids as a carbon sources were also proposed Fig. (**2**) [2, 13, 14].

Chemical composition and molar mass of these biopolyesters highly depend on the bacterial strain as well as the carbon source [15, 16] including renewable resources [17 - 19]. Broad range of PHAs with various compositions and properties were described in the literature [2, 13, 20, 21]. What is important is that PHAs are biodegradable and usually biocompatible and also the products of their degradation are not harmful for natural environment [22 - 24]. Moreover, depending on the composition, PHAs may exhibit different properties including tunable mechanical properties [14, 25, 26]. This feature is driven by the molar mass and crystallinity of the polymer. For instance, bacterial P3HB is a highly crystalline material, and its degree of crystallinity reaches 80%, contrary to a polymer containing 4HB units in the main chain, which possesses relatively low crystallinity [23, 27]. Therefore, properties of the materials can be tailored by the application of respective carbon source and selection of bacterial strain. The possibility of tailoring the properties of PHAs makes PHAs very good candidates for use in many fields [21]. They can be applied as packaging materials; however, one may also use them in regenerative medicine as well as in pharmaceutical applications for instance in drug delivery systems [25, 28 - 30].

Recently, several scientific groups have elaborated catalysts for the synthesis of various β-lactone monomers from carbon oxide, derived from synthesis gas, and respective oxiranes [31 - 33]. Therefore, significant improvement in access to various β-lactones is expected. PHAs can be chemically synthesized through ring-opening polymerization (ROP) of β-lactone monomers, which is a convenient way to obtain PHAs [34 - 37]. By applying coordination or anionic catalytic systems for such processes and depending on the monomers used, respective materials such as homopolymers and/or copolymers with blocky or random microstructures can be obtained [21, 38 - 41]. Moreover, in contrast to natural PHAs containing exclusively R repeating units, there are no such limitations for the synthetic biomimetic polyesters, which can contain various isomeric repeating units, that is, R and S. It is possible to synthesize not only isotactic poly([R]-3-hydroxyalkanoates) [42], as in the case of natural biopolyesters, but also atactic [43] and even syndiotactic polyesters [44] as well as atactic-isotactic block copolymers [45]. Moreover, copolyhydroxybutyrates with various repeating units may also be synthesized [40, 46 - 48]. The most convenient and effective initiators of the anionic ROP of β-lactones are carboxylates with relatively bulky counterion [36].

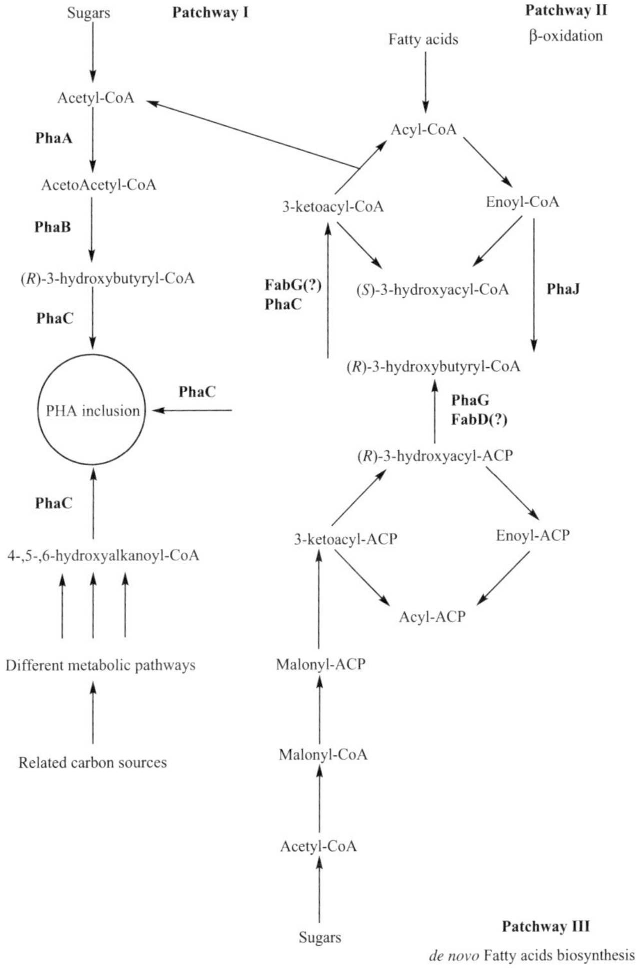

Fig. (2). Polyhydroxyalkanoate biosynthesis from various carbon sources. **PhaA**, β-ketothiolase; **PhaB**, NADPH-dependent acetoacetyl-CoA reductase; **PhaC**, PHA synthase; **PhaG**, 3-hydroxyacyl-ACP-CoA transferase; **PhaJ**, (R)-enoyl-CoA hydratase; **FabD**, malonyl-CoA-ACP transacylase; **FabG**, 3-ketoacyl-CoA reductase.

Recently, ROP of butyrolactone with metal-free organocatalysts was investigated, and the applicability of such systems in the synthesis of well-defined PHB was presented [49 - 51].

The PHAs are also described as a source of biochemicals [52, 53], and macromonomers are obtained by thermal or chemical degradation of high molar mass PHA [54 - 58]. Such macromonomers can be used in the synthesis of many new copolymers that are water soluble, thus being the potential candidates for medical applications [59 - 61].

BIODEGRADABILITY AND BIOCOMPATIBILITY OF PHAs

PHA is biodegraded by various microorganisms such as bacteria and fungi with the formation of water and carbon dioxide or methane under aerobic and anaerobic conditions, respectively [62 - 64]. The biodegradability of P(3HB) has been studied in soil [24], sludge, river water, seawater, and compost.

The investigations of the enzymatic degradation of poly(3-hydroxybutyrate) show that PHA could be degraded inside as well as outside the cells by PHB depolymerases [65 - 67]. A number of PHB depolymerases have been isolated, and their structure and specificity were reviewed [68]. Most of the PHA-producing bacteria are able to degrade the polymer intracellularly. During intracellular degradation, the PHA depolymerase breaks down PHB to produce 3-hydroxybutyric acid [69]. Extracellular depolymerases produced by various microorganisms (bacteria, fungi, and algae) present in the environment hydrolyze P(3HB) to water-soluble oligomers, which can be utilized as nutrients within the cells and metabolized to water and carbon dioxide by these microorganisms [62, 70]. Depolymerase specific for amorphous scl-PHB as well as a depolymerase for synthetic atactic poly([R,S]-3-hydroxybutyrate) was also found and characterized [71]. It is worth to notice that PHB depolymerases produce mainly the monomer (3-hydroxybutyric acid) and a mixture of oligomers (up to hexamer) [71 - 73].

PHAs, in contrast to other polyesters, such as poly(lactic acid) or its copolymers, degrade rather slowly *in vitro* and in mammalian tissues [74]. It has been reported that P(3HB) and poly(3-hydroxybutyrate-*co*-3-hydroxyvalerate) (P(3HB-*co*-3HV)) lost 15%–43% of their initial molar mass after 6 months of implantation. Moreover, only ~2% weight loss was reported for these PHAs [75]. Faster weight loss was reported for disks prepared from poly(3-hydroxybutyrate-*co*-3-hydroxyhexanoate (P(3HB-*co*-3HHx) compared with PHB after implantation in rabbits. After 6 months of implantation, 10% and 6% weight loss was observed, respectively [74]. Moreover, ~40% reduction in weight average molar mass of both P(3HB) and P(3HB-*co*-3HHx) was observed after 6 months of implantation, whereas number average molar mass of P(3HB-*co*-3HHx) and P(3HB) decreased by 80% and 43% of their original weights, respectively. However, PHB films lost 30%–80% of their initial mass in a year [76]. Moreover, P(3HB-*co*-3HV) implants containing hydroxyapatite (HA) as a filler were found to be completely resorbed after 3 months in the subcutaneous region of rabbits [69, 77]. The investigations of properties of injection-molded polyhydroxybutyrate both *in vitro* and *in vivo* demonstrated a slow rate of degradation that may be controlled by filler reinforcement and by the initial molar mass of the polymer. The tissue response to polyhydroxybutyrate alone and that filled with 0.4 volume fraction of hydroxyapatite was favorable with early healing and bone remodeling [78]. It was also shown that the P(3HB)/HA composite favorably affects osteogenic cells [78, 79]. In ectopic bone formation assay, it was proven that the hybrid PHB/HA composites can form scaffolds and facilitate bone tissue development on their surface and in pores.

In vivo investigations showed that the mass loss of monofilaments of PHB and P(3HB-*co*-3HV) that is used to aseptically suture muscular-facial wounds did not exceed 50% and their ultimate strength decreased by just 33%–37% of the initial one during 12 months of experiment [80].

Degradation of P(3HB-*co*-3HV) in the presence of calf serum and pancreatic and synthetic gastric juice was investigated. The degradation ratio was observed as sample weight loss decreases in the following order: bovine serum > pancreatic juice > synthetic gastric juice [81].

The *in vivo* study of electrospun scaffolds P(3HB), P(3HB-*co*-3HV), and P(3HB-*co*-4HV) (containing 7 and 97 mol% of 4HB units) showed that the content and type of the second monomer and the diameter of fiber significantly influence bioabsorption [82].

Materials for medical applications have to be biocompatible, which means that they should not cause acute immune reactions when introduced into soft tissues or blood. Moreover, during degradation in the body, such materials as well as the degradation products must also not induce any immune responses to be considered biocompatible.

PHAs were investigated with respect to the risk of induction of inflammatory response because of their properties and possibility of medical applications. It was found that P(3HB) implanted in the bone of rats did not cause chronic inflammatory reactions in a 12-month follow-up period [78]. Malm *et al.* [83] indicated that PHB patches implanted in the right ventricular outflow tract of sheep heart showed a complete degradation after 12–24 months and that the polymer seemed to be slowly phagocytosed by polynucleated macrophages. Non-porous P(3HB) disks of size 2 × 15 mm and cylinders of size 4 × 7 mm implanted in the muscles of Charles River outbred mice did not cause any adverse changes in the physiological and biochemical parameters over a 6-month observation period. No acute inflammation, abscess formation, or necrosis was observed in tissues adjacent to the implant. Only an insignificant inflammation was observed after 1 month of implantation, which involved mononuclear macrophages, lymphocytes, foreign bodies, and vascularized fibrous capsules [75].

Investigations concerning the possibility of application of P(3HB) membranes in bone regeneration in jaw bone of rats show very little tissue reaction, indicating biocompatibility of the membrane material [84]. It was also shown that the implantation of suture threads made of PHB did not cause any adverse changes in the muscles of rats [85, 86]. Also films made of high molar mass P(3HB) induced no cytotoxic effects on the cultures of mouse cells proliferating *in vitro* [87, 88].

Comparable proliferation data proved the ability of the Zein/P(3HB-*co*-4HB) fiber scaffolds to support viable cell colonization. It was shown that Zein scaffold is more suitable for mouse fibroblast cells (NIH3T3), whereas P(3HB-*co*-4HB) scaffold is more suitable for human osteoblast cells (MG-63). The Zein/P(3HB-*co*-4HB) (60:40) scaffold can be used for both the cells. Authors suggested that observed behavior differences could result from the specific properties of the blends as well as fiber topography [89].

Most experiments indicated that PHAs were tolerated by tissue and blood without the induction of inflammation or tissue necrosis, but some studies mentioned significant inflammatory tissue responses when P(3HB) and P(3HB-*co*-3HV) stents were implanted into animals [90, 91]. However, it was reported that the implantation of suture threads prepared from P(3HB) or P(3HB-*co*-3HV) did not cause any adverse changes in the physiological and biochemical parameters of laboratory animals over a 6-month observation period [92]. Moreover, analysis of the hemocompatibility properties of appropriately purified P(3HB) and P(3HB-*co*-3HV) concluded that these biopolyesters can be used in contact with blood [93]. The study also indicated how important a suitable purification process for these biopolymers is before they are used in medical application.

High molar mass PHAs are biodegraded *in vivo* to oligomers and finally to 3-hydroxybutyric acid through the hydrolysis of ester bonds [94, 95]. The biocompatibility and toxicity of such degradation products were studied by few authors. The degradation products of a P(3HB)-based polyurethane (DegraPol foam), P(3HB) with a number average molar mass $M_n = 2300$, are phagocytized by macrophages and osteoblasts. At low concentrations, particles of PHB failed to induce cytotoxic effects or to activate macrophages. Osteoblasts showed only limited P(3HB) phagocytosis and no signs of any cellular damage [96, 97].

However, these oligomers at high concentrations (>10 μg/cm^3) were toxic to mouse macrophages, primary rat peritoneal macrophages, and primary isolated rat tibia osteoblasts, whereas mouse fibroblasts were resistant to PHB [98].

Several oligo(3-hydroxybutyrates) (OHBs) with M_n ranging from 800 to 2400 have been tested on transformed hamster V79 with fibroblasts and murine melanoma B16(F10) cells using MTT-based drug resistance and clonogenic survival assays. It was shown that 96-h incubation of cells with 1–9 μg/cm^3 of OHBs did not affect cell viability. Incubation of OHBs with rat hepatoma FTO-2B cells stably transfected with chloramphenicol acetyltransferase (CAT) gene ligated to heat-inducible hsp70i gene promoter demonstrated that OHBs also did not induce cellular stress response [99]. Cytotoxicity investigation of chemically synthesized [R,S] OHB with M_n = 400 assessed up to 1000 μg/cm^3 with human colon adenocarcinoma cells HT-29 and human colon carcinoma cells HCT 116 indicated that oligomers at concentrations <100 μg/cm^3 are nontoxic [100].

In vitro studies performed by Ribeiro-Samy *et al.* [101] demonstrated a lack of cytotoxic effect of P(3HB-*co*-3HV) 3D scaffolds and products of their degradation.

The final product of PHA degradation is the respective hydroxyacid. 3-Hydroxybutyric acid formed as a result of P(3HB) biodegradation is a compound belonging to the ketone bodies (products of fatty acids β-oxidation, which is stimulated by severe insulin deficiency). However, such monomeric [R]-hydroxybutyric acid may cause acidosis in organism when the concentration is too high [102]. It has been demonstrated that various 3-hydroxyacids did not affect murine fibroblast L929 cells if present at a concentration of <20 mg/L. However, at higher concentration, these monomers retarded cellular growth and caused subsequent apoptosis, whereas the cytotoxicity of the oligomers decreased inversely with the length of the side chain [103]. Nevertheless, cytotoxicity could be considered to be negligible given that the oligomers never crossed the threshold concentration of 20 mg/L [28]. Table **1** summarizes the selected *in vivo* and *in vitro* studies on the biocompatibility of PHAs.

The impact of [R] 3-hydroxybutyric acid (ketone body) on cell physiology attracts some interest in the context of its possible therapeutic use. [R] 3-hydroxybutyric acid can displace glucose as the predominating fuel for brain, decreasing the need for glucose synthesis in liver (and kidney). [R] 3-hydroxybutyrate is a fuel that produces ATP energy more efficiently than glucose or fatty acid. In a perfused rat heart preparation, it increased contractility and decreased oxygen consumption. It has also protected neuronal cells in tissue culture against exposure to toxins associated with Alzheimer's or Parkinson's disease. This indicates that some neurologic disorders might benefit from ketosis [104 - 107].

Table 1. ***In vitro* and *in vivo* Biocompatibility Study of Polyhydroxyalkanoates.**

Material	Form of application	Studied range of toxicity	Test method/cell line	Ref.
P(3HB-*co*-4HB) and Zein/P(3HB-*co*-4HB) blend	Electrospun fiber scaffold	20 mm diameter and 1 mm height specimens	MTT assay, NIH3T3 and MG-63	[89]
P(3HB)-*b*-DEG	Polymer film	10 mm diameter disks	MTT assay, NIH 3T3 fibroblasts	[108]
BioPEG-ylated P(3HB) P(3HB)-*b*-DEG	Polymer film		OECs	[109]
P(3HB) P(3HB-*co*-3HV) P(3HB-*co*-3HV)-*b*-PEG	Polymer film		XTT assay, 3T3 fibroblasts	[110]
P(3HB-*co*-3HHx) and P(3HB-*co*-3HHx)-*b*-PEG	Nanoparticles	Up to 100 µg/mL	MTT assay, PC3	[111]
P(3HB-*co*-3HV)	Nano- and microparticles	0.5 mg/mL	MTT assay, L929 mouse fibroblast	[112]
P(3HB) and P(3HB-*co*-3HHx)	Nanoparticles	1 mg/mL	MTT assay, macrophages	[113]
P(3HB), P(3HB-*co*-4HB), P(3HB-*co*-3HV), P(3HB-*co*-3HHx)	Microparticles	–	MTT assay, mouse fibroblast NIH 3T3	[114]
P(3HB), P(3HB-*co*-3HHx)	Nanoparticles	0.1–0.01 g/L	NIH/3T3, BT-474, PC3, HCT-116	[115]
P(3HB-*co*-3HV) (12 and 33 mol% of 3HV) and their copolymer with PEG	Nanoparticles	100–400 µg/mL	MTT assay, prenatal rat neuronal hippocampal cells and NIH/3T3	[116]
P(3HB-*co*-3HO), PEG-*b*-P(3HB-*co*-3HO)	Nanoparticles	10 mg/mL	MTT assay, HeLa	[117]

(Table 1) contd.....

Material	Form of application	Studied range of toxicity	Test method/cell line	Ref.
P(3HB), P(3HB)/hydroxyapatite	Rivet-shaped implants (2.3 mm diameter, 5 mm length)	1–6 month of implantation	Implanted into the lateral aspect of the femoral condyles of New Zealand White rabbits	[78]
P(3HB)	Non-porous disks of 2 × 15 mm and cylinders of 4 × 7 mm		Implanted in muscles of Charles River outbred mice	[75]
P(3HB), P(3HB-*co*-3HV)	Suture threads		Implanted 1week up to 1 year into Wistar rats	[85, 86, 92]
P(3HB-*co*-3HV)	3D scaffold	Cylinders with 4 mm diameter and 5 mm length	Minimum essential medium (MEM) extraction and MTS tests with a 1, 7, 14, 21, and 28 days of extraction; mix primary culture of neurons and astrocytes from the hippocampus of P4 Wistar rats	[101]
Oligo(3-hydroxybutanoate)	(R,S) and (R) oligomers with M_n 800, 890, 1650, and 2400 g/mol	1–9 μg/mL	MTT assay, V79 and B16 cells	[99]
	(R,S) oligomers with average number of repeating 4 and 6 units	Up to 1000 μg/mL	MTT assay, HT-29 and HCT 116	[100]
Vanilic acid–oligo(3-hydroxybutanoate) conjugate	Amorphic oligomers with M_n 550 g/mol	1–9 μg/mL	Human cancer KB cells and nontumorigenic HaCaT cell line	[118]
p-Anisilic acid–oligo(3-hydroxybutanoate) conjugate	Amorphic oligomers with M_n 800 g/mol			

(Table 1) contd.....

Material	Form of application	Studied range of toxicity	Test method/cell line	Ref.
Acetylsalicylic acid–oligo(3-hydroxybutanoate) conjugate	(R,S) oligomers in dispersion with carboxmethylcelulose	2000 mg/kg	OECD 420, fixed dose procedure, rats	[119]
Ibuprofen–oligo(3-hydroxybutanoate) conjugate		2000 mg/kg	OECD 420, fixed dose procedure, rats	[120]

BIOMEDICAL DEVICES

The PHAs (natural as well as their synthetic analogs), biodegradable and biocompatible polymers, were studied intensively for biomedical applications that is, scaffolds for tissue engineering. Drug-loaded implants or scaffolds based on these polyesters were also used as drug release systems. Drug delivery systems should provide optimal release profile of active compound to increase therapeutic effect, decrease side effects, and improve patient convenience and compliance. To improve the bioavailability of bioactive substances, increasing interest was recently focused on the development of PHA-based drug carriers.

P(3HB)-based biomedical devices are generally considered biocompatible. Thus, it is expected that surgical devices such as P(3HB) implants and sutures will not cause immune reaction in the organism. Consecutive advantage of PHA biomedical devices is good resistance to sterilization confirmed by stable average molar mass and tensile strength [121]. Surface properties of PHA films showed favorable conditions for proliferation and attachment of cells, proving suitability of PHA as scaffold material [11]. Ellis *et al.* [122] examined the geometry of P(3HB-*co*-3HV) for tissue engineering. Study with laser microperforation showed that it did not inhibit cell proliferation process and migration through the micropores. These results proved that laser microperforation could be used for the production of scaffolds.

Cartilage Tissue Regeneration

PHAs are also used in cartilage tissue engineering. The most important factor for successful regeneration of cartilage chondrocytes was polymer crystallinity. Maturational differentiation of chondrocytes was affected by the amount of P(3HB) in a P(3HB)/P(3HB-*co*-3HHx) blend present on the surface [123]. For cartilage repair, effective scaffolds were produced from poly(3-hydroxybutyrate-*co*-3-hydroxyhexanoate) (P(3HB-*co*-3HHx)) [124]. P(3HB-*co*-3HV) scaffold was compared with collagen containing calcium phosphate. Köse *et al.* [125] showed that poly(3-hydroxybutyrate-*co*-3-hydroxyvalerate) (P(3HB-*co*-

3HV)) scaffolds exhibited better healing properties in the treatment of cartilage impairment in rabbit than collagen scaffolds impregnated with calcium phosphate. P(3HB-*co*-3HV) cartilage scaffolds were implanted in patellar groove on the knees of rabbits into full thickness cartilage defects. Collagen containing calcium phosphate was used as a reference matrix. *In vivo* results at 8 and 20 weeks presented early cartilage formation similar to normal articular cartilage and disclosed minimal foreign body reaction for P(3HB-*co*-3HV) matrices. In collagen matrices containing calcium phosphate fibrocartilage formation was observed in 20 weeks. Thus, P(3HB-*co*-3HV) had better healing response than collagen containing calcium phosphate [125]. P(3HB-*co*-3HHx) and P(3HB-*co*-3HHx)/P(3HB) scaffolds exhibited better conditions for the proliferation of chondrocytes than P(3HB) ones. Wang *et al.* [124] described 3D scaffolds made of P(3HB-*co*-3HHx) for the evaluation of tissue repair effect in rabbit. Scaffold was inoculated with chondrocytes for 10 days before implantation. *In vivo* evaluation of implant was conducted during 16 weeks after implantation. It was found that the defects were filled with white cartilaginous tissues. P(3HB-*co*-3HHx) scaffold inoculated with chondrocytes showed better surface integrality and higher accumulation of extracellular matrix including type II collagen and sulfated glycosaminoglycan.

PHB implants caused stronger tissue response than scaffolds produced from PHA copolymer. This behavior is the result of P(3HB) rigidity. More rigid material exerted stronger influence on the tissues enclosing the implant. Moreover, the bioabsorption rate of the scaffolds formed from PHA copolymers decreased with the 3HB content [82].

Bone Tissue Engineering

Bone tissues have perfect self-regeneration ability. In some cases, bone defects exceed a critical size, forcing a surgical intervention. Bone tissue engineering is a promising alternative to conventional bone transplant, because it avoids the risks of disease transfer and potential site morbidity. PHA substrates favor osteoblast adhesion and proliferation and deposition of calcium [126]. Apart from P(3HB), P(3HB-*co*-3HHx) was also considered as one of the most biocompatible polymers with osteoblasts. For osteoblast proliferation, P(3HB-*co*-3HHx) with lower percentage of 3HHx monomer (12 mol% of 3HHx) is preferred in contrast to fibroblasts, which favored higher content of HHx (20 mol% of 3HHx) [127]. After 12 months implantation of PHB into rabbits, no inflammatory response was observed by Doyle *et al.* [78]. Moreover, PHB produced bone tissue adaptation response. The PHB implant surface was covered with new bone tissue. Relationship between proliferation and mineralization of osteoblast on P(3HB-*co*-3HV) foam with different pore sizes was studied by Köse *et al.* [128].

It was found that cells proliferated better on large pore size foams (300–500 μm) compared with foams with small pore sizes (75–300 μm). The study demonstrated that P(3HB-*co*-3HV) matrices were applicable for osteoblast proliferation and differentiation process including increasing alkaline phosphate activity and osteocalcin excretion. Porous P(3HB-*co*-3HV) scaffold covered with bone marrow stromal cells and implanted into defects in rat exhibited osteogenic differentiation features. Experiment shows distinct bone regeneration in 6 weeks. Blends of PHB and hydroxyapatite (HA) were used as scaffolds to treat bone defects [78, 129]. P(3HB) with hydroxyapatite was applied for hard tissue regeneration to form a bioactive and biodegradable composite [130]. P(3HB-*co*-3HV) (8 mol% of 3HV) composite with 30 wt% of hydroxyapatite showed a mechanical compression strength of ~62 MPa, which is similar to human bones [131]. For the growth and differentiation of murine marrow osteoblasts, P(3HB) blends containing 10 and 20 wt% of hydroxyapatite were the most magnificent [79]. Mineralization levels and inflammatory response were limited by nano-sized hydroxyapatite used as reinforcing of P(3HB-*co*-3HV) [132]. P(3HB-*co*-3HV)/HA scaffolds implanted in rabbit tibias showed lamellar bone formulation at the interface with the assistance of matrix degradation. Thickness of the newly formed bone increased over the experimental period from 130 μm after 1 month to 770 μm after 6 months [133]. Misra *et al.* [134] described PHB foams prepared with bioactive glass particles (45S5 Bioglass). Foams having 85% porosity were adequate for the attachment and proliferation of osteoblast. Scaffold made of P(3HB)/bioactive glass composite was implanted in rat. After 1 week of implantation, no immune response was observed. Wang *et al.* [126] described that P(HB-*co*-HHx) exhibited better conditions for proliferation and differentiation of osteoblasts than P(3HB).

Wang *et al.* [135] described the use of electrospun Ecoflex/P(3HB-*co*-3HV) blend for the preparation of microfibrous bone tissue engineering scaffolds. The authors demonstrate that the obtained mats exhibited increased hydrophilicity and flexibility, acceleration of *in vitro* degradation, and intensity of cellular proliferation on the scaffold. Biocompatibility with human bone marrow stroma cells (hBMSCs) was also improved. Mats containing Ecoflex with P(3HB-*co*-3HV) at mass ratio 30/70, 50/50, and 70/30 showed decreased contact angle, increased weight loss in phosphate-buffered saline, and strain at break with increasing Ecoflex contribution.

Surgical Applications

Polymeric materials used for suture production must exhibit high tensile strength and adequate/applicable rigidity. These properties are significant for effectiveness of materials used in wound closures [92]. PHB and P(3HB-*co*-3HV) sutures were shown to be suitable for muscle wound closures. P(3HB-*co*-3HV) is also used for oral surgery in dogs [136]. Surgical materials are produced from poly(4-hydroxybutyrate) (P(4HB)). Oriented P(4HB) fibers showed higher tensile strength (545 MPa) and lower Young modulus than polypropylene sutures (410–460 MPa) [137].

Materials used for wound dressing should be stable, stress resistant, flexible, and elastic. Easy application and removing is also an important attribute.

Nerve Tissue Engineering

PHA can also be used in nerve tissue engineering. Xu *et al.* [138] described that PHA matrices allow proliferation of neural stem cells. The penetration of stem cells into polymer matrix showed P(3HB-*co*-3HHx). Perfect biodegradable nerve conduit should be characterized by the ability to maintain integrity of tissues, permit cell communication, and allow growth of tissues and their regeneration [139]. PHB has been used as a graft matrix for neuronal regeneration after spinal cord injury in rats [140]. P(3HB) was used as a bridged conduit of long nerve gaps in rabbit peroneal nerves. Application of P(3HB) showed bigger area of regenerating fibers at 42 days compared with nerve autograft group [141]. Authors assumed that P(3HB) conduits are suitable for long-gap nerve injury repair. P(3HB) tubes filled with glial growth factor (GGF) and suspended in alginate hydrogel assisted peripheral nerve regeneration for up to 63 days. This type of PHB tubes with glial growth factor are used for regeneration of 2–4 cm gaps in common peroneal nerve in rabbit. Addition of glial growth factor considerably increased the number of Schwann cells and favored axonal regeneration and muscle reinnervation [142]. These results are important especially for long-term regeneration. Novikova *et al.* [143] used tubular P(3HB) scaffold with predominantly unidirectional fiber orientation after cervical spinal cord injury in rats for axonal regeneration. The scaffold was filled up by adult Schwann cells. In the consequence of addition of Schwann cells, neurofilament-positive axons filled the conduit and became associated with the implanted cells. To increase Schwann cell attachment and proliferation *in vitro*, modification of P(3HB) surface with fibronectin, laminin, or collagen is very advantageous.

The high crystallinity of PHB limits its potential in many applications. Reduction of crystallinity of P(3HB) was obtained by blending with a variety of poly-(ethylene glycols) (PEGs) [144, 145]. Another advantage of PEGs is increased hydrophilicity of modified P(3HB)/PEG blends. The combination of the properties of hydrophilic PEG and hydrophobic P(3HB) compose useful materials for tissue engineering and drug delivery systems. Scaffolds for nerve repair were made of PEG-106-terminated P(3HB)-based biomaterials [109].

Heart Valve Engineering

The most common treatment procedure for end-stage valvular diseases is surgical replacement. In general, surgical replacement is realized by mechanical valves or grafts, which possess good structural durability. However, the mechanical valves have several disadvantages such as prosthetic valve endocarditis and thromboembolic complication caused by their non-physiological surfaces and flow abnormalities [146]. All of the used valves are disable to grow with the patient body, which causes the necessity of surgical replacement of valves in children. Pulmonary valve leaflets and pulmonary artery scaffolds implanted in sheep were produced of the copolymer of poly(glycolic acid) and P3HB [147]. Sodian *et al.* [148] described PHA-based heart valve scaffold implanted into sheep.

Medium chain length PHAs (mcl-PHAs) are flexible materials, which function as leaflets inside the valve. The trileaflet heart valve scaffold consisting of cylindrical stents with the leaflets formed from a 3-hydroxyhexanoate and 3-hydroxyoctanoate copolymer (P(3HHx-*co*-3HO)) with seeded autologous cells was implanted in the pulmonary position in a lamb model [149]. The function of implanted trileaflet valve was maintained up to 120 days with no thrombus formation. Blends can be utilized to improve the performance of PHA to fabricate heart valve scaffolds. Blends of P(3HHx-*co*-3HO) with poly(glycolic acid) (PGA) eliminated nonprogressive valvular regurgitation after 6 months of implantation [150]. Hoerstrup *et al.* [151] reported that trileaflet heart valves made of (P(4HB)) coated with PGA non-woven mesh seeded with autologous ovine myofibroblasts and endothelial cells were grown for 14 days in a pulse duplicator *in vitro* system under progressively increasing flow and pressure. The valves were implanted into lambs, and during 20 weeks of implantation, the size of the inner diameter of the valve constructs at the level of leaflet increased from 19 to 23 mm. These results illustrated the possibility to develop a valve that can grow with the heart valve volume. Adamus *et al.* [45] described a diblock copolymer obtained from poly[(R,S)-3-hydroxybutyrate] (aPHB) and natural poly(3-hydroxyoctanoate) (P(3HO)) for the coating of the vascular prosthesis. The received blend was well penetrated in the outer surface of the prosthesis and demonstrated reduced permeability of vascular prostheses.

The pathology of blood vessels is a serious cause of cardiovascular disorders. This pathology is treated by cardiac and peripheral bypass surgery. Synthetic vascular grafts (*e.g.*, PTFE, Dacron) have been used successfully for large arteries with internal diameter >6 mm. In smaller diameter vessels, they exhibited reduced patency as a consequence of thrombogenicity [152]. Stock *et al.* [153] reported about autologous vascular cells isolated from peripheral veins and seeded on

P(4HB) patches. In the next step, the patches were implanted into the pulmonary artery in a juvenile sheep model. Histology conducted at 169 days demonstrated almost complete resorption of the polymer. Moreover, formation of organized and functional tissues was observed without thrombus or stenosis. Mendelson *et al.* [154] described seeded autologous ovine blood-derived endothelial progenitor cells and bone marrow-derived mesenchymal stem cells onto P(4HB) coated PGA nonwoven biodegradable scaffolds. The scaffold was cultured for 5 days in a laminar fluid flow system. Then, the seeded patches were implanted into sheep pulmonary artery. Two weeks after implantation, seeded patches caused formation of granulation tissue end early pannus. After 4 weeks, the patches contained glycosaminoglycans, collagen, and coverage of the luminal surface by host artery-derived pannus containing alpha-SMA-positive cells and laminated elastin. Almost complete degradation of polymer scaffold was observed during the test period. Wu *et al.* [155] evaluated intravascular biocompatibility of P(3HB-*co*-3HHx). They described implantation of decellularized xenogeneic vascular scaffolds coated with P(3HB-*co*-3HHx) in rabbit abdominal aorta for 12 weeks. The implanted scaffolds maintained original shapes covered by confluent endothelial surface. Uncoated patches were only partially repopulated with endothelial cells, and thrombosis on the surface was observed.

Dermal Tissue Regeneration

Skin regeneration is another application of PHA. Scaffold for skin tissue regeneration was described by Volova *et al.* [156]. Sutures obtained from P(3HB) and P(3HB-*co*-3HV) featured the necessary strength during the healing period. The reaction of tissues to the P(3HB) and P(3HB-*co*-3HV) implantation was characteristic of the wound process and of the reaction on foreign body. There were no adverse effects such as inflammation, necrosis, and calcification after 4–8 weeks of PHA implantation. Electrospun scaffolds were obtained by Ying *et al.* [82]. Poly(3HB-*co*-3HHx) (5 mol% of 3HHx), poly(3HB-*co*-4HB) (7 mol% of 4HB), and poly(3HB-*co*-4HB) (97 mol% of 4HB) were implanted in rat model. The electrospun PHA scaffolds were well tolerated *in vivo* with very mild tissue response. Fig. (**3**) shows the physical appearance of PHA scaffolds before and after implantation. Hybrid nanofibrous mats consisting of P(3HB-*co*-3HV) and chitosan for skin tissue engineering were described by Veleirinho *et al.* [157]. The mats exhibited good adhesion, proliferation of L929 cell line, and noteworthy wound healing process in rat. Kuppan *et al.* [158] evaluated adhesion, proliferation, and gene expression of human skin fibroblasts on P(3HB-*co*-3HV) fibers obtained by electrospinning and 2D P(3HB-*co*-3HV) films. Cell adhesion and proliferation with higher expression of collagen I gene were found on P(3HB-*co*-3HV) fibers ad 2D P(3HB-*co*-3HV) films. The expression profiles were changed after 3 days, which acknowledged cell proliferation. The wound healing process on P(3HB) fibers was estimated in the presence of R-Spondin and angiogenesis-promoting growth factor, which stimulated wound healing process. R-Spondin 1 accelerated wound contraction within 7 days. Fibrous scaffold favored faster bulk degradation compared with the 2D films.

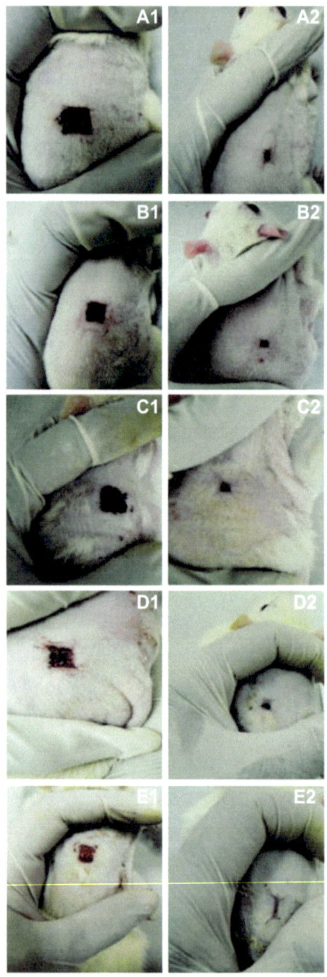

Fig. (3). Macroscopic image of the wound contracture over time for all five groups. (A1) 1 week and (A2) 2 weeks of negative control; (B1) 1 week and (B2) 2 weeks of positive control; (C1) 1 week and (C2) 2 weeks of P(3HB-*co*-3HV) fibers; (D1) 1 week and (D2) 2 weeks of R-Spondin 1; (E1) 1 week and (E2) 2 weeks of P(3HB-*co*-3HV) fibers loaded with R-Spondin 1. Reprinted with permission from Kuppan *et al.* [158].

Miscellaneous Medical Applications

PHB films in scaffold form were used to patch a bowel defect in rats. These material degraded readily *in vivo* than *in vitro* [159].

Wang *et al.* [160] described the blends of flexible and hydrophilic Ecoflex with P(3HB-*co*-3HV) obtained by electrospinning for periodontal tissue engineering. They observed faster adhesion and proliferation of periodontal ligament stem cells (PDLSCs) on blend mat as compared to pure P(3HB-*co*-3HV).

DRUG RELEASING MEDICAL DEVICES

Biodegradable polymers have significant role in numerous clinical applications. The main advantage of biodegradable polyhydroxyalkanoates (PHAs) in medical applications is the possibility to insert PHAs into the human body without the necessity to remove them from the patient body after the treatment [161]. Apart from the applications in biomedical devices, PHAs are also used in drug releasing devices, which is particularly important in surgical perspective. Implantation of scaffolds could lead to bacterial infection, which is the most common complication. Disadvantages connected with infection state delay recovery and may cause non-uniform healing of bone fractures. Infections in extreme cases can lead to implant loosening [162]. To prevent and heal implant-associated infections, antibiotics are often used.

High crystallinity of PHB is the main problem for its use in controlled release devices. This feature may interfere the drug distribution in the structure of the polymer. Low degradation rate of PHB, depending on molar mass and form, which can extend from 1 to 2 years, is another problem [78]. Solution to these PHB-related problems may be application of copolymers containing 3-hydroxyvalerate units. Copolymer P(3HB-*co*-3HV) exhibits lower crystallinity and higher ability for biodegradation. These properties are a consequence of higher amorphicity of P(3HB-*co*-3HV) compared with PHB homopolymer, which generally results in more effective and homogeneous drug distribution. It can be assumed that such behavior can contribute to increased drug release [163].

Li *et al.* [164] reported P(3HB-*co*-3HV) microsphere/45S5 bioactive glass (BG) composite scaffolds with drug release function applied for bone tissue engineering. The P(3HB-*co*-3HV) used in this study contained 12 mol% of 3HV units. Bioactive glass (BG) (45S5 composition) is an object of research for biomedical applications because of the excellent bioactivity [165, 166]. Polymer coating raised the mechanical properties of the brittle bioactive-based scaffolds. BG-based scaffolds with high porosity and interconnected pore structure were coated with P(3HB-*co*-3HV) microspheres with encapsulated vancomycin. Vancomycin is an antibiotic that has good efficacy in the treatment of infections caused by Gram-positive bacteria [167]. P(3HB-*co*-3HV) exhibited lower melting temperature and crystallinity than P(3HB), which makes it more adequate for drug delivery applications [168]. The encapsulated vancomycin was released with a dual release profile involving a burst release [164]. For coated scaffolds, initial burst effect achieved low level of 21% and sustained release after 1 month. Initial high-burst release (77%) and short release period (4 days) was achieved for uncoated scaffolds. Thus, the P(3HB-*co*-3HV) microsphere-coated scaffolds are highly interesting for bone tissue engineering applications because of sustained antibiotic release function.

Osteomyelitis is a disease that demands therapy with systemically administered antibiotic and direct application of antibiotics in the place of infection [169]. P(3HB-*co*-3HV) containing 11.3 mol% of 3HV and P(3HB-*co*-4HB) containing 9.4 mol% of 4-HB units were used to produce implantable rods for the local delivery of antibiotics in osteomyelitis therapy [29]. Sulperazone® (sulbactam-cefoperazone (1:1)) and Duocid® (sulbactam-ampicilin (1:2)) are effective drugs in the therapy of osteomyelitis caused by *Staphylococcus aureus*. Controlled by the drug-loading rate of Sulperazone®, the release from P(3HB-*co*-4-HB) rods was higher than the polymer degradation. Coating rods with the same polymer reduced the initial burst effect compared with the uncoated rods. Duration of antibiotic release from uncoated rods was 1–3 days, whereas the release from coated rods was maintained for over a period of 12 days at constant rate. Moreover, the authors concluded that the drug release from rods with Duocid® was higher than the drug release from the rods with Sulperazone®.

Gursel *et al.* investigated the rods made of P(3HB-*co*-3HV) with different content of 3HV units. P(3HB-*co*-3HV) rods containing 7, 14, and 22 mol% of 3HV units were loaded with sulbactam-cefoperazone (Sulperazone®) or gentamicin. Authors studied the *in vitro* antibiotics release behavior to physiological phosphate buffer. Proper antibiotic therapy demands the minimal effective concentration of antibiotics for at least 6 weeks. P(3HB-*co*-3HV) containing 22 mol% of 3HV units released 60% of Sulperazone in 60 days. Changing the polymer to drug ratio from 2:1 to 20:1 considerably decreased the drug release rate [163]. Gentamicin was released at a rate of 25% in 14 days.

Gursel *et al.* [170] also described antibiotic-loaded rods made from P(3HB-*co*-3HV) containing 11 mol% of 3HV units and P(3HB-*co*-4HB) containing 7.7 mol% of 4HB units carrying 50% (w/w) Sulperazone or Duocid. Rods were implanted into rabbit tibia in implant-related osteomyelitis. Antibiotic was released effectively from both used polymeric matrices. Sulperazone-P(3HB-*co*-4HB) rods provided drug release and ensured treatment for the infection. Rods with Sulperazone implanted in uninfected rabbits showed high antibiotic release. Authors observed that the therapy was efficient despite high release rate. Rods tested *in vitro* were examined by scanning electron microscopy (SEM), which showed that polymeric component was unchanged for 2 weeks after elution of antibiotics. *In vivo* morphology of the implant distinctly changed within 6 weeks after implantation.

Yagmurlu *et al.* [171] described P(3HB-*co*-3HV) rods containing 22 mol% of 3HV units with sulbactam-cefoperazone used in chronic osteomyelitis. The rod was implanted into the infection site of rabbit tibia. After 15 days of implantation, the infection subsided. Almost complete remission was observed after 30 days of implantation.

Orthopedic disks based on P(3HB-*co*-3HV) containing 8 mol% and 12 mol% of 3HV units with gentamicin was described by Rossi *et al.* Antibacterial effectiveness of the obtained complexes was tested with bacteria causing orthopedic infections: *Staphylococcus haemolyticus* and *Staphylococcus aureus*. They found that increasing content of 3HV units lead to faster release of gentamicin. For disks with higher amount of gentamicin, they observed decreased permeability and reduction of the release rate as a consequence of higher homogeneity. Effectiveness of the P(3HB-*co*-3HV) complexes were assessed by the reduction of number of bacteria within 48 h of exposure. The tested complexes exhibited sustained, constant release rate of gentamicin for 6 weeks, above minimum inhibitory concentration of the used bacteria [172].

PHA drug delivery was used as glaucoma drainage implant to limit the generation of fibrotic tissues. In this study, P(3HB) and P(4HB) were used as matrices for the production of drainage tubes containing paclitaxel as an antiproliferative agent and triamcinolone acetonide as an anti-inflammatory agent. Drainage tubes were dip coated in PHB layer, which included drugs. Drainage tubes produced from both the polymers exhibited limited cytotoxicity and moderate vascularization in the cornea and conjunctiva for up to 100 days after the surgery. Higher drug release and degradation rate characterized tubes made of flexible P(4HB) [173].

Matrix for drug-eluting coronary stents was obtained from poly(3-hydroxybutyrate) (P(3HB)) and poly(3-hydroxyoctanoate) P(3HO) 50:50 blend. This blend contained rigid and flexible materials, thus the combined features gave a suitable material for drug-eluting coronary stents. Aspirin is an antithrombotic drug, but its oral bioavailability is poor; hence, it is a challenge to deliver a dosage that releases pharmacological response. Local delivery of antithrombotic drug can reduce the risk of arterial embolism after stent implantation. The blend matrix loaded with aspirin was formed by solvent casting process, which ensured uniform distribution of drug into the matrix. Addition of aspirin elevated roughness of blend film. Aspirin increased the hydrophilic nature of the blend film. This change was manifested by the increased total protein absorption. A weak burst release (~9%) of aspirin on the first day was observed. Aspirin was then released at a constant rate for 20 days. Cumulative release was achieved after a period of 30 days. Hydrolytic stability of aspirin incorporated into hydrophobic matrix increased the delivery [174].

Karpova *et al.* [175] described ultrafine fibers of P(3HB) containing various concentrations (1%, 3%, and 5%) of dipyridamole – antiplatelet agent, angioprotectors, and proofreaders microcirculation, prepared by electrospinning method. A morphological study of the fibrous materials showed the effect of the concentration of dipyridamole on the shape of the fibers.

POLYMER–DRUG CONJUGATES

Polymer–drug conjugates Fig. (**4**) are divided into three types depending on the attachment of therapeutic agent onto polymer chain: the main chain type when the drug is incorporated into polymer backbone; the pendant type when the drug is conjugated as a side group; end-capped type where drug is a terminal group in polymer chain.

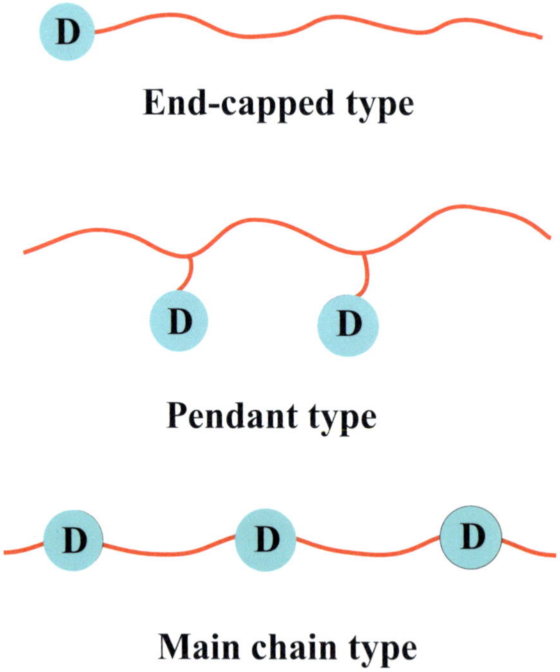

Fig. (4). Schematic representation of polymer–drug conjugate types.

The conjugation of bioactive substance with polymer or oligomer *e.g.* oligo(3-hydroxybutyrate) (OHB), is one of the simplest strategies of drug delivery as the OHB is found in human body [10] and it is nontoxic and biocompatible. One of the first studies that utilized the attachment of drug to an oligomer was the conjugation of penicillin G with OHB [176]. Unfortunately, this study was limited to the presentation of the possibility to obtain the oligomers with bioactive end-groups through the initiation of ROP of β-butyrolactone with appropriate salt (in this case, potassium salt of 6*N*-benzylpenicillanic acid).

The followed study proved that the conjugated drug, doxorubicin with OHB, was successfully delivered to the cells and that it was accumulated in the cytoplasm. Moreover, it did not induce the cytoprotective response [99].

Another example demonstrating positive effect of conjugation of the drug with OHB was acetylsalicylic acid commonly known as aspirin [119]. On average, the studied oligomers had a range of 4–8 repeating units of 3-hydroxybutyric acid. The acetylsalicylic acid–oligo(3-hydroxybutanoate) conjugates did not show any oral cytotoxicity in rats at a level of 2000 mg/kg body weight. The MTT survival assay was conducted on two cancer cell lines: human colon adenocarcinoma cells (HT-29) and human colon carcinoma cells (HCT 116), and it showed a significant decrease of IC_{50} of the conjugate, which lowers the dose to 0.74 mM (HT-29) and 0.4 mM (HCT 116) from the dose of free aspirin 3.8 and 2.8 mM, respectively.

The attachment of OHB to ibuprofen [120] also proved better availability of the drug administrated in the form of conjugate. The IC_{50} for the free drug was 552 and 448 μM for HT-29 and HCT 116 cells, respectively, whereas the same level of drug activity was achieved with conjugated ibuprofen concentration of ~30 μM. Such an increased antiproliferative activity of drug against the studied cells was explained as an enhancement of transport through the cell membrane. This behavior was investigated in the aforementioned study employing the OHB attached to fluorescein [120]. Moreover, this vector-like ability was further proved by using the fluorescein–OHB conjugates to study the transport to mitochondria [9].

The conjugation strategy was also used in the administration of vanillic and anisic acid (antioxidants used in cosmetic formulations) [118]. The vanillic acid–OHB conjugate showed higher antioxidant activity compared with free phenolic acid (3–5 times lower concentration resulted in similar effect). Moreover, the penetration of antioxidant conjugates through the skin was better, but diffusion experiment did not show the penetration of conjugates to blood.

As was described earlier, the conjugates of the bioactive substances and polymer were prepared by ring opening polymerization of β-lactones initiated by bioactive substance in the carboxylate ion form [177] Fig. (**5**). Alternative methods are the polymerization of β-lactone [47] with the drug as a side group or through transesterification [178, 179] Fig. (**5**).

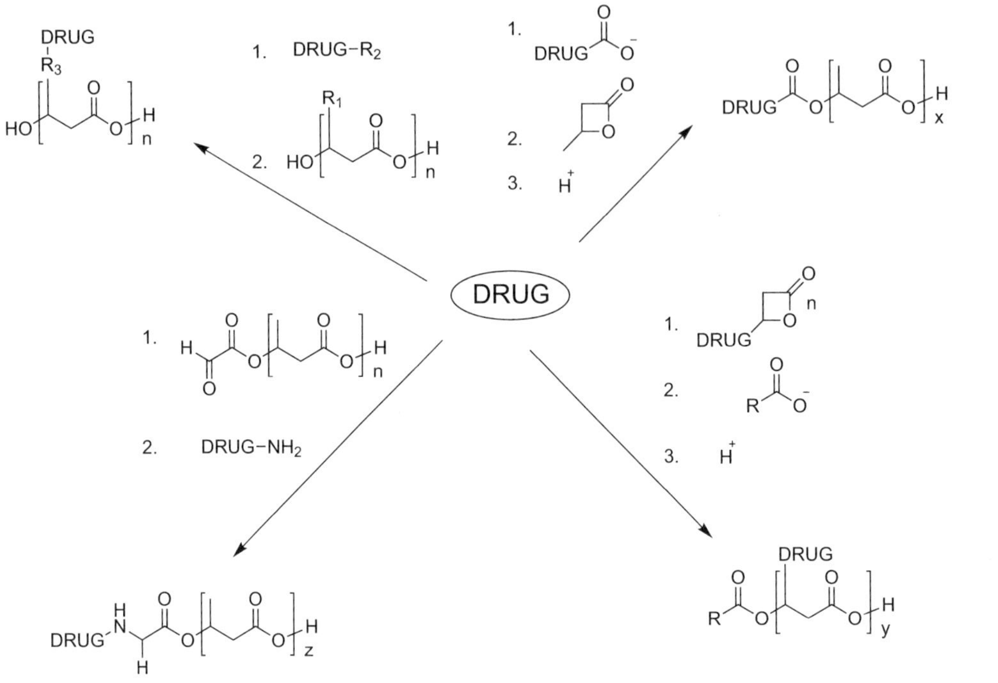

R_1 and R_2 functional groups which could react together, i.e $-N_3$ and triple bond

Fig. (5). Various possible types of PHA-based conjugates described in literature.

The aforementioned anisic acid was also attached to glicydyl, which had further undergone ring expansion in the presence of carbon monoxide to obtain the appropriate β-lactone [46]. Unfortunately, this very interesting option introducing a polymer that contained a drug on each repeating unit as a novel delivery system was only limited to a synthetic study Fig. (**5**).

Additional possibilities to conjugate drugs with polyhydroxyalkanoates are the preparation of polymers with appropriate functions either at the chain ends [180] or as side group [181]. A worth to notice strategy was the preparation of glyoxylate functionalized PHB, which was conjugated with model amine to form imine bond which was pH-sensitive, and therefore, the release of substance differed depending on the conditions it was released in Ref [182]. Fig. (**5**). An alternative to the attachment of bioactive substances to the polymer chain ends is the conjugation of the functional groups in the side chains of poly(3-hydroxyalkanoates). As stated earlier, the PHAs could possess various functionalities in the side chains [3]; however, for the delivery systems, especially two of them could be suitable: main terminal double bond [183] or azide group [184] Fig. (**5**). These functions offer high reactivity and wide possibility of modification through click reaction.

MICRO- AND NANOPARTICLES FOR DRUG DELIVERY

The preparation of particles, nano- as well as micro-, is a popular and quite intensively investigated way to deliver drugs [25, 185, 186]. In the beginning, mainly poly(3-hydroxybutyrate) and its copolymer with 3-hydroxyvaleric acid were used in the preparation of micro- and nanoparticles [187]. Nowadays, the studies are focused more on medium chain length poly(hydroxyalkanoate)s because of their better drug release profile compared with the short chain length PHAs, although the scl-PHAs are not abandoned as interesting materials for drug delivery systems.

The preparation of micro- and nanoparticles from polyhydroxyalkanoates as a method to administrate the drug for different diseases has quite long history. During this long period, some studies were limited to the preparation of particles without conducting further experiments with drugs. Some experiments were extended to study loading, encapsulation, and release of model substances, that is, Nile red. Such studies were usually followed by the evaluation of particles as the delivery systems for specific drugs. The most complex strategy employs not only combining the drug and PHA-based particles but also modification of such particles with targeting molecules and creating a targeted therapy. From numerous examples of particle-based drug delivery systems, only some of the most interesting examples will be discussed in the following section.

Polyhydroxyalkanoate Particles – Model Study

Biocompatibility of *in vivo* and *in vitro* study of poly(3-hydroxybutyrate) microspheres with mean diameter 10 μm was evaluated [188]. The cytotoxicity test performed on the mouse fibroblast cells (NIH 3T3 line) did not induce any toxic response. The *in vivo* test performed on female Wistar rats showed slight inflammation after 24 h reaction, which vanished after 1 week of implementation. There was a strong macrophage response; however, the fibrous response of tissue was not induced.

One of the first studies concerning the use of PHB and P(3HB-*co*-3HV) (9 and 24% of HV units) microparticles as drug delivery systems employed progesterone as the encapsulated substance [189]. The study proved that PHAs could be used to efficiently encapsulate drug with a loading efficiency of >80%. However, the most advantageous releasing profile was achieved for P(3HB-*co*-3HV) microspheres containing 9% of HV units because of the lowest porosity of the particles formed from this material.

Transdermal transport employing the P(3HB-*co*-3HV) (11% of HV units)-based particles loaded with Nile red was performed [112]. The comparison of micro- and nanoparticles was performed by using three different particle sizes: 1900, 426, and 166 nm. The cytotoxicity test showed that the size of the particle did not play any role at the concentration >0.5 mg/mL. However, at the concentration of 1 mg/mL, the microparticles (1900 nm) decreased the proliferation efficiency. Moreover, smaller nanoparticles (166 and 426 nm) showed better cell internalization and were visible in cytoplasm, whereas microparticles did not show such behavior. Nevertheless, the *in vivo* test on BALB/c mice skin showed that all kind of particles penetrated the skin, but again the nano-sized ones had more promising results.

A comparative study of particles prepared from PHB, P(3HB-*co*-3HHx) (containing 12% of HHx units), and polylactide (PLA) loaded with rhodamine B isothiocyanate (RBITC) was performed [113]. Particles of two different sizes (~160 and 250 nm) were prepared from PHAs and particles of 147 nm were formed by the PLA. The PHA-based particles showed better encapsulation efficiency then PLA, because PLA encapsulated 70.8% of RBITC and the PHA particles reached 77% encapsulation efficiency. The intracellular drug release profiles revealed that PHA particles released RBITC at a slower rate than PLA nanoparticles.

The aforementioned model study employed materials for particle formation without any functionalities in the side chains (namely methyl, ethyl, or propyl group in the side chain). The modification of side chains offers more possibilities of application of such modified PHAs. Among many modifications of drug delivery systems [190 - 193], a study presented by Ajellal *et al.* [194] concerned the release of leuprolide acetate, the synthetic non-peptide analog of gonadotropin. However, the formation of nanoparticles from poly-(3HB-*co*-3BL^{allyl}) or its modified version where double bonds were transformed into diols did not have significant impact on the drug release profile.

Evaluation of PHA Particles in Drug Delivery

The microparticles obtained from PHB, P(3HB-*co*-3HV) (6.5, 10.5, 20, and 37 mol% of 3HV units), P(3HB-*co*-3HHx) (7 mol% of HHx units), and P(3HB-*co*-4HB) (6.1 and 16 mol% of 4HB units) were evaluated for the delivery of doxorubicin [114]. The sizes differed depending on the material used for the preparation of the microparticles (emulsion, solvent evaporation method): PHB and P(3HB-*co*-3HV) up to 10 mol% of HV units, had similar sizes ~750 nm, the P(3HB-*co*-3HV) with 20 mol% and more HV units and P(3HB-*co*-3HHx) had the mean diameters ~1200 nm, the P(3HB-*co*-4HB) formed the largest particles ~2500 nm. Doxorubicin was released from the microparticles without burst effect and the drug release kinetics were described by diffusion kinetics equations [195, 196]. The study on the HeLa cells proved the cytotoxic activity of the drug encapsulated in microparticles.

Development of the best method of encapsulation of the anticancer drug achieving controlled delivery and release is one of the main focus concerning the particular delivery systems. Paclitaxel was encapsulated in P(3HB-*co*-3HV) nanoparticles containing 12% of HV units (diameter ~250 nm) [197]. The effectiveness of the drug-loaded nanoparticles to induce cell death was evaluated on Ishikawa and SKOV3 cells. The particles with 5 or 1 μM of encapsulated paclitaxel showed the highest induction of the Ishikawa and SKOV3 cells death, respectively.

P(3HB-*co*-3HV) containing 5, 11, and 15 mol% of HV units was also used for the encapsulation of ellipticine, which inhibits DNA topoisomerase II activity and RNA transcription within the nucleus [198]. The sizes of the particles with encapsulated drugs were in the range of 208–283 nm. Particles obtained from P(3HB-*co*-3HV) (15 mol% of 3HV units) exhibited the highest inhibition of cancer cell line A549, nevertheless in all cases the activity of the polyester particles loaded with ellipticine was two times higher than the activity of free drug.

The P(3HB) and P(3HB-*co*-3HHx) with 5 and 12 mol% of HHx units were used to encapsulate the TGX221 – the inhibitor of phosphoinositide-3-kinases (PI3K), which have poor solubility and short half-life [115]. The anticancer activity was evaluated by using the PC3 cell lines. Reduction of cell growth (15%) was observed when treated with nanoparticles loaded with TGX221 at a concentration of 0.2 and 20 μM of free drug. Nanoparticles containing an equivalent of 20 μM of drug caused 45% of cell growth inhibition. The encapsulation of the TGX221 extended its half-life and improved bioavailability.

The evaluation of application of PHB and P(3HB-*co*-3HV) containing 12 and 50 mol% of 3HV units in photodynamic therapy was performed by using porphyrin (pTHPP) as the encapsulated drug [199]. The particles with the sizes from 157 to 208 nm were tested for photocytotoxicity, employing HT-29 cells, and satisfactory results comparable to free drugs were obtained.

The P(3HB-*co*-3HHx) containing 12 mol% of 3HHx units was used to deliver the platelet-derived growth factor-BB (PDGF-BB) for the long-term stimulation of human mesenchymal stem cells (hMSCs) [200]. The nanoparticles loaded with PDGF-BB where compared with drug-free nanoparticles and nanoparticles prepared from bovine albumin serum. All the particles had an average diameter of

~150 nm. Such nanoparticles were used for the growth of hMSCs in 2D and 3D culture. The study in 2D culture shows that the presence of particles containing growth factor improved cell proliferation. This observation was confirmed in the 3D culture of hMSCs cells, where the presence of nanoparticles loaded with PDGF-BB strongly enhanced the cell growth.

Copolymers of PHA with PEG are quite interesting material to be used in drug delivery systems. P(3HB-*co*-3HV) containing 12 and 33 mol% of HV units and P(3HB-*co*-4HB) containing 6 and 20 mol% of 4HB units are interesting materials for the preparation of particles for drug delivery systems, and they were coupled with PEG (M_n = 2000 g/mol) through transesterification in the presence of bis(2-ethylhexanoate) tin catalyst [116]. The obtained nanoparticles (average diameter ~120 nm) were used to encapsulate a thymoquinone, anticancer drug, in which the hydrophobic nature limits its clinical application. The *in vitro* cell viability studies indicated that the core–shell structured nanoparticles obtained from PHA–PEG copolymers show compatibility in biological environment and provide a safe and nontoxic system for the loading of drugs without producing any significant toxic effects on the cell.

The nanoparticle delivery of rapamycin, the kinase inhibitor with poor bioavailability and limited half-life, was investigated by using the P(3HB-*co*-3HHx) and its copolymer with PEG [111]. The human prostate cancer (PC3) cell line was chosen to evaluate the efficiency of drug delivery system. The treatment of PC3 cells with the rapamycin-loaded nanoparticles showed a significant decrease in cell proliferation compared with free drug.

The block copolymer of poly(3-hydroxyvalerate-*co*-4-hydroxybutyrate) (P(3HV-*co*-4HB)) containing 58 mol% of 4HB units with PEG (M_n = 5000 g/mol) was used to prepare nanoparticles (diameter 155 nm, PDI = 0.154) loaded with cisplatin [201]. The *in vitro* release was stable during the whole experiment. The cytotoxicity was evaluated by using DU145 human prostate cancer cell line in which the drug loaded to nanoparticles showed higher inhibition of cells proliferation.

The NuBCP-9 peptide (FSRSLHSLL) targeted the Bcl-2 antiapoptotic activity in cancer cells and was loaded to P3HB-b-PEG (with masses 72 000 and 4000 g/mol, respectively) with a mean diameter of 126 nm [202]. The *in vitro* studies performed on MCF-7 breast cancer cell line showed IC_{50} to be 1.6 μM in 72 h, whereas free peptide did not show cytotoxicity at the concentration of 15 μM, as it was unable to enter the cell. Also, apoptosis assessment showed that 85% of cancer cells were in the apoptosis phase. The *in vivo* evaluation of possible tumor regression after administration of nanoparticles with drug on Balb/c mice showed that the tumor volume decreased by 90%.

Targeted Therapy Based on PHA Particles

Evaluation of the modified particles for targeted drug delivery systems (TDDS) was performed in two ways: the modification of particles through the chemical methods, that is, attachment of folic acid [117] or by the biosynthesis of PHA particles with attached targeting protein (i.e., RGD4C (α_v-integrin binding peptide) [203]). In addition, there is also a strategy combining the aforementioned method where in the first step the particle is synthesized by the standard procedure followed by the attachment of short chain of PHB conjugated with protein (i.e., hypermannosylated rhAGP-PhaP) [204].

Poly(3-hydroxybutyrate-*co*-3-hydroxyoctanoate) (P(3HB-*co*-3HO)) containing 10 mol% of 3HO units was used to prepare doxorubicin (DOX)-loaded particles with folic acid as targeting ligand [117]. The attachment of folic acid to polyester was obtained through a two-stage process employing the Steglich esterification: the folic acid was modified with PEG-bis-amine, which was further attached to P(3HB-*co*-3HO). Such copolymers were used to prepare the nanoparticles through solvent extraction/evaporation method to obtain particles with diameter 241 nm and PDI 0.24. The *in vitro* cytotoxicity of the nanoparticles modified with folic acid loaded with doxorubicin was 3 times higher than the cytotoxicity of the free drug (IC_{50} 0.87 to 2.8 μM, respectively). Also, the folic acid–modified particles had 32 times higher activity than folic acid–free particles. The superiority of the doxorubicin-loaded particles with attached folic acid comparable to free DOX was proved by *in vivo* test on BALB/c nude mice bearing HeLa tumor. As was shown, the tumor volumes after 14 days were significantly smaller than in any other group (control and free DOX).

The P(3HB-*co*-3HHx) containing 12 mol% of HHx was also used to prepare TDDS with folic acid as the targeting molecule [205]. However, in this case, the nanoparticles loaded with etoposide (topoisomerase II inhibitor; used in the therapy of lung, stomach, ovarian, testicular cancers, and lymphomas) were prepared through solvent extraction/evaporation method as the first step followed by the attachment of folic acid through the carbodiimide method. The conjugation of folic acid to nanoparticles doubled the *in vitro* effectiveness of etoposide action in comparison with free drug, expressed by apoptosis and necrosis of cells.

Poly(3HB-*co*-3HHx) containing the same amount (12 mol%) of 3HHx units was used to deliver curcumin in breast cancer therapy with concanavalin A (ConA) as a targeting ligand [206]. Similarly, the attachment of ConA was performed after the formation of nanoparticles by using EDC/NHS methodology. The nanoparticles had diameters ~260 nm and PDI ~0.3. Nanoparticles with curcumin and attached ligand caused decrease of MDA-MB 231 cells viability *in vitro* by 53% and 21% compared with the control and cells incubated with unmodified P(3HB-*co*-3HHx) nanoparticles with curcumin, respectively. An additional test showed that TDDS therapy using nanoparticles with attached ConA exhibited high cell internalization and high apoptotic activity compared with free curcumin and non-targeted nanoparticles with drug.

Poly(3-hydroxyalkanoate)s are synthesized in enzymatic polymerization by the PHA-synthases employing the 3-hydroxybutyryl-CoA (or other 3-hydroxyalkanoate-CoA) as the monomer [2, 3, 15]. This process could be made *in vitro* using PHA synthase and appropriate 3-hydroxyalkanoate-CoA [207]. However, the most important part of this process is that the PHA synthase is covalently bond to the surface of the synthesized particles, and the polymer inside the particles is amorphous. Moreover, as shown by Kim *et al.* [203], the recombination of gene and synthesis of recombinant PHA synthases with the attached peptide being targeting ligand or imaging moieties is possible. In the aforementioned work, the targeting ligand was RGD4C (Cys-Asp-Cys-Arg-Gly-Asp-Cys-Phe-Cys) to target the $\alpha_v\beta_3$ integrins, which are highly expressed in various cancers. The nanoparticles used in the study of targeted delivery have an average diameter of 233 nm; however, researchers report that it was possible to obtain particles in the range of 70–600 nm by tuning the substrate-to-enzyme ratio. The study using the Nile red dye shows that particles with ligand attached to the MDA-MB 231 breast cancer cells are contrary to the non-modified particles.

The advancement of this strategy was to attach two kinds of moieties (targeting and imaging) on the same particles to achieve diagnostic and therapeutic action. Kwon *et al.* [208] presented PHB nanoparticles, which were synthesized with PHA synthase fused with green fluorescent protein (GFP) and antigen-binding domain of the monoclonal antibody (mAb) A33 (A33scFv) specific to colon cancer loaded with Nile red. The nanoparticles were tested on A33-positive SW1222 colon cancer cells line and HT29, A33 negative. As was shown, the nanoparticles were visible in SW1222 cells contrary to HT29, which proved the effectiveness of targeting ligand A33scFv.

The development of the biosynthesis strategy is combining the synthesis of nanoparticles and later the creation of the outer layer. This is realized by the formation of PHB with conjugated PHA synthases fused with other proteins. The main reason of this attempt is to reduce the cost of particles, because the PHAs are commercially available and have relatively low price but the 3-hydroxybutyrate-CoA is still quite expensive. Biomodification of the surface of the PHB nanoparticles obtained through the emulsion – solvent evaporation method was presented by Lee *et al.* [209]. The RGD4C was used as a targeting molecule fused with PHB particles loaded with the Nile red prior to biofunctionalization to follow its activity. Very good internalization with MDA-MB 231 cancer cells was achieved.

A similar strategy was employed for nanoparticles prepared from P(3HB-*co*-3HHx) containing 12 mol% of HHx units loaded with rhodamine B isothiocyanate [204]. The targeted ligand was mannosylated human α1-acid glycoprotein (hAGP) or human epidermal growth factor (hEGF), which were receptors of macrophages and hepatocellular carcinoma cells. The receptor-mediated DDS was selectively taken up by macrophages (hAGP), BEL7402 hepatocellular carcinoma cells *in vitro*, and hepatocellular carcinoma cells *in vivo* (hEGF).

CONCLUSIONS AND OUTLOOK

Bacterial or microbial polyesters, polyhydroxyalkanoates, have evoked a huge research interest because of their biobased origin, biodegradability, and generally good biocompatibility in combination with large versatility in the form of structures and properties. Originally altering the monomer composition and the length of side chain enabled the production of PHA polymers with a wide range of mechanical properties ranging from rigid and brittle to elastomeric. Later, the introduction of synthetic analogs and novel functionalities (*e.g.*, introduction of unsaturation in main chain or side chains, bromination, chlorination, epoxidation, hydroxylation, carboxylation, and crosslinking) has further increased the diversity of this material group. This diversification makes it possible to tune in detail the thermal and mechanical properties, morphology, chemical and biological functionality, hydrophilicity, and degradation behaviors. An interesting material group under development is also the PHA-based water soluble polymers produced by functionalization or block-copolymerisation of PHAs with polar functional groups or hydrophilic segments, respectively. Other special advantages of PHA materials are the biodegradability under a broad range of conditions as well as the optical purity of the polymers because of the stereospecificity of PHA synthase. New cheap carbon sources and recombinant bacteria or mixed cultures as well as new extraction and purification technologies have been introduced to decrease the production cost, which is still high for commodity applications. However, the cost has less significance for materials aimed for advanced biomedical applications.

PHA-based systems have already been successfully tested in numerous biomedical applications. In general, good biocompatibility was confirmed from chemical point of view although there could be smaller variations depending on rigidity or crystallinity of the products. The successful applications include bioresorbable sutures and scaffolds for cartilage, bone, nerve, heart valve, dermal tissue regeneration, orthopedic pins, stents, wound dressing, drug releasing implants, and micro- and nanoparticles for controlled and/or targeted drug delivery. One interesting approach is the utilization of polymer–drug conjugates, where the drug is conjugated at the chain ends, in the side groups, or along the main chain, to increase the effect and bioavailability of the drug substances. PHAs degrade through surface erosion, which is generally considered an advantage for controlled drug delivery. The development of new PHA structures, especially mcl-PHAs and the new possibilities of additional functionalization have enabled future development of PHA-based micro- and nanoparticle drug delivery systems aiming at improved drug release profiles and/or inclusion of targeting and imaging functionalities. Examples of targeting functionalities include attachment of folic acid by chemical synthesis or biosynthesis of PHA particles with proteins attached on the surface of particles. As imaging agents, for example, fluorescent proteins and Nile red were reported. The already reported results from numerous *in vitro* and *in vivo* studies demonstrating the potential of this material group in large number of biomedical applications as well as the recent developments in diversification of functionalities and properties give clear promise of enormous future potential. It is especially important to solve the challenges of all biomass/biopolymer-based products before commercialization, such as continuous and large-enough production scale in combination with reasonable price, repeatable quality and purity of the samples.

CONFLICT OF INTEREST

The authors confirm that they have no conflict of interest to declare for this publication.

ACKNOWLEDGEMENTS

This work was partially supported by Polish National Science Centre grant no. 2011/03/B/ST5/01478 (P.K).

REFERENCES

[1] Rocha RC, da Silva LF, Taciro MK, Pradella JG. Production of poly(3-hydroxybutyrate-c--3-hydroxyvalerate) P(3HB-co-3HV) with a broad range of 3HV content at high yields by Burkholderia sacchari IPT 189. World J Microbiol Biotechnol 2008; 24: 427-31. [http://dx.doi.org/10.1007/s11274-007-9480-x]

[2] Sudesh K, Abe H, Doi Y. Synthesis, structure and properties of polyhydroxyalkanoates: Biological polyesters. Prog Polym Sci 2000; 25: 1503-55. [http://dx.doi.org/10.1016/S0079-6700(00)00035-6]

[3] Zinn M, Witholt B, Egli T. Occurrence, synthesis and medical application of bacterial polyhydroxyalkanoate. Adv Drug Deliv Rev 2001; 53(1): 5-21. [http://dx.doi.org/10.1016/S0169-409X(01)00218-6] [PMID: 11733115]

[4] Bresan S, Sznajder A, Hauf W, Forchhammer K, Pfeiffer D, Jendrossek D. Polyhydroxyalkanoate (PHA) Granules Have no Phospholipids. Sci Rep 2016; 6: 26612.
[http://dx.doi.org/10.1038/srep26612] [PMID: 27222167]

[5] Reusch RN, Sadoff HL. Putative structure and functions of a poly-beta-hydroxybutyrate/calcium polyphosphate channel in bacterial plasma membranes. Proc Natl Acad Sci USA 1988; 85(12): 4176-80.
[http://dx.doi.org/10.1073/pnas.85.12.4176] [PMID: 2454464]

[6] Reusch RN. Low molecular weight complexed poly(3-hydroxybutyrate): a dynamic and versatile molecule in vivo. Can J Microbiol 1995; 41 (Suppl. 1): 50-4.
[http://dx.doi.org/10.1139/m95-167] [PMID: 7606668]

[7] Seebach D, Fritz MG. Detection, synthesis, structure, and function of oligo(3-hydroxyalkanoates): contributions by synthetic organic chemists. Int J Biol Macromol 1999; 25(1-3): 217-36.
[http://dx.doi.org/10.1016/S0141-8130(99)00037-9] [PMID: 10416670]

[8] Das S, Kurcok P, Jedlinski Z, Reusch RN. Ion Channels Formed by Biomimetic Oligo-(R)-3-hydroxybutyrates and Inorganic Polyphosphates in Planar Lipid Bilayers. Macromolecules 1999; 32: 8781-5.
[http://dx.doi.org/10.1021/ma991105t]

[9] Elustondo PA, Angelova PR, Kawalec M, *et al.* Polyhydroxybutyrate targets mammalian mitochondria and increases permeability of plasmalemmal and mitochondrial membranes. PLoS One 2013; 8(9): e75812.
[http://dx.doi.org/10.1371/journal.pone.0075812] [PMID: 24086638]

[10] Dedkova EN, Blatter LA. Role of B-hydroxybutyrate, its polymer poly-B-hydroxybutyrate and inorganic polyphosphate in mammalian health and disease. Front Physiol 2014; 5: 1-22.
[http://dx.doi.org/10.3389/fphys.2014.00260] [PMID: 24478714]

[11] Misra SK, Valappil SP, Roy I, Boccaccini AR. Polyhydroxyalkanoate (PHA)/inorganic phase composites for tissue engineering applications. Biomacromolecules 2006; 7(8): 2249-58.
[http://dx.doi.org/10.1021/bm060317c] [PMID: 16903667]

[12] Lemoigne M. Études sur l'autolyse microbienne acidification sur formation d'acide b-oxobutyrique. Ann Inst Pasteur (Paris) 1925; 39: 144-73.

[13] Crosa JH, Brenner DJ, Ewing WH, Falkow S. Molecular relationships among the Salmonelleae. J Bacteriol 1973; 115(1): 307-15.
[PMID: 4717519]

[14] Kai D, Loh XJ. Polyhydroxyalkanoates: Chemical modifications toward biomedical applications. ACS Sustain Chem& Eng 2014; 2: 106-19.
[http://dx.doi.org/10.1021/sc400340p]

[15] Chen G-Q, Hazer B, Steinbüchel A, Philip S, Keshavarz T, Roy I, *et al.* A microbial polyhydroxyalkanoates (PHA) based bio- and materials industry. Chem Soc Rev 2009; 38(8): 2434-46.
[http://dx.doi.org/10.1039/b812677c] [PMID: 19623359]

[16] Jiang G, Hill DJ, Kowalczuk M, *et al.* Carbon sources for polyhydroxyalkanoates and an integrated biorefinery. Int J Mol Sci 2016; 17(7): 1157.
[http://dx.doi.org/10.3390/ijms17071157] [PMID: 27447619]

[17] Verlinden RA, Hill DJ, Kenward MA, Williams CD, Piotrowska-Seget Z, Radecka IK. Production of polyhydroxyalkanoates from waste frying oil by Cupriavidus necator. AMB Express 2011; 1(1): 11.
[http://dx.doi.org/10.1186/2191-0855-1-11] [PMID: 21906352]

[18] Muhr A, Rechberger EM, Salerno A, Reiterer A, Schiller M, Kwiecień M, *et al.* Biodegradable latexes from animal-derived waste: Biosynthesis and characterization of mcl-PHA accumulated by Ps. citronellolis. React Funct Polym 2013; 73: 1391-8. [http://dx.doi.org/10.1016/j.reactfunctpolym.2012.12.009]

[19] Spekreijse J, Le Nôtre J, Sanders JP, Scott EL. Conversion of polyhydroxybutyrate (PHB) to methyl crotonate for the production of biobased monomers. J Appl Polym Sci 2015; 132: 42462. [http://dx.doi.org/10.1002/app.42462]

[20] Lenz RW, Marchessault RH. Bacterial polyesters: biosynthesis, biodegradable plastics and biotechnology. Biomacromolecules 2005; 6(1): 1-8. [http://dx.doi.org/10.1021/bm049700c] [PMID: 15638495]

[21] Li SY, Dong CL, Wang SY, Ye HM, Chen G-Q. Microbial production of polyhydroxyalkanoate block copolymer by recombinant Pseudomonas putida. Appl Microbiol Biotechnol 2011; 90(2): 659-69. [http://dx.doi.org/10.1007/s00253-010-3069-2] [PMID: 21181145]

[22] Anderson AJ, Dawes EA. Occurrence, metabolism, metabolic role, and industrial uses of bacterial polyhydroxyalkanoates. Microbiol Rev 1990; 54(4): 450-72.

[23] Valappil SP, Misra SK, Boccaccini AR, Roy I. Biomedical applications of polyhydroxyalkanoates: an overview of animal testing and in vivo responses. Expert Rev Med Devices 2006; 3(6): 853-68. [http://dx.doi.org/10.1586/17434440.3.6.853] [PMID: 17280548]

[24] Rychter P, Biczak R, Herman B, *et al.* Environmental degradation of polyester blends containing atactic poly(3-hydroxybutyrate). Biodegradation in soil and ecotoxicological impact. Biomacromolecules 2006; 7(11): 3125-31. [http://dx.doi.org/10.1021/bm060708r] [PMID: 17096541]

[25] Nigmatullin R, Thomas P, Lukasiewicz B, Puthussery H, Roy I. Polyhydroxyalkanoates, a family of natural polymers, and their applications in drug delivery. J Chem Technol Biotechnol 2015; 90: 1209-21. [http://dx.doi.org/10.1002/jctb.4685]

[26] Chen G-Q, Wu Q. The application of polyhydroxyalkanoates as tissue engineering materials. Biomaterials 2005; 26(33): 6565-78. [http://dx.doi.org/10.1016/j.biomaterials.2005.04.036] [PMID: 15946738]

[27] van der Walle GA, de Koning GJ, Weusthuis RA, Eggink G. Properties. Modifications and Applications of Biopolyesters, Springer Berlin Heidelberg 2001; pp. 263-91.

[28] Ali I, Jamil N. Polyhydroxyalkanoates: Current applications in the medical field. Front Biol (Beijing) 2016; 11: 19-27. [http://dx.doi.org/10.1007/s11515-016-1389-z]

[29] Türesin F, Gürsel I, Hasirci V. Biodegradable polyhydroxyalkanoate implants for osteomyelitis therapy: in vitro antibiotic release. J Biomater Sci Polym Ed 2001; 12(2): 195-207. [http://dx.doi.org/10.1163/156856201750180924] [PMID: 11403236]

[30] Chen G, Wang Y. Medical applications of biopolyesters polyhydroxyalkanoates. Chin J Polym Sci 2013; 31: 719-36. [http://dx.doi.org/10.1007/s10118-013-1280-1]

[31] Kramer JW, Lobkovsky EB, Coates GW. Practical β-lactone synthesis: epoxide carbonylation at 1 atm. Org Lett 2006; 8(17): 3709-12. [http://dx.doi.org/10.1021/ol061292x] [PMID: 16898798]

[32] Schmidt JA, Lobkovsky EB, Coates GW. Chromium(III) octaethylporphyrinato tetracarbonylcobaltate: a highly active, selective, and versatile catalyst for epoxide carbonylation. J Am Chem Soc 2005; 127(32): 11426-35. [http://dx.doi.org/10.1021/ja051874u] [PMID: 16089471]

[33] Bałakier T, Chaładaj W, Jurczak J, Adamus G, Kowalczuk M. An effective protocol for the synthesis enantiomerically pure 4-substituted oxetane-2-ones. Tetrahedron 2013; 69: 4990-3. [http://dx.doi.org/10.1016/j.tet.2013.04.020]

[34] Carpentier JF. Discrete metal catalysts for stereoselective ring-opening polymerization of chiral Racemic β-Lactones. Macromol Rapid Commun 2010; 31(19): 1696-705. [http://dx.doi.org/10.1002/marc.201000114] [PMID: 21567583]

[35] Jedliński Z, Kowalczuk M, Kurcok P. Anionic ring opening polymerization by alkali metal solutions. Makromol Chemie Macromol Symp. 277-93. [http://dx.doi.org/10.1002/masy.19860030121]

[36] Kurcok P, Śmiga M, Jedliński Z. Beta-Butyrolactone polymerization initiated with tetrabutylammonium carboxylates: A novel approach to biomimetic polyester synthesis. J Polym Sci A Polym Chem 2002; 40: 2184-9. [http://dx.doi.org/10.1002/pola.10285]

[37] Brulé E, Gaillard S, Rager M-N, Roisnel T, Guérineau V, Nolan SP, *et al.* Polymerization of Racemic β-Butyrolactone Using Gold Catalysts: A Simple Access to Biodegradable Polymers. Organometallics 2011; 30: 2650-3. [http://dx.doi.org/10.1021/om200271q]

[38] Jedliński Z, Kowalczuk M, Kurcok P, Brzoskowska L, Franek J. Anionic block polymerization of β-lactones initiated by potassium solutions, 1. Synthesis of poly(4-methyl-2-oxetanone-block- 2-oxetanone). Makromol Chem 1987; 188: 1575-82. [http://dx.doi.org/10.1002/macp.1987.021880704]

[39] Kawalec M, Śmiga-Matuszowicz M, Kurcok P. Counterion and solvent effects on the anionic polymerization of β-butyrolactone initiated with acetic acid salts. Eur Polym J 2008; 44: 3556-63. [http://dx.doi.org/10.1016/j.eurpolymj.2008.09.008]

[40] Adamus G. Molecular Level Structure of (R,S)-3-Hydroxybutyrate /(R,S)-3-Hydroxy- 4-ethoxybutyrate Copolyesters with Dissimilar Architecture. Analysis 2009; 42: 4547-57. [http://dx.doi.org/10.1021/ma900349u]

[41] Hori Y, Takahashi Y, Yamaguchi A, Nishishita T. Ring-opening copolymerization of optically active. beta.-butyrolactone with several lactones catalyzed by distannoxane complexes: synthesis of new biodegradable polyesters. Macromolecules 1993; 26: 4388-90. [http://dx.doi.org/10.1021/ma00068a053]

[42] Jedlinski Z, Kurcok P, Lenz RW. First Facile Synthesis of Biomimetic Poly-(R)-3-hydroxybutyrate via Regioselective Anionic Polymerization of (S)-b-Butyrolactone. Macromolecules 1998; 31: 6718-20. [http://dx.doi.org/10.1021/ma980663p]

[43] Kurcok P, Matuszowicz A, Jedliński Z. Anionic polymerization of β-lactones initiated with potassium hydride. A convenient route to polyester macromonomers. Macromol Rapid Commun 1995; 16: 201-6. [http://dx.doi.org/10.1002/marc.1995.030160308]

[44] Jedliński Z, Kowalczuk M, Kurcok P, Adamus G, Matuszowicz A, Sikorska W, *et al.* Stereochemical Control in the Anionic Polymerization of β-Butyrolactone Initiated with Alkali-Metal Alkoxides. Macromolecules 1996; 29: 3773-7. [http://dx.doi.org/10.1021/ma951888s]

[45] Adamus G, Sikorska W, Janeczek H, Kwiecień M, Sobota M, Kowalczuk M. Novel block copolymers of atactic PHB with natural PHA for cardiovascular engineering: Synthesis and characterization. Eur Polym J 2012; 48: 621-31. [http://dx.doi.org/10.1016/j.eurpolymj.2011.12.017]

[46] Maksymiak M, Bałakier T, Jurczak J, Kowalczuk M, Adamus G. Bioactive (co)oligoesters with antioxidant properties-synthesis and structural characterization at the molecular level. RSC Advances 2016; 6: 57751-61.
[http://dx.doi.org/10.1039/C6RA09870C]

[47] Kwiecień I, Bałakier T, Jurczak J, Kowalczuk M, Adamus G. Molecular architecture of novel potentially bioactive (co)oligoesters containing pesticide moieties established by electrospray ionization multistage mass spectrometry. Rapid Commun Mass Spectrom 2015; 29(6): 533-44.
[http://dx.doi.org/10.1002/rcm.7133] [PMID: 26160419]

[48] Barouti G, Guillaume SM, Ulery BD, Nair LS, Laurencin CT, Tian H, *et al.* Polyhydroxybutyrate (PHB)-based triblock copolymers: synthesis of hydrophobic PHB/poly(benzyl β-malolactonate) and amphiphilic PHB/poly(malic acid) analogues by ring-opening polymerization. Polym Chem 2016; 7: 4603-8.
[http://dx.doi.org/10.1039/C6PY00910G]

[49] Kawalec M, Coulembier O, Gerbaux P, Sobota M, De Winter J, Dubois P, *et al.* Traces do matter - Purity of 4-methyl-2-oxetanone and its effect on anionic ring-opening polymerization as evidenced by phosphazene superbase catalysis. React Funct Polym 2012; 72: 509-20.
[http://dx.doi.org/10.1016/j.reactfunctpolym.2012.04.013]

[50] Jaffredo CG, Carpentier J-F, Guillaume SM. Controlled ROP of β-butyrolactone simply mediated by amidine, guanidine, and phosphazene organocatalysts. Macromol Rapid Commun 2012; 33(22): 1938-44.
[http://dx.doi.org/10.1002/marc.201200410] [PMID: 22887774]

[51] Jaffredo CG, Carpentier J-F, Guillaume SM. Organocatalyzed controlled ROP of β-lactones towards poly(hydroxyalkanoate)s: from β-butyrolactone to benzyl β-malolactone polymers. Polym Chem 2013; 4: 3837-50.
[http://dx.doi.org/10.1039/c3py00401e]

[52] Schweitzer D, Snell KD. Acrylates via Metathesis of Crotonates. Org Process Res Dev 2015; 19: 715-20.
[http://dx.doi.org/10.1021/op5003006]

[53] Yang X, Odelius K, Hakkarainen M. Microwave-Assisted Reaction in Green Solvents Recycles PHB to Functional Chemicals. ACS Sustain Chem& Eng 2014; 2: 2198-203.
[http://dx.doi.org/10.1021/sc500397h]

[54] Kawalec M, Adamus G, Kurcok P, *et al.* Carboxylate-induced degradation of poly(3-hydroxybutyrate)s. Biomacromolecules 2007; 8(4): 1053-8.
[http://dx.doi.org/10.1021/bm061155n] [PMID: 17330956]

[55] Nishida H, Ariffin H, Shirai Y, Hass M. Precise Depolymerization of Poly(3-hydoxybutyrate) by Pyrolysis. Biopolymers 2010; 61: 1382-6.
[http://dx.doi.org/10.5772/10270]

[56] Ariffin H, Nishida H, Shirai Y, Hassan MA. Determination of multiple thermal degradation mechanisms of poly(3-hydroxybutyrate). Polym Degrad Stabil 2008; 93: 1433-9.
[http://dx.doi.org/10.1016/j.polymdegradstab.2008.05.020]

[57] Kawalec M, Sobota M, Scandola M, Kowalczuk M, Kurcok P. A convenient route to PHB macromonomers via anionically controlled moderate-temperature degradation of PHB. J Polym Sci A Polym Chem 2010; 48: 5490-7.
[http://dx.doi.org/10.1002/pola.24357]

[58] Yang X, Clénet J, Xu H, Odelius K, Hakkarainen M. Two step extrusion process: From thermal recycling of PHB to plasticized PLA by reactive extrusion grafting of PHB degradation products onto PLA chains. Macromolecules 2015; 48: 2509-18.
[http://dx.doi.org/10.1021/acs.macromol.5b00235]

[59] Li Z, Loh XJ. Water soluble polyhydroxyalkanoates: future materials for therapeutic applications. Chem Soc Rev 2015; 44(10): 2865-79. [http://dx.doi.org/10.1039/C5CS00089K] [PMID: 25788317]

[60] Hazer B. Amphiphilic Poly(3-hydroxy alkanoate)s: Potential Candidates for Medical Applications Int J Polym Sci. 2010. Article ID 423460. [http://dx.doi.org/10.1155/2010/423460.]

[61] Ke Y, Zhang XY, Ramakrishna S, He LM, Wu G. Synthetic routes to degradable copolymers deriving from the biosynthesized polyhydroxyalkanoates: A mini review. Express Polym Lett 2016; 10: 36-53. [http://dx.doi.org/10.3144/expresspolymlett.2016.5]

[62] Tokiwa Y, Calabia BP. Degradation of microbial polyesters. Biotechnol Lett 2004; 26(15): 1181-9. [http://dx.doi.org/10.1023/B:BILE.0000036599.15302.e5] [PMID: 15289671]

[63] Federle TW, Barlaz MA, Pettigrew CA, *et al.* Anaerobic biodegradation of aliphatic polyesters: poly(3-hydroxybutyrate-co-3-hydroxyoctanoate) and poly(ε-caprolactone). Biomacromolecules 2002; 3(4): 813-22. [http://dx.doi.org/10.1021/bm025520w] [PMID: 12099827]

[64] Weng Y-X, Wang Y, Wang X-L, Wang Y-Z. Biodegradation behavior of PHBV films in a pilot-scale composting condition. Polym Test 2010; 29: 579-87. [http://dx.doi.org/10.1016/j.polymertesting.2010.04.002]

[65] Jendrossek D, Handrick R. Microbial degradation of polyhydroxyalkanoates. Annu Rev Microbiol 2002; 56: 403-32. [http://dx.doi.org/10.1146/annurev.micro.56.012302.160838] [PMID: 12213937]

[66] Jendrossek D. Extracellular polyhydroxyalkanoate (PHA) depolymerases: The key enzymes of PHA degradation In: Doi Y, Steinbüchel A, editors Biopolym Online, Weinheim, Germany: Wiley-VCH Verlag GmbH and Co KGaA. 2005; pp. 41-51. [http://dx.doi.org/10.1002/3527600035.bpol3b03.]

[67] Merrick JM, Steger R, Dombroski D. Hydrolysis of native poly(hydroxybutyrate) granules (PHB), crystalline PHB, and artificial amorphous PHB granules by intracellular and extracellular depolymerases. Int J Biol Macromol 1999; 25(1-3): 129-34. [http://dx.doi.org/10.1016/S0141-8130(99)00026-4] [PMID: 10416659]

[68] Jendrossek D, Schirmer A, Schlegel HG. Biodegradation of polyhydroxyalkanoic acids. Appl Microbiol Biotechnol 1996; 46(5-6): 451-63. [http://dx.doi.org/10.1007/s002530050844] [PMID: 9008883]

[69] Philip S, Keshavarz T, Roy I. Polyhydroxyalkanoates: biodegradable polymers with a range of applications. J Chem Technol Biotechnol 2007; 82: 233-47. [http://dx.doi.org/10.1002/jctb.1667]

[70] Doi Y. Microbial Polyesters. New York: VCHPublishers 1990.

[71] Handrick R, Reinhardt S, Focarete ML, *et al.* A new type of thermoalkalophilic hydrolase of Paucimonas lemoignei with high specificity for amorphous polyesters of short chain-length hydroxyalkanoic acids. J Biol Chem 2001; 276(39): 36215-24. [http://dx.doi.org/10.1074/jbc.M101106200] [PMID: 11457823]

[72] Jendrossek D. Microbial Degradation of Polyesters. Springer Berlin Heidelberg 2001; pp. 293-325.

[73] Papageorgiou AC, Hermawan S, Singh CB, Jendrossek D. Structural basis of poly(3-hydroxybutyrate) hydrolysis by PhaZ7 depolymerase from Paucimonas lemoignei. J Mol Biol 2008; 382(5): 1184-94. [http://dx.doi.org/10.1016/j.jmb.2008.07.078] [PMID: 18706425]

[74] Qu X-H, Wu Q, Zhang K-Y, Chen GQ. In vivo studies of poly(3-hydroxybutyrate-c--3-hydroxyhexanoate) based polymers: biodegradation and tissue reactions. Biomaterials 2006; 27(19): 3540-8.
[http://dx.doi.org/10.1016/j.biomaterials.2006.02.015] [PMID: 16542719]

[75] Gogolewski S, Jovanovic M, Perren SM, Dillon JG, Hughes MK. Tissue response and in vivo degradation of selected polyhydroxyacids: polylactides (PLA), poly(3-hydroxybutyrate) (PHB), and poly(3-hydroxybutyrate-co-3-hydroxyvalerate) (PHB/VA). J Biomed Mater Res 1993; 27(9): 1135-48.
[http://dx.doi.org/10.1002/jbm.820270904] [PMID: 8126012]

[76] Duvernoy O, Malm T, Ramström J, Bowald S. A biodegradable patch used as a pericardial substitute after cardiac surgery: 6- and 24-month evaluation with CT. Thorac Cardiovasc Surg 1995; 43(5): 271-4.
[http://dx.doi.org/10.1055/s-2007-1013226] [PMID: 8610286]

[77] Jones N, Cooper J, Waters R, Williams D. Resorption profile and biological response of calcium phosphate filled PLLA and PHB7V. ASTM Spec Tech Publ 2000; 1396: 69-82.
[http://dx.doi.org/10.1520/STP15301S.]

[78] Doyle C, Tanner ET, Bonfield W. In vitro and in vivo evaluation of polyhydroxybutyrate and of polyhydroxybutyrate reinforced with hydroxyapatite. Biomaterials 1991; 12(9): 841-7.
[http://dx.doi.org/10.1016/0142-9612(91)90072-I] [PMID: 1764555]

[79] Shishatskaya EI, Khlusov IA, Volova TG. A hybrid PHB-hydroxyapatite composite for biomedical application: production, in vitro and in vivo investigation. J Biomater Sci Polym Ed 2006; 17(5): 481-98.
[http://dx.doi.org/10.1163/156856206776986242] [PMID: 16800151]

[80] Shishatskaya EI, Volova TG, Gordeev SA, Puzyr AP. Degradation of P(3HB) and P(3HB-co-3HV) in biological media. J Biomater Sci Polym Ed 2005; 16(5): 643-57.
[http://dx.doi.org/10.1163/1568562053783678] [PMID: 16001722]

[81] Atkins TW, Peacock J. The incorporation and release of bovine serum albumin from poly-hydroxybutyrate-hydroxyvalerate microcapsules. J Microencapsul 1996; 13(6): 709-17.
[http://dx.doi.org/10.3109/02652049609026054] [PMID: 8933356]

[82] Ying TH, Ishii D, Mahara A, *et al.* Scaffolds from electrospun polyhydroxyalkanoate copolymers: fabrication, characterization, bioabsorption and tissue response. Biomaterials 2008; 29(10): 1307-17.
[http://dx.doi.org/10.1016/j.biomaterials.2007.11.031] [PMID: 18155139]

[83] Malm T, Bowald S, Bylock A, Busch C. Prevention of postoperative pericardial adhesions by closure of the pericardium with absorbable polymer patches. An experimental study. J Thorac Cardiovasc Surg 1992; 104(3): 600-7.
[PMID: 1513149]

[84] Kostopoulos L, Karring T. Guided bone regeneration in mandibular defects in rats using a bioresorbable polymer. Clin Oral Implants Res 1994; 5(2): 66-74.
[http://dx.doi.org/10.1034/j.1600-0501.1994.050202.x] [PMID: 7918911]

[85] Shishatskaya EI, Volova TG, Gitelson II. In vivo toxicological evaluation of polyhydroxyalkanoates. Dokl Biol Sci 2002; 383: 109-11.
[http://dx.doi.org/10.1023/A:1015325504494] [PMID: 12053558]

[86] Shishatskaya EI, Volova TG, Puzyr AP, Mogilnaya OA, Efremov SN, Gitelson II. Tissue morphogenesis under the conditions of implantation of polyhydroxybutyrate, a biodegradable polymer. Dokl Biol Sci 2002; 383: 123-6.
[http://dx.doi.org/10.1023/A:1015333706311] [PMID: 12053561]

[87] Shishatskaya EI, Eremeev AV, Gitelzon II, Setkov NA, Volova TG. Cytotoxicity of polyhydroxyalkanoates in animal cell cultures. Dokl Biol Sci 2000; 374: 539-42.
[PMID: 11103339]

[88] Köse GT, Kenar H, Hasirci N, Hasirci V. Macroporous poly(3-hydroxybutyrate-co-3-hydroxyvalerate) matrices for bone tissue engineering. Biomaterials 2003; 24(11): 1949-58. [http://dx.doi.org/10.1016/S0142-9612(02)00613-0] [PMID: 12615485]

[89] Zhijiang C, Qin Z, Xianyou S, Yuanpei L. Zein/Poly(3-hydroxybutyrate-co-4-hydroxybutyrate) electrospun blend fiber scaffolds: Preparation, characterization and cytocompatibility. Mater Sci Eng C 2016; 58: 757-67. [http://dx.doi.org/10.1016/j.msec.2015.09.048] [PMID: 27987775]

[90] van der Giessen WJ, Lincoff AM, Schwartz RS, *et al.* Marked inflammatory sequelae to implantation of biodegradable and nonbiodegradable polymers in porcine coronary arteries. Circulation 1996; 94(7): 1690-7. [http://dx.doi.org/10.1161/01.CIR.94.7.1690] [PMID: 8840862]

[91] Unverdorben M, Spielberger A, Schywalsky M, *et al.* A polyhydroxybutyrate biodegradable stent: preliminary experience in the rabbit. Cardiovasc Intervent Radiol 2002; 25(2): 127-32. [http://dx.doi.org/10.1007/s00270-001-0118-3] [PMID: 11901431]

[92] Shishatskaya EI, Volova TG, Puzyr AP, Mogilnaya OA, Efremov SN. Tissue response to the implantation of biodegradable polyhydroxyalkanoate sutures. J Mater Sci Mater Med 2004; 15(6): 719-28. [http://dx.doi.org/10.1023/B:JMSM.0000030215.49991.0d] [PMID: 15346741]

[93] Sevastianov VI, Perova NV, Shishatskaya EI, Kalacheva GS, Volova TG. Production of purified polyhydroxyalkanoates (PHAs) for applications in contact with blood. J Biomater Sci Polym Ed 2003; 14(10): 1029-42. [http://dx.doi.org/10.1163/156856203769231547] [PMID: 14661877]

[94] Sultana N, Wang M. Fabrication of HA/PHBV composite scaffolds through the emulsion freezing/freeze-drying process and characterisation of the scaffolds. J Mater Sci Mater Med 2008; 19(7): 2555-61. [http://dx.doi.org/10.1007/s10856-007-3214-3] [PMID: 17665100]

[95] Nair LS, Laurencin CT. Biodegradable polymers as biomaterials. Prog Polym Sci 2007; 32: 762-98. [http://dx.doi.org/10.1016/j.progpolymsci.2007.05.017]

[96] Saad B, Ciardelli G, Matter S, *et al.* Degradable and highly porous polyester urethane foam as biomaterial: effects and phagocytosis of degradation products in osteoblasts. J Biomed Mater Res 1998; 39(4): 594-602. [http://dx.doi.org/10.1002/(SICI)1097-4636(19980315)39:4<594::AID-JBM14>3.0.CO;2-7] [PMID: 9492221]

[97] Saad B, Neuenschwander P, Uhlschmid GK, Suter UW. New versatile, elastomeric, degradable polymeric materials for medicine. Int J Biol Macromol 1999; 25(1-3): 293-301. [http://dx.doi.org/10.1016/S0141-8130(99)00044-6] [PMID: 10416677]

[98] Saad B, Ciardelli G, Matter S, Welti M, Uhlschmid GK, Neuenschwander P, *et al.* Cell response of cultured macrophages, fibroblasts, and co-cultures of Kupffer cells and hepatocytes to particles of short-chain poly[(R)-3-hydroxybutyric acid]. J Mater Sci Mater Med 1996; 7: 56-61. [http://dx.doi.org/10.1007/BF00121191]

[99] Piddubnyak V, Kurcok P, Matuszowicz A, *et al.* Oligo-3-hydroxybutyrates as potential carriers for drug delivery. Biomaterials 2004; 25(22): 5271-9. [http://dx.doi.org/10.1016/j.biomaterials.2003.12.029] [PMID: 15110478]

[100] Zawidlak-Wegrzyńska B, Kawalec M, Bosek I, *et al.* Synthesis and antiproliferative properties of ibuprofen-oligo(3-hydroxybutyrate) conjugates. Eur J Med Chem 2010; 45(5): 1833-42. [http://dx.doi.org/10.1016/j.ejmech.2010.01.020] [PMID: 20171760]

[101] Ribeiro-Samy S, Silva NA, Correlo VM, *et al.* Development and characterization of a PHB-HV-based 3D scaffold for a tissue engineering and cell-therapy combinatorial approach for spinal cord injury regeneration. Macromol Biosci 2013; 13(11): 1576-92. [http://dx.doi.org/10.1002/mabi.201300178] [PMID: 24038969]

[102] Tasaki O, Hiraide A, Shiozaki T, Yamamura H, Ninomiya N, Sugimoto H. The dimer and trimer of 3-hydroxybutyrate oligomer as a precursor of ketone bodies for nutritional care. JPEN J Parenter Enteral Nutr 1999; 23(6): 321-5. [http://dx.doi.org/10.1177/0148607199023006321] [PMID: 10574479]

[103] Sun J, Dai Z, Zhao Y, Chen G-Q. In vitro effect of oligo-hydroxyalkanoates on the growth of mouse fibroblast cell line L929. Biomaterials 2007; 28(27): 3896-903. [http://dx.doi.org/10.1016/j.biomaterials.2007.05.011] [PMID: 17574664]

[104] Veech RL, Chance B, Kashiwaya Y, Lardy HA, Cahill GF Jr. Ketone bodies, potential therapeutic uses. IUBMB Life 2001; 51(4): 241-7. [International Union Biochem Mol Biol Life]. [http://dx.doi.org/10.1080/152165401753311780] [PMID: 11569918]

[105] Cahill GF, Veech RL. Ketoacids? Good medicine? Trans Am Clin Climatol Assoc 2003; 114: 149-61. discussion 162-3. [PMID: 12813917]

[106] Kashiwaya Y, Takeshima T, Mori N, Nakashima K, Clarke K, Veech RL. D-beta-hydroxybutyrate protects neurons in models of Alzheimers and Parkinsons disease. Proc Natl Acad Sci USA 2000; 97(10): 5440-4. [http://dx.doi.org/10.1073/pnas.97.10.5440] [PMID: 10805800]

[107] Murray AJ, Knight NS, Cole MA, *et al.* Novel ketone diet enhances physical and cognitive performance. FASEB J 2016; 30(12): 4021-32. [http://dx.doi.org/10.1096/fj.201600773R] [PMID: 27528626]

[108] Volova T, Zhila N, Kiselev E, Shishatskaya E. A study of synthesis and properties of poly-- -hydroxybutyrate/diethylene glycol copolymers. Biotechnol Prog 2016; 32(4): 1017-28. [http://dx.doi.org/10.1002/btpr.2267] [PMID: 27037961]

[109] Chan RT, Russell RA, Marçal H, Lee TH, Holden PJ, Foster LJ. BioPEGylation of polyhydroxybutyrate promotes nerve cell health and migration. Biomacromolecules 2014; 15(1): 339-49. [http://dx.doi.org/10.1021/bm401572a] [PMID: 24299034]

[110] Bonartsev A, Yakovlev S, Boskhomdzhiev A, *et al.* The terpolymer produced by Azotobacter chroococcum 7B: effect of surface properties on cell attachment. PLoS One 2013; 8(2): e57200. [http://dx.doi.org/10.1371/journal.pone.0057200] [PMID: 23468935]

[111] Lu X-Y, Li M-C, Zhu X-L, Fan F, Wang L-L, Ma J-G. Microbial synthesized biodegradable PHBHHxPEG hybrid copolymer as an efficient intracellular delivery nanocarrier for kinase inhibitor. BMC Biotechnol 2014; 14: 4. [http://dx.doi.org/10.1186/1472-6750-14-4] [PMID: 24438107]

[112] Eke G, Kuzmina AM, Goreva AV, Shishatskaya EI, Hasirci N, Hasirci V. In vitro and transdermal penetration of PHBV micro/nanoparticles. J Mater Sci Mater Med 2014; 25(6): 1471-81. [http://dx.doi.org/10.1007/s10856-014-5169-5] [PMID: 24510225]

[113] Xiong Y-C, Yao Y-C, Zhan X-Y, Chen G-Q. Application of polyhydroxyalkanoates nanoparticles as intracellular sustained drug-release vectors. J Biomater Sci Polym Ed 2010; 21(1): 127-40. [http://dx.doi.org/10.1163/156856209X410283] [PMID: 20040158]

[114] Murueva AV, Shishatskaya EI, Kuzmina AM, Volova TG, Sinskey AJ. Microparticles prepared from biodegradable polyhydroxyalkanoates as matrix for encapsulation of cytostatic drug. J Mater Sci Mater Med 2013; 24(8): 1905-15. [http://dx.doi.org/10.1007/s10856-013-4941-2] [PMID: 23674057]

[115] Lu XY, Ciraolo E, Stefenia R, Chen GQ, Zhang Y, Hirsch E. Sustained release of PI3K inhibitor from PHA nanoparticles and in vitro growth inhibition of cancer cell lines. Appl Microbiol Biotechnol 2011; 89(5): 1423-33.
[http://dx.doi.org/10.1007/s00253-011-3101-1] [PMID: 21286711]

[116] Shah M, Naseer MI, Choi MH, Kim MO, Yoon SC. Amphiphilic PHA-mPEG copolymeric nanocontainers for drug delivery: preparation, characterization and in vitro evaluation. Int J Pharm 2010; 400(1-2): 165-75.
[http://dx.doi.org/10.1016/j.ijpharm.2010.08.008] [PMID: 20713137]

[117] Zhang C, Zhao L, Dong Y, Zhang X, Lin J, Chen Z. Folate-mediated poly(3-hydroxybutyrate-c--3-hydroxyoctanoate) nanoparticles for targeting drug delivery. Eur J Pharm Biopharm 2010; 76(1): 10-6.
[http://dx.doi.org/10.1016/j.ejpb.2010.05.005] [PMID: 20472060]

[118] Maksymiak M, Debowska R, Bazela K, *et al.* Designing of Biodegradable and Biocompatible Release and Delivery Systems of Selected Antioxidants Used in Cosmetology. Biomacromolecules 2015; 16(11): 3603-12.
[http://dx.doi.org/10.1021/acs.biomac.5b01065] [PMID: 26444385]

[119] Juzwa M, Rusin A, Zawidlak-Wegrzyńska B, Krawczyk Z, Obara I, Jedliński Z. Oligo(3-hydroxybutanoate) conjugates with acetylsalicylic acid and their antitumour activity. Eur J Med Chem 2008; 43(8): 1785-90.
[http://dx.doi.org/10.1016/j.ejmech.2007.11.004] [PMID: 18162262]

[120] Zawidlak-Wegrzyńska B, Kawalec M, Bosek I, *et al.* Synthesis and antiproliferative properties of ibuprofen-oligo(3-hydroxybutyrate) conjugates. Eur J Med Chem 2010; 45(5): 1833-42.
[http://dx.doi.org/10.1016/j.ejmech.2010.01.020] [PMID: 20171760]

[121] Shishatskaya EI, Volova TG. A comparative investigation of biodegradable polyhydroxyalkanoate films as matrices for in vitro cell cultures. J Mater Sci Mater Med 2004; 15(8): 915-23.
[http://dx.doi.org/10.1023/B:JMSM.0000036280.98763.c1] [PMID: 15477744]

[122] Ellis G, Cano P, Jadraque M, *et al.* Laser microperforated biodegradable microbial polyhydroxyalkanoate substrates for tissue repair strategies: an infrared microspectroscopy study. Anal Bioanal Chem 2011; 399(7): 2379-88.
[http://dx.doi.org/10.1007/s00216-011-4653-8] [PMID: 21240671]

[123] Zheng Z, Bei F-F, Tian H-L, Chen G-Q. Effects of crystallization of polyhydroxyalkanoate blend on surface physicochemical properties and interactions with rabbit articular cartilage chondrocytes. Biomaterials 2005; 26(17): 3537-48.
[http://dx.doi.org/10.1016/j.biomaterials.2004.09.041] [PMID: 15621244]

[124] Wang Y, Bian Y-Z, Wu Q, Chen G-Q. Evaluation of three-dimensional scaffolds prepared from poly(3-hydroxybutyrate-co-3-hydroxyhexanoate) for growth of allogeneic chondrocytes for cartilage repair in rabbits. Biomaterials 2008; 29(19): 2858-68.
[http://dx.doi.org/10.1016/j.biomaterials.2008.03.021] [PMID: 18406457]

[125] Köse GT, Korkusuz F, Özkul A, *et al.* Tissue engineered cartilage on collagen and PHBV matrices. Biomaterials 2005; 26(25): 5187-97.
[http://dx.doi.org/10.1016/j.biomaterials.2005.01.037] [PMID: 15792546]

[126] Wang Y-W, Wu Q, Chen G-Q. Attachment, proliferation and differentiation of osteoblasts on random biopolyester poly(3-hydroxybutyrate-co-3-hydroxyhexanoate) scaffolds. Biomaterials 2004; 25(4): 669-75.
[http://dx.doi.org/10.1016/S0142-9612(03)00561-1] [PMID: 14607505]

[127] Wang Y-W, Yang F, Wu Q, *et al.* Effect of composition of poly(3-hydroxybutyrate-c--3-hydroxyhexanoate) on growth of fibroblast and osteoblast. Biomaterials 2005; 26(7): 755-61.
[http://dx.doi.org/10.1016/j.biomaterials.2004.03.023] [PMID: 15350780]

[128] Köse GT, Ber S, Korkusuz F, Hasirci V. Poly(3-hydroxybutyric acid-co-3-hydroxyvaleric acid) based tissue engineering matrices. J Mater Sci Mater Med 2003; 14(2): 121-6. [http://dx.doi.org/10.1023/A:1022063628099] [PMID: 15348483]

[129] Knowles JC, Hastings GW, Ohta H, Niwa S, Boeree N. Development of a degradable composite for orthopaedic use: in vivo biomechanical and histological evaluation of two bioactive degradable composites based on the polyhydroxybutyrate polymer. Biomaterials 1992; 13(8): 491-6. [http://dx.doi.org/10.1016/0142-9612(92)90099-A] [PMID: 1321677]

[130] Ni J, Wang M. In vitro evaluation of hydroxyapatite reinforced polyhydroxybutyrate composite. Mater Sci Eng C 2002; 20: 101-9. [http://dx.doi.org/10.1016/S0928-4931(02)00019-X]

[131] Galego N, Rozsa C, Sánchez R, Fung J. Analía Vázquez, Santo Tomás J. Characterization and application of poly(β-hydroxyalkanoates) family as composite biomaterials. Polym Test 2000; 19: 485-92. [http://dx.doi.org/10.1016/S0142-9418(99)00011-2]

[132] Cool SM, Kenny B, Wu A, *et al.* Poly(3-hydroxybutyrate-co-3-hydroxyvalerate) composite biomaterials for bone tissue regeneration: in vitro performance assessed by osteoblast proliferation, osteoclast adhesion and resorption, and macrophage proinflammatory response. J Biomed Mater Res A 2007; 82(3): 599-610. [http://dx.doi.org/10.1002/jbm.a.31174] [PMID: 17315229]

[133] Luklinska ZB, Schluckwerder H. In vivo response to HA-polyhydroxybutyrate/polyhydroxyvalerate composite. J Microsc 2003; 211(Pt 2): 121-9. [http://dx.doi.org/10.1046/j.1365-2818.2003.01204.x] [PMID: 12887706]

[134] Misra SK, Ansari TI, Valappil SP, *et al.* Poly(3-hydroxybutyrate) multifunctional composite scaffolds for tissue engineering applications. Biomaterials 2010; 31(10): 2806-15. [http://dx.doi.org/10.1016/j.biomaterials.2009.12.045] [PMID: 20045554]

[135] Wang A, Gan Y, Yu H, *et al.* Improvement of the cytocompatibility of electrospun poly[(R)---hydroxybutyrate-co-(R)-3-hydroxyvalerate] mats by Ecoflex. J Biomed Mater Res A 2012; 100(6): 1505-11. [http://dx.doi.org/10.1002/jbm.a.34034] [PMID: 22408070]

[136] Leenstra TS, Kuijpers-Jagtman AM, Maltha JC. The healing process of palatal tissues after palatal surgery with and without implantation of membranes: an experimental study in dogs. J Mater Sci Mater Med 1998; 9(5): 249-55. [http://dx.doi.org/10.1023/A:1008848509911] [PMID: 15348880]

[137] Martin DP, Williams SF. Medical applications of poly-4-hydroxybutyrate: a strong flexible absorbable biomaterial. Biochem Eng J 2003; 16: 97-105. [http://dx.doi.org/10.1016/S1369-703X(03)00040-8]

[138] Xu X-Y, Li X-T, Peng S-W, *et al.* The behaviour of neural stem cells on polyhydroxyalkanoate nanofiber scaffolds. Biomaterials 2010; 31(14): 3967-75. [http://dx.doi.org/10.1016/j.biomaterials.2010.01.132] [PMID: 20153524]

[139] Oh SH, Kim JH, Song KS, *et al.* Peripheral nerve regeneration within an asymmetrically porous PLGA/Pluronic F127 nerve guide conduit. Biomaterials 2008; 29(11): 1601-9. [http://dx.doi.org/10.1016/j.biomaterials.2007.11.036] [PMID: 18155135]

[140] Novikov LN, Novikova LN, Mosahebi A, Wiberg M, Terenghi G, Kellerth J-O. A novel biodegradable implant for neuronal rescue and regeneration after spinal cord injury. Biomaterials 2002; 23(16): 3369-76. [http://dx.doi.org/10.1016/S0142-9612(02)00037-6] [PMID: 12099279]

[141] Young RC, Wiberg M, Terenghi G. Poly-3-hydroxybutyrate (PHB): a resorbable conduit for long-gap repair in peripheral nerves. Br J Plast Surg 2002; 55(3): 235-40. [http://dx.doi.org/10.1054/bjps.2002.3798] [PMID: 12041978]

[142] Simon MA, Chalifoux LV, Ringler DJ. Pathologic features of SIV-induced disease and the association of macrophage infection with disease evolution. AIDS Res Hum Retroviruses 1992; 8(3): 327-37. [http://dx.doi.org/10.1089/aid.1992.8.327] [PMID: 1571193]

[143] Novikova LN, Pettersson J, Brohlin M, Wiberg M, Novikov LN. Biodegradable poly--hydroxybutyrate scaffold seeded with Schwann cells to promote spinal cord repair. Biomaterials 2008; 29(9): 1198-206. [http://dx.doi.org/10.1016/j.biomaterials.2007.11.033] [PMID: 18083223]

[144] Chan RTH, Marçal H, Russell RA, Holden PJ, Foster LJR. Application of polyethylene glycol to promote cellular biocompatibility of polyhydroxybutyrate films. Int J Polym Sci 2011; 2011 Article ID 473045. [http://dx.doi.org/10.1155/2011/473045]

[145] Winnacker M, Rieger B. Copolymers of polyhydroxyalkanoates and polyethylene glycols: recent advancements with biological and medical significance. Polym Int 2017; 66: 497-503. [http://dx.doi.org/10.1002/pi.5261]

[146] Senthilnathan V, Treasure T, Grunkemeier G, Starr A. Heart valves: which is the best choice? Cardiovasc Surg 1999; 7(4): 393-7. [http://dx.doi.org/10.1016/S0967-2109(99)00026-5] [PMID: 10430519]

[147] Shum-Tim D, Stock U, Hrkach J, *et al.* Tissue engineering of autologous aorta using a new biodegradable polymer. Ann Thorac Surg 1999; 68(6): 2298-304. [http://dx.doi.org/10.1016/S0003-4975(99)01055-3] [PMID: 10617020]

[148] Sodian R, Sperling JS, Martin DP, Stock U, Mayer JE Jr, Vacanti JP. Tissue engineering of a trileaflet heart valve-early in vitro experiences with a combined polymer. Tissue Eng 1999; 5(5): 489-94. [http://dx.doi.org/10.1089/ten.1999.5.489] [PMID: 10586103]

[149] Sodian R, Sperling JS, Martin DP, *et al.* Fabrication of a trileaflet heart valve scaffold from a polyhydroxyalkanoate biopolyester for use in tissue engineering. Tissue Eng 2000; 6(2): 183-8. [http://dx.doi.org/10.1089/107632700320793] [PMID: 10941212]

[150] Stock UA, Degenkolbe I, Attmann T, Schenke-Layland K, Freitag S, Lutter G. Prevention of device-related tissue damage during percutaneous deployment of tissue-engineered heart valves. J Thorac Cardiovasc Surg 2006; 131(6): 1323-30. [http://dx.doi.org/10.1016/j.jtcvs.2006.01.053] [PMID: 16733165]

[151] Hoerstrup SP, Sodian R, Daebritz S, *et al.* Functional living trileaflet heart valves grown in vitro. Circulation 2000; 102(19) (Suppl. 3): III44-9. [http://dx.doi.org/10.1161/01.CIR.102.suppl_3.III-44] [PMID: 11082361]

[152] Cassell OC, Hofer SO, Morrison WA, Knight KR. Vascularisation of tissue-engineered grafts: the regulation of angiogenesis in reconstructive surgery and in disease states. Br J Plast Surg 2002; 55(8): 603-10. [http://dx.doi.org/10.1054/bjps.2002.3950] [PMID: 12550111]

[153] Stock UA, Sakamoto T, Hatsuoka S, *et al.* Patch augmentation of the pulmonary artery with bioabsorbable polymers and autologous cell seeding. J Thorac Cardiovasc Surg 2000; 120(6): 1158-67. [http://dx.doi.org/10.1067/mtc.2000.109539] [PMID: 11088041]

[154] Mendelson K, Aikawa E, Mettler BA, *et al.* Healing and remodeling of bioengineered pulmonary artery patches implanted in sheep. Cardiovasc Pathol 2007; 16(5): 277-82. [http://dx.doi.org/10.1016/j.carpath.2007.03.008] [PMID: 17868878]

[155] Wu S, Liu Y, Cui B, Tang Y, Wang Q, Qu X, *et al.* Intravascular biocompatibility of poly (3-hydroxybutyrate-co-3-hydroxyhexanoate, PHBHHx) for cardiovascular tissue engineering. Chin J Biotechnol 2008; 24: 610-6.
[http://dx.doi.org/10.1016/S1872-2075(08)60030-8]

[156] Volova T, Shishatskaya E, Sevastianov V, Efremov S, Mogilnaya O. Results of biomedical investigations of PHB and PHB/PHV fibers. Biochem Eng J 2003; 16: 125-33.
[http://dx.doi.org/10.1016/S1369-703X(03)00038-X]

[157] Veleirinho B, Coelho DS, Dias PF, Maraschin M, Ribeiro-do-Valle RM, Lopes-da-Silva JA. Nanofibrous poly(3-hydroxybutyrate-co-3-hydroxyvalerate)/chitosan scaffolds for skin regeneration. Int J Biol Macromol 2012; 51(4): 343-50.
[http://dx.doi.org/10.1016/j.ijbiomac.2012.05.023] [PMID: 22652216]

[158] Kuppan P, Vasanthan KS, Sundaramurthi D, Krishnan UM, Sethuraman S. Development of poly(3-hydroxybutyrate-co-3-hydroxyvalerate) fibers for skin tissue engineering: effects of topography, mechanical, and chemical stimuli. Biomacromolecules 2011; 12(9): 3156-65.
[http://dx.doi.org/10.1021/bm200618w] [PMID: 21800891]

[159] Freier T, Kunze C, Nischan C, *et al.* In vitro and in vivo degradation studies for development of a biodegradable patch based on poly(3-hydroxybutyrate). Biomaterials 2002; 23(13): 2649-57.
[http://dx.doi.org/10.1016/S0142-9612(01)00405-7] [PMID: 12059014]

[160] Wang A, Gan Y, Qu J, Cheng B, Wang F, Yu H. Application of electrospun poly[(R)-3-hydroxybutyrate-co-(R)-3-hydroxyvalerate]-ecoflex mats in periodontal regeneration:a primary study. 2012 Int Conf Biomed Eng Biotechnol. 972-5.
[http://dx.doi.org/10.1109/iCBEB.2012.78]

[161] Jirage AS, Baravkar VS, Kate VK, Payghan SA, Disouza JI. Poly-β-hydroxybutyrate : intriguing biopolymer in biomedical applications and pharma formulation trends. Int J Pharm Biol Arch 2013; 4: 1107-18.

[162] Goodman SB, Yao Z, Keeney M, Yang F. The future of biologic coatings for orthopaedic implants. Biomaterials 2013; 34(13): 3174-83.
[http://dx.doi.org/10.1016/j.biomaterials.2013.01.074] [PMID: 23391496]

[163] Gursel I, Yagmurlu F, Korkusuz F, Hasirci V. In vitro antibiotic release from poly(3-hydroxybutyrat--co-3-hydroxyvalerate) rods. J Microencapsul 2002; 19(2): 153-64.
[http://dx.doi.org/10.1080/02652040110065413] [PMID: 11837970]

[164] Li W, Ding Y, Rai R, Roether JA, Schubert DW, Boccaccini AR. Preparation and characterization of PHBV microsphere/45S5 bioactive glass composite scaffolds with vancomycin releasing function. Mater Sci Eng C Mater Biol Appl 2014; 41: 320-8.
[http://dx.doi.org/10.1016/j.msec.2014.04.052] [PMID: 24907766]

[165] Gorustovich AA, Roether JA, Boccaccini AR. Effect of bioactive glasses on angiogenesis: a review of in vitro and in vivo evidences. Tissue Eng Part B Rev 2010; 16(2): 199-207.
[http://dx.doi.org/10.1089/ten.teb.2009.0416] [PMID: 19831556]

[166] Rahaman MN, Day DE, Bal BS, *et al.* Bioactive glass in tissue engineering. Acta Biomater 2011; 7(6): 2355-73.
[http://dx.doi.org/10.1016/j.actbio.2011.03.016] [PMID: 21421084]

[167] Xie Z, Liu X, Jia W, Zhang C, Huang W, Wang J. Treatment of osteomyelitis and repair of bone defect by degradable bioactive borate glass releasing vancomycin. J Control Release 2009; 139(2): 118-26.
[http://dx.doi.org/10.1016/j.jconrel.2009.06.012] [PMID: 19545593]

[168] Hazer DB, Kılıçay E, Hazer B. Poly(3-hydroxyalkanoate)s: Diversification and biomedical applications. Mater Sci Eng C 2012; 32: 637-47.
[http://dx.doi.org/10.1016/j.msec.2012.01.021]

[169] Dirschl DR, Almekinders LC. Osteomyelitis. Common causes and treatment recommendations. Drugs 1993; 45(1): 29-43.
[http://dx.doi.org/10.2165/00003495-199345010-00004] [PMID: 7680983]

[170] Gürsel I, Korkusuz F, Türesin F, Alaeddinoglu NG, Hasirci V. In vivo application of biodegradable controlled antibiotic release systems for the treatment of implant-related osteomyelitis. Biomaterials 2001; 22(1): 73-80.
[http://dx.doi.org/10.1016/S0142-9612(00)00170-8] [PMID: 11085386]

[171] Yagmurlu MF, Korkusuz F, Gürsel I, Korkusuz P, Örs U, Hasirci V. Sulbactam-cefoperazone polyhydroxybutyrate-co-hydroxyvalerate (PHBV) local antibiotic delivery system: in vivo effectiveness and biocompatibility in the treatment of implant-related experimental osteomyelitis. J Biomed Mater Res 1999; 46(4): 494-503.
[http://dx.doi.org/10.1002/(SICI)1097-4636(19990915)46:4<494::AID-JBM7>3.0.CO;2-E] [PMID: 10398010]

[172] Rossi S, Azghani AO, Omri A. Antimicrobial efficacy of a new antibiotic-loaded poly(hydroxybutyric-co-hydroxyvaleric acid) controlled release system. J Antimicrob Chemother 2004; 54(6): 1013-8.
[http://dx.doi.org/10.1093/jac/dkh477] [PMID: 15537698]

[173] Löbler M, Sternberg K, Stachs O, *et al.* Polymers and drugs suitable for the development of a drug delivery drainage system in glaucoma surgery. J Biomed Mater Res B Appl Biomater 2011; 97(2): 388-95.
[http://dx.doi.org/10.1002/jbm.b.31826] [PMID: 21432996]

[174] Basnett P, Ching KY, Stolz M, Knowles JC, Boccaccini AR, Smith C, *et al.* Aspirin-loaded P(3HO)/P(3HB) blend films: potential materials for biodegradable drug-eluting stents. Bioinspired. Biomim Nanobiomaterials 2013; 2: 141-53.
[http://dx.doi.org/10.1680/bbn.13.00009]

[175] Karpova SG, Olkhov AA, Shilkina NG, Popov AA, Filatova AG, Kucherenko EL, *et al.* 2017.

[176] Jedliński Z, Kowalczuk M, Adamus G, Sikorska W, Rydz J. Novel synthesis of functionalized poly(3-hydroxybutanoic acid) and its copolymers. Int J Biol Macromol 1999; 25(1-3): 247-53.
[http://dx.doi.org/10.1016/S0141-8130(99)00039-2] [PMID: 10416672]

[177] Kwiecień I, Adamus G, Kowalczuk M. Electrospray ionisation mass spectrometry molecular-level structural characterisation of novel phenoxycarboxylic acid-oligo(3-hydroxybutyrate) conjugates with potential agricultural applications. Rapid Commun Mass Spectrom 2012; 26(23): 2673-82.
[http://dx.doi.org/10.1002/rcm.6391] [PMID: 23124657]

[178] Kwiecień I, Adamus G, Bartkowiak A, Kowalczuk M. Synthesis and structural characterization at the molecular level of oligo(3-hydroxybutyrate) conjugates with antimicrobial agents designed for food packaging materials. Des Monomers Polym 2014; 17: 311-21.
[http://dx.doi.org/10.1080/15685551.2013.840505]

[179] Kwiecień I, Radecka I, Kowalczuk M, Adamus G. Transesterification of PHA to oligomers covalently bonded with (bio)active compounds containing either carboxyl or hydroxyl functionalities. PLoS One 2015; 10(3): e0120149.
[http://dx.doi.org/10.1371/journal.pone.0120149] [PMID: 25781908]

[180] Michalak M, Kawalec M, Kurcok P. Reactive mono- and di-epoxy-functionalized poly(3-hydroxybutyrate)s. Synthesis and characterization. Polym Degrad Stabil 2012; 97: 1861-70.
[http://dx.doi.org/10.1016/j.polymdegradstab.2012.05.007]

[181] Hazer B. Simple synthesis of amphiphilic poly(3-hydroxy alkanoate)s with pendant hydroxyl and carboxylic groups via thiol-ene photo click reactions. Polym Degrad Stabil 2015; 119: 159-66.
[http://dx.doi.org/10.1016/j.polymdegradstab.2015.04.024]

[182] Michalak M, Marek AA, Zawadiak J, Kawalec M, Kurcok P. Synthesis of PHB-based carrier for drug delivery systems with pH-controlled release. Eur Polym J 2013; 49: 4149-56. [http://dx.doi.org/10.1016/j.eurpolymj.2013.09.021]

[183] Hazer B, Steinbüchel A. Increased diversification of polyhydroxyalkanoates by modification reactions for industrial and medical applications. Appl Microbiol Biotechnol 2007; 74(1): 1-12. [http://dx.doi.org/10.1007/s00253-006-0732-8] [PMID: 17146652]

[184] Pinto A, Ciesla JH, Palucci A, Sutliff BP, Nomura CT. Chemically intractable no more: in vivo incorporation of "click"-ready fatty acids into poly-[(R)-3-hydroxyalkanoates] in Escherichia coli. ACS Macro Lett 2016; 5: 215-9. [http://dx.doi.org/10.1021/acsmacrolett.5b00823]

[185] Shrivastav A, Kim H-Y, Kim Y-R. Advances in the applications of polyhydroxyalkanoate nanoparticles for novel drug delivery system. BioMed Res Int 2013; 2013 Article ID 581684. [http://dx.doi.org/10.1155/2013/581684]

[186] Masood F. Polymeric nanoparticles for targeted drug delivery system for cancer therapy. Mater Sci Eng C Mater Biol Appl 2016; 60: 569-78. [http://dx.doi.org/10.1016/j.msec.2015.11.067] [PMID: 26706565]

[187] Lu X-Y, Wu D-C, Li Z-J, Chen G-Q. Polymer nanoparticles. Prog Mol Biol Transl Sci 2011; 104: 299-323. [http://dx.doi.org/10.1016/B978-0-12-416020-0.00007-3.]

[188] Shishatskaya EI, Voinova ON, Goreva AV, Mogilnaya OA, Volova TG. Biocompatibility of polyhydroxybutyrate microspheres: in vitro and in vivo evaluation. J Mater Sci Mater Med 2008; 19(6): 2493-502. [http://dx.doi.org/10.1007/s10856-007-3345-6]] [PMID: 18253816]

[189] Gangrade N, Price JC. Poly(hydroxybutyrate-hydroxyvalerate) microspheres containing progesterone: preparation, morphology and release properties. J Microencapsul 1991; 8(2): 185-202. [http://dx.doi.org/10.3109/02652049109071487] [PMID: 1765899]

[190] Kurth N, Renard E, Brachet F, Robic D, Guerin P, Bourbouze R. Poly(3-hydroxyoctanoate) containing pendant carboxylic groups for the preparation of nanoparticles aimed at drug transport and release. Polymer (Guildf) 2001; 43: 1095-101. [http://dx.doi.org/10.1016/S0032-3861(01)00692-9]

[191] Renard E, Ternat C, Langlois V, Guerin P. Synthesis of Graft Bacterial Polyesters for Nanoparticles Preparation. Macromol Biosci 2003; 3: 248-52. [http://dx.doi.org/10.1002/mabi.200390033]

[192] Barouti G, Jarnouen K, Cammas-Marion S, Loyer P, Guillaume SM. Polyhydroxyalkanoate-based amphiphilic diblock copolymers as original biocompatible nanovectors. Polym Chem 2015; 6: 5414-29. [http://dx.doi.org/10.1039/C5PY00831J]

[193] Vene E, Barouti G, Jarnouen K, *et al.* Opsonisation of nanoparticles prepared from poly(β-hydroxybutyrate) and poly(trimethylene carbonate)-b-poly(malic acid) amphiphilic diblock copolymers: Impact on the in vitro cell uptake by primary human macrophages and HepaRG hepatoma cells. Int J Pharm 2016; 513(1-2): 438-52. [http://dx.doi.org/10.1016/j.ijpharm.2016.09.048] [PMID: 27640247]

[194] Ajellal N, Thomas CM, Aubry T, Grohens Y, Carpentier J-F. Encapsulation and controlled release of l-leuprolide from poly([small beta]-hydroxyalkanoate)s: impact of microstructure and chemical functionalities. New J Chem 2011; 35: 876-80. [http://dx.doi.org/10.1039/c0nj00998a]

[195] Goreva AV, Shishatskaya EI, Volova TG, Sinskey AJ. Characterization of polymeric microparticles based on resorbable polyesters of oxyalkanoic acids as a platform for deposition and delivery of drugs. Polym Sci Ser A 2012; 54: 94-105. [http://dx.doi.org/10.1134/S0965545X12020022]

[196] Livshits VA, Bonartsev AP, Iordanskii AL, Ivanov EA, Makhina TA, Myshkina VL, *et al.* Microspheres based on poly(3-hydroxy)butyrate for prolonged drug release. Polym Sci Ser B 2009; 51: 256-63. [http://dx.doi.org/10.1134/S1560090409070082]

[197] Vilos C, Morales FA, Solar PA, *et al.* Paclitaxel-PHBV nanoparticles and their toxicity to endometrial and primary ovarian cancer cells. Biomaterials 2013; 34(16): 4098-108. [http://dx.doi.org/10.1016/j.biomaterials.2013.02.034] [PMID: 23465827]

[198] Masood F, Chen P, Yasin T, Fatima N, Hasan F, Hameed A. Encapsulation of Ellipticine in poly-(- -hydroxybutyrate-co-3-hydroxyvalerate) based nanoparticles and its in vitro application. Mater Sci Eng C Mater Biol Appl 2013; 33(3): 1054-60. [http://dx.doi.org/10.1016/j.msec.2012.11.025] [PMID: 23827542]

[199] Pramual S, Assavanig A, Bergkvist M, *et al.* Development and characterization of bio-derived polyhydroxyalkanoate nanoparticles as a delivery system for hydrophobic photodynamic therapy agents. J Mater Sci Mater Med 2016; 27(2): 40. [http://dx.doi.org/10.1007/s10856-015-5655-4] [PMID: 26712706]

[200] Dong CL, Webb WR, Peng Q, *et al.* Sustained PDGF-BB release from PHBHHx loaded nanoparticles in 3D hydrogel/stem cell model. J Biomed Mater Res A 2015; 103(1): 282-8. [http://dx.doi.org/10.1002/jbm.a.35149] [PMID: 24610890]

[201] Shah M, Ullah N, Choi MH, Kim MO, Yoon SC. Amorphous amphiphilic P(3HV-co-4HB)-b-mPEG block copolymer synthesized from bacterial copolyester via melt transesterification: nanoparticle preparation, cisplatin-loading for cancer therapy and in vitro evaluation. Eur J Pharm Biopharm 2012; 80(3): 518-27. [http://dx.doi.org/10.1016/j.ejpb.2011.11.014] [PMID: 22178562]

[202] Kapoor S, Gupta D, Kumar M, *et al.* Intracellular delivery of peptide cargos using polyhydroxybutyrate based biodegradable nanoparticles: Studies on antitumor efficacy of BCL-2 converting peptide, NuBCP-9. Int J Pharm 2016; 511(2): 876-89. [http://dx.doi.org/10.1016/j.ijpharm.2016.07.077] [PMID: 27492021]

[203] Kim H-N, Lee J, Kim H-Y, Kim Y-R. Enzymatic synthesis of a drug delivery system based on polyhydroxyalkanoate-protein block copolymers. Chem Commun (Camb) 2009; 7345(46): 7104-6. [http://dx.doi.org/10.1039/b912871a] [PMID: 19920997]

[204] Yao Y-C, Zhan X-Y, Zhang J, *et al.* A specific drug targeting system based on polyhydroxyalkanoate granule binding protein PhaP fused with targeted cell ligands. Biomaterials 2008; 29(36): 4823-30. [http://dx.doi.org/10.1016/j.biomaterials.2008.09.008] [PMID: 18824258]

[205] Kılıçay E, Demirbilek M, Türk M, Güven E, Hazer B, Denkbas EB. Preparation and characterization of poly(3-hydroxybutyrate-co-3-hydroxyhexanoate) (PHBHHX) based nanoparticles for targeted cancer therapy. Eur J Pharm Sci 2011; 44(3): 310-20. [http://dx.doi.org/10.1016/j.ejps.2011.08.013] [PMID: 21884788]

[206] Kilicay E, Karahaliloglu Z, Hazer B, Tekin IÖ, Denkbas EB. Concanavaline A conjugated bacterial polyester-based PHBHHx nanoparticles loaded with curcumin for breast cancer therapy. J Microencapsul 2016; 33(3): 274-85. [http://dx.doi.org/10.3109/02652048.2016.1169325] [PMID: 27049468]

[207] Nobes GA, Jurasek L, Marchessault RH, Martin DP, Putaux JL, Chanzy H. Growth and kinetics of in vitro poly([R]-(-)-3-hydroxybutyrate) granules interpreted as particulate polymerization with coalescence. Macromol Rapid Commun 2000; 21: 77-84. [http://dx.doi.org/10.1002/(SICI)1521-3927(20000201)21:2<77::AID-MARC77>3.0.CO;2-6]

[208] Kwon H-S, Jung S-G, Kim H-Y, Parker S, Batt C, Kim Y-R. A multi-functional polyhydroxybutyrate nanoparticle for theranostic applications. J Mater Chem B Mater Biol Med 2014; 2: 3965-71. [http://dx.doi.org/10.1039/c4tb00304g]

[209] Lee J, Jung S-G, Park C-S, Kim H-Y, Batt CA, Kim Y-R. Tumor-specific hybrid polyhydroxybutyrate nanoparticle: surface modification of nanoparticle by enzymatically synthesized functional block copolymer. Bioorg Med Chem Lett 2011; 21(10): 2941-4. [http://dx.doi.org/10.1016/j.bmcl.2011.03.058] [PMID: 21489794]

SUBJECT INDEX

A

Abiraterone 134, 147, 149, 158
Ablative therapies 67, 82
Acid suppressive therapy (AST) 65, 67, 115
Activity 6, 16, 20, 28, 37, 40, 42, 158, 177, 187, 204, 205, 206, 207, 209, 210, 214, 215, 216, 218, 219, 226, 228, 267, 271
  telomerase 42, 177
Acute lymphoblastic leukemia 1, 5, 24, 43
Adenocarcinoma 52, 53, 60, 62, 64, 67, 68, 74, 83, 96, 105, 106, 115, 134, 175, 177, 185
  esophageal 52, 53, 74, 83, 105, 106, 115
Adjuvant chemotherapy (AC) 93, 94
Agents 4, 6, 9, 14, 15, 16, 25, 30, 31, 42, 90, 104, 110, 111, 115, 134, 144, 147, 159, 194, 196, 202, 205, 206, 209, 210, 231
  antimitotic 196
  chemoprotective 209, 210
Alkylating agents 9, 90, 198, 202
Anamorelin 114, 115
Anaplastic large cell lymphoma (ALCL) 1, 16, 18, 20, 31, 33, 34
Androgens 135, 140, 141, 142, 148, 149, 150, 154, 158, 159, 178, 223, 224
  blockade, total 141, 149, 150
  receptor (AR) 135, 141, 142, 148, 158, 159, 178, 223, 224
Anemia 3, 7, 32, 33, 37, 39, 40, 41, 42, 43, 156, 176, 198
Angiogenesis 38, 69, 106, 108, 174, 205, 207, 223, 224, 226, 228
Antiandrogen 141, 143, 145, 209
Anti-androgens 134, 142, 143, 145, 148, 150
Antibody drug conjugate (ADC) 18, 19
Anticancer 172, 174, 189, 196, 201, 202, 203, 204, 205, 207, 209, 210, 211, 219, 222, 225, 228, 267
  activity 201, 204, 211, 219, 222, 225, 228, 267
  agents 174, 189, 196, 202, 203, 204, 205, 207, 209, 219
  compounds 174, 203
  drug development 172, 174, 203, 205, 209, 210
Anticancer drugs 172, 173, 174, 195, 200, 201, 202, 204, 205, 206, 207, 208, 209, 210, 222, 230, 231, 267, 268
  derived 222
  ideal 173
  modern 231
  new 208
  potential 207
  research 172, 173, 174
  target-based potent 204
  targeted 206
  targets of 200, 201
Antiproliferative activity 225, 227, 229
Apoptosis 18, 22, 30, 35, 37, 38, 63, 70, 148, 154, 178, 188, 189, 194, 196, 197, 205, 223, 225, 228, 229, 230, 249, 269
Argon plasma coagulation (APC) 67, 82, 209
Asparaginase Erwinia 27, 28
Asparagines 27, 202
Aspirin 72, 213, 261, 262, 263
Assays, mechanism-based 218, 219
ASXL1 mutation 43

B

Barrett's esophagus 52, 55, 60, 62, 63, 64, 65, 66, 67, 71, 77, 82, 115
Barrett's metaplasia (BM) 62, 64
B-cell, refractory 26, 27
Bcl-2 antiapoptotic activity in cancer cells 268
Belinostat 35, 36
Bicalutamide 138, 142, 143, 144, 146, 148, 151, 155
Bignoniaceae 221, 222
Bioactive 242, 254, 259, 262, 263, 264
  glass (BG) 254, 259
  substances 242, 262, 263, 264
Bleomycin 17, 20, 200, 222
Blinatumomab 25, 26, 27, 31, 43
Bloom syndrome 24, 56, 57
Bone marrow 1, 3, 15, 16, 20, 24, 31, 32, 175, 176, 185
  transplant 1
Bone tissues 253, 259, 260
Bortezomib 21, 22, 23, 39

Bosutinib 4, 5, 16
Brachytherapy 111, 112, 113, 138, 155, 194
Breast cancer 174, 184, 185, 194, 196, 198, 201, 204, 209, 210, 226
  treatment of 184, 198, 201, 226
Brentuximab 18, 19, 20
Bruton's tyrosine kinase (BTK) 11, 13

C

Cancer 24, 31, 32, 44, 55, 79, 97, 98, 114, 115, 155, 177, 182, 183, 184, 185, 187, 194, 198, 199, 204, 219, 226, 269
  advanced 97, 98, 114, 115
  aggressive 24, 31, 155
  bladder 183, 184, 185, 198
  cervical 55, 185, 187, 226
  chronic blood 32, 44
  human 183, 199, 204, 219
  liver 183, 184
  neck 55, 194
  pancreatic 177, 182, 183, 194
  residual 79
  testicular 194, 198, 199, 269
Cancer and acute leukemia group B (CALGB) 139
Cancer cells 18, 22, 30, 69, 78, 79, 135, 138, 141, 142, 146, 147, 158, 173, 177, 178, 179, 180, 182, 189, 194, 195, 199, 202, 203, 204, 205, 206, 211, 219, 226, 228, 229, 230, 263, 268, 270, 271
  breast 270
  cluster 78
  hematologic 22
  hollow fiber assay 219
  human 230
  lines 199, 203, 204, 205, 211, 226, 228, 229, 263
  lymphatic 202
  metastatic 180, 189
  prostate 135, 141, 142, 146, 147, 158
  rare small groups of 79
Cancer chemotherapeutic drugs 172
Cancer development 173, 182, 186, 190, 192
  stages of 173, 190
Cancer of the prostate strategic urologic research endeavour (CaPSURE) 154
Cancerous cells 177, 178, 187, 196, 198, 202, 204, 205, 206, 207, 215
Cancerous tissues 67, 207
Capecitabine 89, 90, 91, 96, 98, 99, 103, 104, 105, 106, 108, 116
Carbon sources 244, 245
Carboplatin 21, 88, 89, 91, 96, 97, 98, 104
Carcinogenesis 54, 55, 109, 177, 178, 186, 189, 190
Carcinogenic agents 185
Carcinomas 60, 64, 65, 66, 67, 68, 77, 78, 79, 82, 175, 186
  intramucosal 64, 65, 66, 67, 82
  residual 78, 79
Carfilzomib 36, 37
Castrate-resistant prostate cancer (CRPC) 147, 148, 149, 158
Catalase 190, 191
Cell cycle 18, 30, 31, 35, 37, 62, 67, 68, 79, 178, 179, 180, 187, 195, 197, 199, 227, 228, 229, 230
  arrest 18, 35, 37, 197, 199, 227, 229
Cells 7, 8, 11, 13, 16, 22, 24, 26, 30, 31, 32, 33, 38, 41, 62, 63, 78, 89, 108, 173, 174, 175, 178, 179, 180, 182, 187, 188, 189, 190, 192, 195, 196, 206, 207, 209, 215, 219, 225, 246, 248, 249, 251, 252, 254, 256, 257, 263, 268, 269, 270
  columnar 62
  daughter 195, 196
  endothelial 108, 178, 207, 256, 257
  infected 188
  initiated 178
  preneoplastic 178
  single 79
  spindle 67, 68
  therapy 30, 31
Central nervous system (CNS) 24, 25
Characteristic features of cancer cells 178
Chemoradiation 77, 83, 84, 96, 97, 112
Chemoresistance 80, 81
Chemotherapeutic agents 1, 44, 88, 89, 90, 103, 104, 172, 194, 195, 198, 204, 206, 210
Chemotherapy 1, 17, 18, 20, 21, 24, 25, 30, 52, 76, 77, 81, 84, 88, 89, 90, 92, 93, 94, 95, 103, 104, 108, 113, 115, 139, 147, 149, 158, 172, 184, 194, 198, 210

arm 30
concurrent 88
neoadjuvant 52, 76, 81, 92, 93, 94, 95
regimens, multidrug 18
Chlorambucil 8, 10, 15, 198, 202
Chondrocytes 252, 253
Chromosomes 2, 24, 56, 57, 179, 195, 196
Chronic lymphocytic leukemia (CLL) 1, 2, 3, 4, 5, 6, 7, 8, 9, 10, 11, 13, 14, 15, 16, 23, 43, 176
myelogenous leukemia (CML) 2, 3, 4, 5, 6, 7, 15, 16, 176
myeloid leukemia 1, 4, 15
Cisplatin 21, 88, 89, 90, 91, 92, 95, 96, 98, 99, 103, 104, 105, 108, 115, 116, 148, 196, 202, 268
Classification, 3-Tiered 79
CLL, untreated 8, 10, 12
CML, chronic phase 4, 5, 6, 7
Cohort 86, 93, 99, 100, 101
Collagen 180, 243, 252, 253, 255, 257
Colon cancers 175, 270
Combination therapy 82, 88, 105, 143, 150, 151, 206, 209, 229
Comorbidities 8, 14, 82, 84, 113
Complete remission (CR) 19, 20, 22, 23, 25, 27, 29, 30, 36, 261
Complications, postoperative 85, 87
Crassulaceae 220, 221
Creatinine clearance 10, 14, 157
CRT, definitive 88, 92, 98
CT scans 99, 101, 192
Cutaneous T-cell lymphoma (CTCL) 31, 33, 34, 35, 36, 43
Cyclophosphamide 17, 18, 21, 25, 35, 37, 198, 202
Cyproterone acetate 141, 151, 156
Cytarabine 21, 25, 30, 199
Cytoplasm 177, 181, 182, 190, 191, 263, 266
Cytotoxic effects 198, 230, 248, 249
Cytotoxicity 190, 249, 268, 269

D

Dasatinib 4, 5, 15, 25
Degarelix 134, 144, 145
Development of antibodies 208
Dexamethasone 21, 37, 39, 42
Diarrhea 7, 12, 13, 14, 90, 104, 142, 149, 151
Disease 2, 3, 4, 9, 11, 13, 15, 16, 17, 19, 21, 22, 29, 36, 43, 57, 75, 78, 84, 85, 87, 88, 91, 93, 94, 95, 96, 97, 98, 99, 100, 101, 103, 108, 109, 146, 150, 151, 152, 154, 172, 173, 192, 203, 204, 208, 212, 213, 214, 215, 260, 265
-free-survival (DFS) 78, 85
localized 17, 91, 98, 152
relapsed 21
residual nodal 94, 95
systemic 86, 94
unresectable 98, 103
progression 3, 4, 11, 19, 36, 109, 150
Distant metastases 73, 84, 91, 95, 97, 99, 100, 137, 153
DNA replication in cancerous cells 196
Docetaxel 90, 93, 99, 103, 104, 106, 137, 139, 147, 158, 196, 199
addition of 104, 137, 139
Dolastatin 227, 228, 230
Doxorubicin 17, 18, 21, 35, 90, 173, 196, 200, 222, 263, 266, 267, 269
process of anticancer 210
Drugs 18, 19, 20, 22, 23, 26, 35, 40, 89, 104, 136, 139, 140, 143, 146, 148, 152, 156, 158, 172, 173, 174, 196, 197, 198, 199, 201, 204, 205, 206, 208, 209, 210, 211, 212, 213, 215, 216, 218, 219, 231, 242, 243, 244, 252, 255, 259, 261, 262, 263, 264, 265, 266, 267, 268, 270, 271, 272
antimitotic 196, 197
antithrombotic 261
delivery systems 242, 243, 244, 252, 255, 265, 266, 268
development 172, 173, 174, 204, 212, 218, 219
encapsulated 267
Dysphagia 72, 97, 100, 106, 111, 112, 113, 114
Dysplasia 61, 62, 63, 64, 65, 66, 69, 71, 72, 73, 77, 81, 108, 116
high-grade 61, 64, 66, 73, 77
low-grade 61, 64, 66
squamous 61, 71

E

Early stage esophageal cancer 67, 81, 84
E.coli asparaginase 27, 28
EGJ adenocarcinomas 93, 95, 106
Either squamous cell carcinoma (ESCC) 52, 53, 54, 55, 56, 57, 58, 61, 67, 68, 69, 70, 71, 81, 88, 91, 92, 94, 107, 111, 116
Endometrial cancer 201, 209
Endoscopic 52, 63, 65, 66, 67, 77, 81, 82, 83, 84, 100, 112, 116
  ablation 65, 66
  mucosal resection (EMR) 52, 63, 66, 67, 81, 82, 116
  palliation 112
  resection 77, 82, 83, 84
  submucosal dissection (ESD) 52, 67, 81, 82, 116
  surveillance 66, 100
  therapy 63, 66, 81, 82, 83
Endoscopy 52, 61, 64, 65, 66, 71, 72, 88, 99, 103, 113
Enobosarm 114, 115
Enzalutamide 134, 147, 148, 149, 158, 159
Epidermal growth factor (EGF) 52, 58, 69, 116, 208, 223, 271
  receptor (EGFR) 52, 58, 69, 110, 116, 208, 223
Epirubicin 90, 95, 96, 103, 104
ESCC 54, 55, 69, 70
  development of 54, 55, 69
  risk of 54, 55, 70
Esophageal cancer (EC) 52, 53, 54, 55, 56, 58, 60, 62, 63, 64, 67, 68, 69, 70, 71, 72, 75, 76, 77, 80, 81, 82, 83, 84, 85, 86, 89, 90, 91, 96, 97, 99, 103, 104, 105, 106, 110, 111, 113, 114, 115
  advanced 75, 103
  resectable 84, 96
Esophageal mucosa 54, 80
Esophagectomy 66, 82, 83, 84, 86, 98, 99, 100, 101, 102
Esophagogastric junction 60, 73, 96, 99, 104, 106
  cancer 96, 99, 104, 106
Esophagus, thoracic 75, 85, 96
Estrogens 135, 136, 140, 141, 146, 156, 210
European organization for research and treatment of cancer (EORTC) 136, 150, 151, 152, 153
EUS 66, 72, 75
  accuracy of 75
Evaluation 28, 63, 72, 75, 78, 79, 202, 204, 205, 219, 253, 265, 267, 269
  pathologic 63, 78, 79
Extensive disease in prostate cancer 139
External beam radiation therapy (EBRT) 89, 97, 113, 115

F

Failure-free survival (FFS) 18, 137
Familial Barrett's esophagus (FBE) 57
Fanconi anemia (FA) 24, 57, 116
Fibroblasts 249, 250, 253
Finasteride 135, 142
Fistulas 97, 112, 113, 114
  tracheoesophageal 97, 112, 113
Flashes, hot 141, 143, 151, 155, 156
Fluid retention 141, 142, 143
Fluoropyrimidine 89, 90, 96, 98, 99, 103, 104, 105, 108, 109, 115
  therapy 105, 109
Flutamide 137, 138, 141, 142, 146, 150, 151, 152, 156, 201
Folic acid 196, 199, 242, 269, 272
  attachment of 242, 269, 272

G

Galeterone 158, 159
Gastric cancers 105, 108, 188
Genome-wide association studies (GWAS) 56, 70, 116
Gentamicin 260, 261
Gleason score 138, 152
Glial growth factor (GGF) 255
Glutathione peroxidases 190, 191, 223
Glycoproteins 179, 180, 271
GnRH agonists 137, 143, 144, 145
Gonadotropin-releasing hormone 134, 201
Goserelin 136, 142, 144, 151, 152
Grade Tumor Location 73, 74
Graft-versus-host disease (GVHD) 41

Groups 81, 211, 262, 263, 264, 272
side 262, 263, 264, 272
small 81, 211
Growth factors 40, 107, 177, 178, 180, 181, 182, 207, 210
Gynecomastia 140, 141, 157, 158

H

Halichondrins 229, 230
Hematopoietic cell transplantation (HCT) 9, 13, 15, 34, 251, 263
Hepatitis 9, 21, 184, 187
Hepatocellular carcinoma cells 271
Hereditary cancer syndromes 52, 55
High-grade dysplasia (HGD) 61, 63, 64, 65, 66, 71, 73, 74, 77, 81, 82, 116
Hodgkin lymphoma (HL) 1, 14, 16, 17, 18, 19, 20, 175
Hormonal therapy 136, 138, 149, 150, 155, 156, 159, 193, 209, 210
Human cancer KB cells and nontumorigenic HaCaT cell line 251
Hydrogen peroxide 190, 191
Hydroxyapatite 247, 251, 254
3-hydroxybutyric acid 246, 248, 249, 263

I

Ibrutinib 11, 12, 13, 15, 16, 21, 23, 43
Idelalisib 13, 14, 15, 16
group 14
Imatinib 2, 4, 5, 7, 15, 25
Imetelstat 42, 43
Immune response 179, 208, 209, 247, 254
Induction chemotherapy 92
Infusional FU 90, 91
Infusion reactions 8, 9, 10, 26, 27
continuous 26, 27
Inhibitors, histone deacetylase 31, 33, 35, 39, 43
Inotuzumab ozogamicin 30, 31
Intensity modulated radiotherapy (IMRT) 89
Intermittent ADT 150, 154, 155, 156
Invasive esophagectomies 86
Ionizing radiations 184, 185, 194
Irinotecan 96, 98, 99, 104, 105, 106, 110, 116, 200
Irinotecan and cisplatin 96, 99, 105, 106

J

JAK2 mutation 43
Janus associated kinases (JAKs) 32, 39, 41

K

Ketoconazole 147, 148

L

β-lactones 244, 245, 263
Lamina propria, tumor invades 73
Lenalidomide 21, 22, 23, 42
Leucovorin 90, 92, 93, 98, 105, 116
Leukemia 1, 2, 24, 27, 30, 57, 176, 183, 185, 198, 202, 204, 228
chronic 1, 2
cells 24, 27, 30, 202
Leuprolide 142, 144, 145, 150, 152
group 144
LHRH analogs 143, 144, 145, 155
Line therapy, second 105, 106, 108, 109, 110, 143
Long-term hormones (LTH) 138
Low-grade dysplasia (LGD) 61, 63, 64, 65, 66, 71, 116
Lung cancer 174, 176, 177, 183, 184, 185, 194, 196, 198, 226
Luteinizing hormone (LH) 141, 142, 143, 155
-releasing hormone (LHRH) 141, 142, 143, 151, 155
Lymph node metastasis, regional 73, 75, 84
Lymphocytes 16, 17, 20, 24, 59, 248
Lymphomas 3, 16, 21, 30, 175, 177, 198, 199, 202, 269

M

Macrophages 248, 250, 271
Major molecular response (MMR) 4, 5
Malignancies 2, 3, 7, 52, 55, 56, 57, 58, 62, 81
Malignant cells 3, 94, 173, 179, 180

Mantle cell lymphoma (MCL) 1, 11, 20, 21, 22, 23
Matrix metalloproteinases 178, 206, 207
Maximum androgen blockade (MAB) 150, 151, 270
Maximum tolerated dose (MTD) 38
Mechanical tumor obstruction 113
Medicinal plants 172, 212, 213, 220, 231
Membranous reactivity, lateral 78
Metabolites 11, 208
Metastasis 69, 73, 76, 109, 134, 143, 147, 151, 154, 173, 174, 178, 189, 205, 206, 207
Metastatic disease 75, 83, 97, 98, 103, 104, 106, 135, 140, 142, 145, 147, 149, 150, 151, 153, 154, 155
  esophageal cancer 104, 106
  prostate cancer 135, 147, 149, 150, 151, 153, 154, 155
Methotrexate 21, 25, 196, 199
Mitogen activated protein kinase (MAPK) 178, 223, 224
Monoclonal antibodies 7, 16, 17, 20, 25, 31, 42, 110, 270
Monotherapy 10, 15, 42, 84, 88, 105, 143, 150, 151
Mucositis 33, 90, 113
Multi-drug resistance (MDR) 209, 210
Multimodality assessment of esophageal cancer 60, 76
Multiple myeloma 1, 31, 32, 36, 37, 38, 39, 42, 44
Mutations 4, 5, 6, 7, 15, 24, 32, 43, 56, 57, 62, 63, 68, 69, 158, 159, 177, 178, 179, 180, 182, 186, 189, 190, 192, 207
  genetic 4, 56, 158, 159
Mycosis fungoides (MF) 31, 33
Myelofibrosis 1, 31, 32, 39, 40, 42, 43, 44

N

Narrow-band imaging (NBI) 71, 116
National comprehensive cancer network (NCCN) 96, 99, 102, 104, 106, 108
NCCN consensus, uniform 96, 99, 104, 106
Neoadjuvant CRT 87, 91, 92, 93, 95
Neutropenia 5, 7, 8, 10, 33, 35, 36, 37, 38, 39, 42, 43, 104, 105
Non-Hodgkin lymphoma (NHL) 14, 18, 20, 21, 23, 31
Novel anticancer agents 198, 210, 220
Nucleotides 196, 199

O

Obinutuzumab 9, 10, 15, 16
Ofatumumab 7, 8, 9, 10, 15, 16
  role of 9
Oligomers 246, 248, 249, 251, 252, 262, 263
Omacetaxine 6, 7, 16
Oncogenes 177, 181, 186, 207
Oncogenic mutations 182
Orchiectomy 134, 140, 141, 143, 144, 150, 151, 153
Osteoblasts 248, 253, 254
Osteoporosis 67, 142, 156, 157
Ovarian cancer 182, 184, 194, 196, 201, 209, 226
Overall response rate (ORR) 8, 10, 12, 13, 19, 20, 22, 23, 29, 34, 36, 37, 38, 39, 111
Oxaliplatin 89, 90, 91, 96, 98, 103, 104, 105, 116
Oxidative damages 190, 192

P

Paclitaxel 88, 90, 91, 96, 97, 98, 99, 104, 106, 109, 196, 267
Panobinostat 37, 39
Pathogenesis of esophageal cancer 52, 54
Pathologic response, complete 93, 94, 95
Pegaspargase 27, 28
Perioperative chemotherapy 95
Peripheral T-cell Lymphoma (PTCL) 31, 33, 34, 35, 36, 43
PET scans 75, 76, 79, 99, 101
  role of 79
PHA particles 242, 266, 269, 272
Pharmacogenetics 208, 210
PHA synthase 245, 270, 271
PHB 246, 270
  depolymerases 246
  nanoparticles 270
Philadelphia chromosome 2, 3, 16, 24, 25
Photosensitizers 209, 210

Plant extracts 212, 216, 218
Plasminogen activators 206, 207
Poly-ADP ribose polymerase (PARP) 159, 224
Polyesters 242, 243, 246, 252, 269
Polymer, natural 242, 243
Polymerase chain reaction (PCR) 56, 116
Polymer 250, 262, 264, 272
  chain 262, 264
  –drug conjugates 262, 272
  film 250
Polymeric nanoparticles 243
Polymerization 198, 199, 223, 263
Pomalidomide 32, 37, 38, 39
Pomalidomide and dexamethasone 37, 39
Ponatinib 5, 6, 16, 25
Postoperative chemotherapy 93, 95
Potent anticancer activity 173, 228, 229
  drugs 173
Precursor lesions 55, 61, 71
Prednisone 9, 17, 18, 21, 35, 39, 147, 149
Preoperative CRT 79, 92, 95
Preparation of micro- and nanoparticles 265
Prior therapies 6, 11, 19, 22, 23, 29, 33, 35, 37, 39, 106, 110
Progression 22, 32, 37, 44, 55, 61, 63, 65, 70, 104, 117, 137, 151, 153, 154, 155, 157, 178, 189, 195
  neoplastic 61, 63, 65
Progression-free survival (PFS) 7, 8, 10, 12, 13, 14, 19, 20, 37, 42, 92, 97, 105, 111, 116, 146, 148, 149, 152, 159
  improved 10, 12
Prostate cancer 134, 135, 136, 137, 138, 139, 148, 151, 158
  advanced 136, 139
  intermediate risk 139
  intermediate-risk 135, 138
  resistant 134, 148, 158
  treatment 136, 137
  trialists' collaborative group meta-analysis 151
Prostate-specific 134, 151
Prostate specific antigen (PSA) 135, 138, 141, 143, 145, 146, 147, 151, 152, 154, 155
Prostatic cancer 134, 136
Proteins 19, 58, 62, 180, 182, 186, 187, 189, 190, 192, 195, 205, 226, 243, 269, 270, 272
Proton beam therapy (PBT) 89
Proton pump inhibitors (PPIs) 63, 67, 72, 114, 116
Proto-oncogene 107, 181, 188
PSA levels 147, 155
Psammaplins 225, 227
Pyrexia 12, 13, 14

R

Radiation 17, 20, 21, 25, 52, 84, 87, 88, 89, 97, 98, 106, 112, 113, 114, 134, 135, 136, 137, 138, 147, 159, 194
  esophagitis 89, 97, 113, 114
  therapy 17, 25, 97, 98, 113, 137, 159, 194
Radiation therapy oncology group (RTOG) 88, 97, 138, 149, 153
Radiotherapy 32, 44, 88, 89, 97, 98, 116, 134, 136, 137, 138, 139, 149, 152, 153, 156, 157
  dose-escalated 139, 149, 153
  external beam 138, 153
Rainbow trial 109
Ramucirumab 105, 106, 108, 109, 110
Randomised androgen deprivation and radiotherapy (RADAR) 139
RAS mutations 110
Reactive oxygen species (ROS) 189, 190, 192, 224
Red blood cells (RBC) 176
Refractory HL 19, 20
Regorafenib 110, 111
Relapse 4, 15, 17, 20, 21, 23, 25, 29, 39
Relapsed/refractory 33, 34, 35, 36, 37, 38, 42, 43
  AITL 34, 35
  PTCL 33, 35, 36
Relapse-free survival (RFS) 93, 94, 116
Relief, immediate 112, 113
Resection 52, 66, 77, 79, 81, 83, 84, 85, 92, 93, 94, 99, 140
  surgical 52, 79, 83, 92, 93
Residual disease 93, 94, 95

Response 10, 14, 19, 20, 22, 23, 25, 27, 29, 30, 33, 34, 35, 36, 38, 39, 40, 41, 42, 43, 78, 79, 91, 99, 108, 143, 146, 147, 158, 174, 178, 189, 190, 247, 253, 254
  inflammatory 190, 247, 253, 254
  median duration of 10, 19, 22, 23, 27, 29, 33, 34, 36, 43
  median time to 22, 34, 36, 38
Ring-opening polymerization (ROP) 244, 246, 263
Risk factors 17, 24, 54, 55, 56, 57, 62, 66, 67, 71, 72, 81, 184, 188
  independent 55, 81
Rituximab 9, 10, 11, 14, 21, 23
Romidepsin 33, 34, 35
ROS Molecules 190, 191
Ruxolitinib 39, 40, 41

S

Schwann cells 255
Semisynthetic 196, 216, 229, 230
Sezary syndrome (SS) 31, 33, 34
Short-term hormones (STH) 138
Signaling pathways 68, 81, 107, 109, 172, 178, 181, 182, 189, 198, 218
Skin cancer 176, 183, 185, 187
Small lymphocytic lymphoma (SLL) 3, 11, 14
Southwest oncology group (SWOG) 135, 143
Specialized surgeries 194
Spinal cord compression 143, 144, 154, 157, 160
Squamous cell carcinoma 52, 53, 57, 61, 67, 68, 71, 73, 116, 175, 177, 185, 187
Squamous epithelium, normal 61, 62
Stampede trial 137, 139
Standard uptake value (SUV) 76, 79, 116
Stem bark and wood 221, 222
Stem cell transplant 17, 18, 19, 20, 21, 23, 25, 36
  autologous 17, 18, 19, 21
Studied range of toxicity 250, 251, 252
Superoxide dismutases (SOD) 190, 191
Supportive cancer-care agents 209, 210
Surgery, salvage 99, 101
Surveillance, epidemiology, and end results (SEER) 53, 140
Surveillance endoscopy 65, 66, 99, 101
Synthesis 6, 16, 33, 90, 195, 196, 197, 199, 200, 201, 211, 213, 215, 222, 226, 228, 244, 246, 270
  of DNA 199, 226
  of nucleic acids 196, 200, 201, 226
  protein 6, 16, 33, 228
Systems 16, 20, 22, 24, 71, 175, 212, 214, 246
  immune 16, 20, 22, 24, 175
  traditional 212, 214

T

Target, molecular 29, 205, 206, 210
Targeted 20, 42, 44, 58, 104, 107, 110
  agents 20, 42, 44, 104, 107, 110
  therapies in esophageal cancer 58
Targeting ligand 269, 270
Tasman radiation oncology group (TROG) 139
Taxanes 90, 103, 105, 173, 196, 197, 199, 207, 216, 222
T-cell Lymphomas 1, 18, 31, 33, 43
Testicles 24, 149
Testosterone 140, 143, 144, 145, 146, 147, 151, 155
Testosterone surge 144
Therapeutic agents 15, 44, 174, 184, 185, 188, 204, 209, 211, 212, 213, 214, 222, 262
Therapies 1, 2, 3, 4, 6, 7, 9, 11, 15, 20, 21, 23, 25, 27, 28, 29, 30, 31, 32, 35, 39, 40, 41, 43, 44, 52, 60, 66, 67, 76, 79, 83, 84, 98, 106, 107, 108, 110, 111, 136, 147, 154, 155, 185, 193, 231, 260, 265, 269
  continuous 155
  targeted 1, 11, 21, 23, 25, 31, 43, 44, 52, 106, 107, 110, 111, 136, 193, 265
  trimodality 84, 108
Therapies in esophageal cancer 104
Thrombocytopenia 3, 6, 7, 10, 14, 33, 35, 36, 38, 39, 40, 41, 43, 105
Tissues 37, 42, 59, 81, 173, 175, 185, 189, 193, 194, 198, 206, 242, 248, 252, 253, 255, 257, 265
  connective 59, 175
Topoisomerase II 223, 224, 228

Toxic effects 198, 201, 205, 206, 208, 209, 211, 228
Toxicities 4, 19, 22, 33, 35, 36, 37, 38, 40, 93, 104, 105, 106, 139, 159, 206, 208, 211, 216, 231, 248, 250, 251, 252
dose-limiting 35
Transhiatal esophagogastrectomy 85, 117
Trastuzumab 104, 105, 107, 108
Tumor 68, 72, 75, 77, 78, 79, 177, 180, 182, 187, 208, 268, 269
invasion 75, 77
-node-metastasis (TNM) 72
regression 78, 79, 208, 268
regression score 79
suppressor genes 68, 177, 180, 182, 187
volumes 269
Tumor cell(s) 31, 70, 78, 89, 146, 177, 205, 207, 209
markers 177
Tylosis esophageal cancer 58
Tyrosine kinase inhibitor (TKI) 2, 4, 5, 6, 7, 15, 16, 23, 25, 31, 110, 117

V

Vascular endothelial growth factor (VEGF) 5, 69, 70, 108, 109, 110, 117, 178, 207, 223, 224, 226, 228
Vinblastine 17, 197, 198, 199, 224
Vinca alkaloids 173, 197, 199, 222, 227
Vincristine 17, 18, 21, 29, 35, 197, 198, 199, 224
Vindesine 197, 198, 199
Virus, human papiloma 185, 187

W

White blood cells (WBC) 16, 25, 175, 176
Whole exome sequencing (WES) 68, 117, 148

Z

Zoledronic acid 136, 137, 139, 140, 147, 148

Made in the USA
Las Vegas, NV
04 November 2026

57425979R00186